A Geography of Infection

Previous volumes by one or more of the authors exploring the interface between epidemiology and geography include:

Spatial Autocorrelation (1973)
Elements of Spatial Structure (1975)
Spatial Diffusion: An Historical Geography of Epidemics in an Island Community (1981)
Spatial Processes (1981)
Spread of Measles in Fiji and the Pacific (1985)
Spatial Aspects of Influenza Epidemics (1986)
Atlas of Disease Distributions (1988)
London International Atlas of AIDS (1992)
Measles: An Historical Geography of a Major Human Viral Disease (1993)
Deciphering Global Epidemics (1998)
Island Epidemics (2000)
The Geographical Structure of Epidemics (2000)
World Atlas of Epidemic Diseases (2004)
War Epidemics (2004)
Poliomyelitis: A World Geography (2006)
Infectious Diseases: A Geographical Analysis (2009)
Atlas of Epidemic Britain (2012)
Infectious Disease Control: A Geographical Analysis (2013)
Atlas of Refugees, Displaced Populations, and Epidemic Diseases (2018)

A Geography of Infection

SPATIAL PROCESSES AND PATTERNS IN EPIDEMICS AND PANDEMICS

Matthew Smallman-Raynor
University of Nottingham

Andrew Cliff
University of Cambridge

Keith Ord
Georgetown University

Peter Haggett
University of Bristol

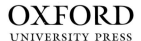
OXFORD
UNIVERSITY PRESS

OXFORD
UNIVERSITY PRESS

Great Clarendon Street, Oxford, OX2 6DP,
United Kingdom

Oxford University Press is a department of the University of Oxford.
It furthers the University's objective of excellence in research, scholarship,
and education by publishing worldwide. Oxford is a registered trade mark of
Oxford University Press in the UK and in certain other countries

© Oxford University Press 2022

The moral rights of the authors have been asserted

First Edition published in 2022

Impression: 1

Published in the United States of America by Oxford University Press
198 Madison Avenue, New York, NY 10016, United States of America

British Library Cataloguing in Publication Data
Data available

Library of Congress Control Number: 2021945595

ISBN 978–0–19–284839–0

DOI: 10.1093/med/9780192848390.001.0001

Printed in Great Britain by
Bell & Bain Ltd., Glasgow

Oxford University Press makes no representation, express or implied, that the
drug dosages in this book are correct. Readers must therefore always check
the product information and clinical procedures with the most up-to-date
published product information and data sheets provided by the manufacturers
and the most recent codes of conduct and safety regulations. The authors and
the publishers do not accept responsibility or legal liability for any errors in the
text or for the misuse or misapplication of material in this work. Except where
otherwise stated, drug dosages and recommendations are for the non-pregnant
adult who is not breast-feeding

Links to third party websites are provided by Oxford in good faith and
for information only. Oxford disclaims any responsibility for the materials
contained in any third party website referenced in this work.

In grateful memory of six old friends who, during their busy lives, found time to encourage us to explore the links between epidemiology and geography:

Dr Norman Bailey (World Health Organization, Geneva)
Professor Torsten Hägerstrand (Lund University)
Dr Edgar Hope-Simpson (Cirencester GP Practice)
Professor David Kendall FRS (University of Cambridge)
Dr Steve Thacker (US Centers for Disease Control and Prevention, Atlanta)
Dr David Tyrrell FRS (MRC Common Cold Research Unit, Salisbury).

Preface

I: A Genealogical Note

Books, no less than individuals, may have complex family histories. The genealogy of *A Geography of Infection* is no exception. Its immediate roots lie in an invitation to one of us, then newly retired, to deliver the first endowed Clarendon Lectures in Geography and Environmental Studies. Four lectures were duly given in the University of Oxford's School of Geography in the Michaelmas Term 1999 and subsequently published by Oxford University Press (OUP) in a small book entitled *The Geographical Structure of Epidemics* (Haggett, 2000).

In a superficial sense, the present volume may be seen as an updated and revised version of that book, but one whose format, page size, and use of colour allows maps with greater clarity and effectiveness to be used. The preceding volume was deliberately confined to a broad discussion of principles, to a non-mathematical presentation, and to using only a narrow range of infectious diseases, notably those (such as measles) which had played a key role in nineteenth- and twentieth-century modelling of disease spread.

The present book retains much of the organizational structure of the original book and its emphasis on clear graphics. But AD 2021 is several orders of magnitude more challenging than AD 2000 and a still further generation away from the euphoria of smallpox eradication in the 1970s. Even before the epoch-making onslaught of coronavirus disease 2019 (COVID-19), the growing rumbles from new diseases (Ebola in West Africa, severe acute respiratory syndrome in East Asia, and Middle East respiratory syndrome in the Middle East), the mounting resistance of old diseases to standard therapies, and the exponential increases in the speed of disease movement were already darkening the skies. As they did so, the epidemiological world responded, not just in the search for new vaccines but in mathematical modelling of the ways in which epidemic diseases spread through vulnerable populations. Once a rare sideline, mathematical modelling of epidemics now finds a place in scores of university departments around the world.

So, in this new book on the geography of epidemics and pandemics, the crew has been increased from one to four, with a far wider range of experience and skills than the original single author. All have collaborated over the years since the accidental meeting between two of its members on a Lake Michigan shore in 1966 and our first joint volume in 1975. In this volume we have followed our usual practice of changing positions within the boat as demands change, so our youngest member has now moved up to stroke and our oldest (at 88) acts out a less energetic but vociferous role as cox.

II: COVID-19

As we write, COVID-19 is at our doors in Cambridge, the Chew Valley, Nottingham, and Washington, DC. 'Lockdown' in the United Kingdom and the United States has meant hasty revision of earlier drafts, and we have had to meet remotely, like so many others, both to write and sign off manuscript and illustrations. COVID-19 began as an *outbreak* in Wuhan city in December 2019, spread as a China-wide *epidemic* in the next 2 months, and became a full-blown global *pandemic* from March 2020. The small geographically localized storm moved quickly through the gears to become a global epidemiological hurricane that continues to rage.

Worldwide, up to the end of March 2021, there have been over 125 million confirmed cases of COVID-19, including nearly 3 million deaths, reported to the World Health Organization, affecting 223 countries and territories. Although vaccine development and rollout is now proceeding apace, lighting a way out of the pandemic, COVID-19 ranks as one of the great epidemiological catastrophes of the last one hundred years. Whatever the final death toll, the need for spatial separation ('social distancing') and lockdown has already triggered the biggest peacetime economic downturn since the Great Depression of the 1930s.

As this volume goes to press, it remains unclear whether COVID-19 will grow to be one of the really large pandemics of infectious diseases which, from time to time, have swept from continent to continent around the inhabited world. If it does, then the pages that follow will show it keeps good company. Plague in the fourteenth to seventeenth centuries, cholera in the nineteenth, influenza in the first half of the twentieth century, and HIV/AIDS from the 1980s have all shared the capacity to move quickly through the human population, creating a bow-wave of anxiety and apprehension in advance of the illnesses and deaths that followed. With each pandemic, the population has reeled but, given time, it has bounced back from every new microbiological onslaught.

Although we have an understandable focus on COVID-19 in this book, we have tried to set it in context by bringing together work on a wide range of the great epidemic diseases that have assaulted the human population over the last five thousand years. Our emphasis is on deciphering the spatial processes by which infectious diseases move from place to place, and mapping the disease patterns they produce. In the first chapter, we define and discuss the various statistical models that have been used to study the geographical spread of infectious diseases. Subsequent chapters then use multiple examples, drawn mainly from the authors' own work in medical geography over the last half a century, to illustrate how epidemics and pandemics of these diseases emerge and diffuse in time and space. The examples we have selected span centuries of time, geographical locations from the local to the global, and environments ranging from the tropical to the Arctic. In organizing the material, we have opted to do so by geographical scale, beginning with the local and national in Chapter 2 and then moving, by way of international epidemics in Chapter 3, to the great global pandemics of past and present times in Chapters 4 and 5. Having spent four chapters explaining how infectious diseases spread in time and space, we conclude in Chapter 6 on a positive note by studying ways in which the spread of epidemic diseases can be controlled by isolation, quarantine, and spatially targeted vaccination schemes, all crucially informed by adequate surveillance and infection reporting systems.

Some of the topics we cover have formed the central themes of our earlier books, monographs, and atlases. Our aim here has been to reassemble and synthesize relevant materials in such a way that they shed fresh light on an age-old problem. The materials in Chapters 3, 4, and 6, in particular, draw freely on two of our previous OUP books, *Infectious Diseases: Emergence and Re-Emergence* (2009) and *Infectious Disease Control* (2013). All our diagrams have been drawn or redrawn for the present work, with most appearing in colour for the first time.

III: Thanks

A book of this kind, with examples drawn from a 50-year assemblage of case studies, could not have been completed during the current lockdown without help from many quarters over a long period of time. We mention on the dedication page (v), six who are no longer with us. They include a geographer, two mathematicians, and three practising physicians including one, David Tyrrell, credited with June Almeida, of taking the first picture of a coronavirus. We are also grateful to Brian Berry, then at the University of Chicago, for encountering an influenza virus in 1971 that allowed epidemiology into PH's research life where it has grown for five decades. In Berry's own words:

> 1970 was a very busy year for other reasons. I was appointed a member of the Scientific Group on Research in Epidemiology and Communications Science at the World Health Organization. I handed the baton to Peter Haggett in 1971 when influenza laid me low before one important session. I called Peter in Bristol and asked whether he could replace me. 'When?' 'Tomorrow.' 'Where?' 'Geneva.' Good trooper that he is, he went. (Berry, 2006, p. 140)

And, as they say, the rest is history.

For the authors, this volume is part of a much larger map on which we have all been working for two generations. There has been a series of epidemic monographs which focus on specific infectious diseases (notably measles, influenza, and poliomyelitis), on specific epidemiological sources (the United States consular records of disease), and on specific themes (such as island epidemiology and the role of conflict in epidemic generation), and there have been atlases—on AIDS, displaced populations and disease, and disease mapping. Like all scientists, we recognize the truth of Bernard of Chartres's (d. c.1130) remark, repeated by Isaac Newton in a letter to Robert Hooke in 1675, that to see further we 'stand on the shoulders of giants' who have worked on similar themes before us. We have been particularly blessed by the resources made available to us by successive head librarians, notably and currently, Tomas Allen, at the library of the World Health Organization; and Donna Stroup, for many years based in the Epidemiology Program Office of the United States Centers for Disease Control. They placed resources at our disposal to complement the British collections on epidemic history in our own university libraries and medical schools. Likewise, we want to thank Sharon Messenger and Melissa White, then in the library and archives of the Royal College of General Practitioners, for piloting us through the volumes of material generated by the College's first President, William Pickles, when he was a general practitioner in Wensleydale in the first half of the last century. Pickles's unique records of infections in a single rural practice are analysed in Chapter 2. Finally, we also record with gratitude the Wellcome Trust and the Leverhulme Trust who, through their grant schemes, have supported our work for many years.

The Department of Geography at Cambridge has provided, crucially for the kinds of publications we have produced, cartographic help. Philip Stickler, sometime Head of the Cartographic Unit in the Department, has sustained the authors for a quarter of a century with his superb maps, graphs, and diagrams, and he has continued to do so in retirement. OUP has now published eight of our books. We have been especially indebted to Nicola Wilson, currently Editor-in-Chief and Senior Commissioning Editor of Medical Publishing at OUP who, along with Rachel Goldsworthy, Senior Assistant Commissioning Editor, has overseen the complex task of integrating illustrations with the text for the current project. The design team must have wept on more than one occasion with the high image to text ratio—a problem not helped by the size of many of the graphics files so that moving them around was, even in this computing day and age, like watching paint dry.

Manuscript preparation is always an individual affair, and two of the authors have had a base for several years now at the Bull and Swan in Stamford where, in normal times, we met regularly to exchange material—generally monthly which, for a time, was as frequently as the inn changed hands! In these extraordinary times, the Bull and Swan has gone into suspended animation, but we hope all will be resumed ere long—there is light at the end of what has been a very long and depressingly dark tunnel.

On so many occasions, our joint ventures have given the four of us the pleasure of writing together and have ensured enduring affection and companionship between us. But inevitably the demands of four different universities on two continents has meant that, for a number of years, one or another of us would have commitments, personal or academic, which led to someone standing aside for a particular project. So, it is an especial pleasure on this occasion for us to be back in harness together once more.

Finally, a note for our families and friends. Those closest to us have inevitably borne the brunt of our obsession with research, with its periods of preoccupied expressions and all-too-frequent grumpy reactions. We let this book stand as a token of our deep thanks to all of them.

Matthew Smallman-Raynor
Andrew Cliff
Keith Ord
Peter Haggett
Feast of St Quirinus of Neuss
30 April 2021

Contents

Abbreviations

AIDS	acquired immunodeficiency syndrome
AHF	Argentine haemorrhagic fever
CDC	Centers for Disease Control and Prevention
CI	confidence interval
CP	contact probabilities
CoV	coronavirus
COVID-19	coronavirus disease 2019
DALY	disability-adjusted life year
ENSO	El Niño–Southern Oscillation
EDM	epidemic data matrix
EPI	Expanded Programme on Immunization
FE	following edge
FMD	foot-and-mouth disease
GP	general practitioner
GRO	General Register Office
GOARN	Global Outbreak Alert and Response Network
GPEI	Global Polio Eradication Initiative
HPS	hantavirus pulmonary syndrome
HIV	human immunodeficiency virus
IPCC	Intergovernmental Panel on Climate Change
UNAIDS	Joint United Nations Programme on HIV/AIDS
LE	leading edge
MIF	mean information field
MMR	measles, mumps, and rubella
MERS	Middle East respiratory syndrome
MST	minimum spanning tree
MDS	multidimensional scaling
NHS	National Health Service
OIHP	Office International d'Hygiène Publique
RCGP	Royal College of General Practitioners
SARS	severe acute respiratory syndrome
SARS-CoV-2	severe acute respiratory syndrome coronavirus 2
SIR	susceptible–infective–recovered
TB	tuberculosis
WHO	World Health Organization

Note on Conventions

This book necessarily includes reference to some scores of infectious diseases. There is neither space nor intention to give a detailed clinical view of each. The interested reader is referred to the American Public Health Association's *Control of Communicable Diseases Manual*, first published in 1917 and now in its 20th edition (D.L. Heymann, editor), and the *International Classification of Diseases* list available at https://icd.who.int/browse10/2019/en. For readers interested in the history of each disease, *The Cambridge World History of Human Disease* (Kiple, 1993) remains a useful starting point. A geographical view of major diseases is provided in our *World Atlas of Epidemic Diseases* (Cliff et al., 2004).

Note on names of Icelandic medical districts: names of medical districts in Iceland appear as either the stem or the genitive case. As examples, Reykjavík, Akureyri, and Ísafjörður refer to places, while Reykjavíkur, Akureyrar, and Ísafjarðar refer to the medical districts based on these centres.

1

Epidemics as Diffusion Waves

1.1 Introduction

Is it ketching*? Why, how you talk. Is a harrow ketching? If you don't hitch on to one tooth, you're bound to on another, ain't you? … and it ain't no slouch of a harrow, nuther.*

Mark Twain [on measles],
The Adventures of Huckleberry Finn,
New York: Harpers, 1884.

Exactly 40 years ago, in the spring of 1981, Cambridge University Press published an obscure monograph entitled *Spatial Diffusion*. It

was anchored in a study of some 120 years of measles outbreaks in the North Atlantic island of Iceland. Its opening paragraph has an oddly prescient ring in a year when a large epidemiological 'boulder' (rather than a pebble) has just splashed so disastrously into the Earth's human population:

> A stone is tossed into a pond. The consequent splash forms a large wave immediately around the entry point. Within a second, waves are starting to move out in a circular pattern across the surface of the water. Some seconds later, very small ripples are disturbing the weeds on the far side of the pond.
>
> Information is tossed into a communication system. An American president is killed by a sniper's bullet at 12.31 p.m. on 22 November 1963 on a Dallas road. Information is tossed into a communication system. It is beamed out on radio and television around the world, is passed by word of mouth from one listener to the rest of his family, or is told by the garage man to the motorist stopping for petrol.
>
> A virus is tossed into a susceptible population. Passengers arriving at an Icelandic port from Copenhagen in the early summer of 1907 include a few known to be suffering from measles infection. One escapes the island's quarantine procedures, and joins the local population, some of whom are off to the capital city, Reykjavík, to join the crowds gathering for a visit by the King of Denmark. The virus is transmitted between some neighbours in the crowd. Within 16 months, an epidemic has spread through the whole island infecting over 7,000 people and killing 354. (Cliff et al., 1981, p. 1)

Although the stone, the assassination, and the epidemic are, in most respects, wholly dissimilar phenomena, one being trivial, the other two historic, all share something in common.

The movement through a population—of water particles in the first case; of worldwide listeners, viewers, and readers in the second; and of susceptible islanders in the third—is termed *spatial diffusion*. It frequently takes a wave-like form. Each wave moves outward through its medium away from single or multiple centres, each dissipating as it runs out of kinetic energy, or boredom, or susceptible victims. In the case of the stone, the wave pattern is simple and circular and can be readily observed and recorded. The other two need to be pieced together from hard-won research. Their waves may follow many branching pathways, move at different velocities, and move in an intensely complex pattern. This process is called diffusion waves.

Another basic commonality is that all three—the water particles, the information, and the virus—involve Mark Twain's harrow, that touching process we call *contagion*. The term was first used in

English for diseases in 1398,[1] being derived from two Latin words *con* (with) and *tangere* (to touch). As we shall see shortly in section 1.3, that touching process can take complex forms. With diseases moving between humans, it may be a cough, a kiss, a sexual act, or a contaminated door handle. It may be passed on via such direct person-to-person transfer or an indirect move involving fleas, mosquitos, lice, or rodents, in a complex choreography of moves. We have tried to map a wide range of these moves in our *World Atlas of Epidemic Diseases* (Cliff et al., 2004), but here we pay particular—although by no means exclusive—attention to what a leading epidemiologist of the last century dubbed *crowd diseases* (Greenwood, 1935). These include many of the common childhood fevers (measles, rubella, whooping cough, etc.), the great classic plagues of the medieval world, and the newer plagues of influenza and the coronaviruses including the deadly coronavirus disease 2019 (COVID-19).

Just a century separates two significant events in the study of epidemics. In 1889, a St Petersburg mathematician published a brief study of measles outbreaks in a local girls' boarding school and proposed a simple but elegant model of how the observed pattern of infection might have been generated (Dietz, 1988). In 1994, the newly founded Isaac Newton Institute for Mathematical Sciences at the University of Cambridge held its first world symposium on epidemic modelling (Mollison, 1995). Between these two events, and even more so in the decades which followed, the literature on epidemics has exploded from a niche area of applied mathematics to an industry in which few universities lack a specialist in that field.

In the social sciences, the modelling of diffusion processes draws on a range of disciplines. Pioneering work was conducted in economics by Lösch (1954) in modelling price waves in the United States and later by a Bristol University team (Cliff et al., 1975) in tracking business cycles in South West England. Rogers (1995) provides a wide survey of diffusion research throughout the social sciences.

This book focuses on the diffusion of diseases in the form of epidemic waves over a wide spatial range from local cases and outbreaks within general practitioner (GP) practices to pandemics on a global scale. It draws on a large geographical and statistical literature and on our own joint research over the last half century. It tries to unravel the ways in which many infectious diseases move through human populations. However, it is *not* a medical book about epidemic diseases nor is it a mathematical manual for disease modellers. Major works abound for both and are referenced at appropriate points in this book. We have had the privilege to work alongside outstanding professionals from both fields (see 'Preface'), but our main focus here is on the specifics of the quantitative geography of infection.

Such a focus is not new. It stretches back over the millennia to the physician Hippocrates of Kos (*c*.460–370 BC) whose *Airs, Waters and Places* provided a start for epidemiological studies. As chief librarian at Alexandria, Eratosthenes of Kyrene (*c*.240 BC), the first mathematical geographer, would have been familiar with Hippocrates's

works. They may have influenced his three-volume *Geografika* (Roller, 2010). Eratosthenes made important contributions to earth science (computing the size of our planet) and to mathematics (via number theory), as well as establishing the geographical discipline itself. Both scholars worked on a broad canvas and we hope they would have been sympathetic to the recommendations a half century ago to place World Health Organization (WHO) epidemiology on a broader disciplinary framework (Cassel et al., 1969).

1.2 Building Blocks: Infection, Contagion, Disease

In this section, we review the three main terms which underlie much of the analysis of epidemic processes in the rest of this book. We look in turn at infection (section 1.2.1), at contagion (section 1.2.2), and at disease, both its definition and data and the measures of the burdens it imposes (section 1.2.3). Infection, contagion, and disease are very old words in English and their usage over the centuries has twisted and clouded their meaning.

1.2.1 Infection Dynamics

Infection comes from the preposition *in*, the Latin verb *inficere*, and the Old French *infeccion*, meaning to 'dip in', 'taint', 'poison', 'spoil', or 'stain'. It was used from the time of Hippocrates in the fourth century BC to describe a disease that was communicated through the agency of air or water. It came into English usage in the late fourteenth century in the sense of both 'a contaminated condition' and 'infectious disease'. From 1540, infection was sometimes distinguished from contagion (section 1.2.2) in the sense of body-to-body communication.

Infection: definitions and examples

In biological terms, infection may be defined as 'the invasion of one organism by a smaller (infecting) organism' (Fine, in Vynnycky and White, 2010, p. 1). Set in these general terms, infection is a broad, even ubiquitous phenomenon in nature, with all plants and animals carrying a cargo of microorganisms on their journey through life. Some will be long-term passengers, some brief and threatening visitors. Jonathan Swift's memorable lines remind us that species of plants or animals carry pests of one form or another and these continue all the way up from microbes to whales:

> So, naturalists observe, a flea
> Has smaller fleas that on him prey;
> And these have smaller still to bite 'em;
> And so proceed ad infinitum.
>
> Jonathan Swift, *On Poetry: A Rhapsody*, 1733.

Nor is infection necessarily a harmful process. Although this book is about the geography of the *pathogenic* impacts of infection in the form of epidemics in human populations, it could be argued that many infections are neutral. Humans may simply act as hosts or carriers. Indeed, infections may be helpful to the health of the larger infected organisms. Research on gut bacteria, for example, shows them forming an essential part of the digestion process in the human host (Mosley, 2018).

Infectious agents may be classified in many ways but Table 1.1 shows one of the most useful. This arranges, on the left, the six main

---

[1] J. Trevisa tr. Bartholomew de Glanville *De Proprietatibus Rerum* (1495) vii. lxiv. 281, 'Lepra also comith of fader and moder, and so this contagyon passyth in to the chylde as it were by lawe of herytage'.

Table 1.1 Some major infectious diseases classified by causative agent

Causative agents	Subdivisions	Virus divisions (alphabetical order)	Major human infectious diseases
1. Prions			Creutzfeldt–Jakob disease, kuru
2. Viruses	2A. DNA viruses	*Hepnadaviridae* *Herpesviridae* *Poxviridae*	Hepatitis B Chickenpox, Epstein–Barr Smallpox
	2B. RNA viruses	*Arenaviridae* *Bunyaviridae* *Coronaviridae* *Filoviridae* *Flaviviridae* *Orthomyxoviridae* *Paramyxoviridae* *Picornaviridae* *Retroviridae* *Rhabdoviridae* *Togaviridae*	Lassa fever, South American haemorrhagic fever Korean haemorrhagic fever, Rift Valley fever COVID-19, Middle East respiratory syndrome (MERS), SARS, common cold Ebola, Marburg disease Dengue, yellow fever, hepatitis C Influenza Measles, mumps, parainfluenza Poliomyelitis HIV/AIDS Rabies Rubella
3. Rickettsia			Louse-borne typhus fever, Rocky Mountain spotted fever
4. Bacteria	Bacilli		Cholera, plague, diphtheria, typhoid, whooping cough, Legionnaires' disease, anthrax
	Cocci		Scarlet fever, meningitis, gonorrhoea
	Spirochaetes		Relapsing fever, syphilis, yaws, leptospirosis, Lyme disease
	Mycobacteria		Leprosy, tuberculosis
5. Protozoa			Malaria, Chagas' disease, sleeping sickness, leishmaniasis, cryptosporidiosis
6. Helminths			Filariasis, Guinea worm, hookworm, river blindness, schistosomiasis

Source: Data from Cliff, A.D., Haggett, P., Smallman-Raynor, M.R. (2004). *World Atlas of Epidemic Diseases*. London: Arnold.

biological groups from which agents are drawn in size from immeasurably small and simple prions through to large visible helminths. On the right are examples of the resulting human diseases (using their common names). Evidently, viruses are one of the classes from which many human diseases are drawn.

Infection: the infectious process

The processes that link an infectious disease agent to the human body are of immense complexity. Here we simply take one example, the RNA paramyxovirus which causes the common childhood disease of measles, a disease which still kills 200,000 children worldwide each year. This one disease has played a key role in shaping research on epidemics. So, it is useful to take as our example in **Figure 1.1** the collision between the small measles virus (only visible under an electron microscope) and the familiar contours of a human body.

Disease spread at the individual level is shown in **Figure 1.1A**, giving a typical time profile of measles infection in a host individual. Note that the horizontal scale is non-linear with breaks and different scales for time duration within each phase of the overall measles host lifespan. This includes some months of maternal antibody protection, followed by some childhood years as susceptible (S) until the child meets another infected person, usually another child. When the virus is passed on, primarily via the respiratory tract, the key infection period begins with a latent period (L) while virus numbers build up and the first signs of infection begin to be recognized at the end of the latent period. This leads on to a period of full infection where the child is capable of passing on the virus. **Table 1.2** gives examples for ten common diseases of the length of the serial interval (the time between onset of symptoms in an index case and a secondary case directly infected by the index case) and the ability to pass infection that ranges from 2 days for influenza to months or years for tuberculosis.

The infection process is depicted as a chain structure in **Figure 1.1B**. The average or typical chain length of 14 days for measles is illustrated. The process of chains interlinking is captured by Mark Twain's harrow metaphor in the chapter head quotation.

Figure 1.1C shows a transition in time and scale using Burnet's classic view of a typical epidemic (Burnet and White, 1972). Each circle here represents an infected person, and the connecting lines indicate transfer from one case to the next. Bright red circles indicate individuals who fail to infect others and so break the chain. Three periods are shown (from left to right), the first when practically the whole population is susceptible; the second at the height of the epidemic; and the third at the close, when most individuals are immune. The proportions of susceptible (yellow) and immune (blue) individuals are indicated in the rectangles beneath the main diagram.

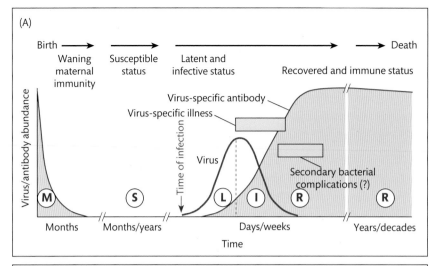

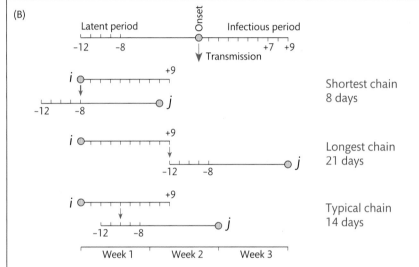

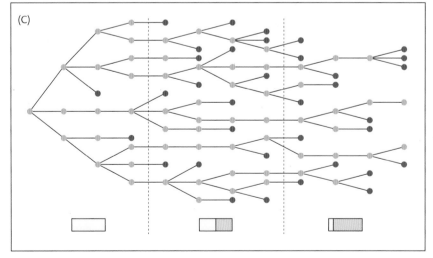

Figure 1.1 The measles infection process at the individual level. (A) Typical time profile of infection in a host individual. Note the time breaks and different scales for time duration within each phase of the overall life-span. The circled red letters indicate the different phases: *M* = mother-conferred immunity; *S* = susceptible to infection; *L* = latent period of infection; *I* = infected; *R* = recovered. (B) The infection process as a chain structure. The typical chain length of 14 days characteristic of measles is shown. (C) Burnet and White's (1972) view of a typical epidemic in a community of people, where each pale red circle represents an infection and the connecting lines indicate transfer from one case to the next. Bright red circles indicate individuals who fail to infect others. Three periods are shown by the rectangles beneath the main diagram. The first is when practically the whole population is susceptible; the second is at the height of the epidemic; and the third is at the close when most individuals are immune. The proportions of susceptible (yellow) and immune (blue) individuals are indicated in the rectangles.

Reproduced from Haggett, P. (2000). *The Geographical Structure of Epidemics*. Oxford: Clarendon Press.

Table 1.2 Infection values for some common infectious diseases

Disease	Serial interval[a] (range in days)	Herd immunity threshold[b] (%)
Influenza	2–4	50–75
Diphtheria	2–30	85
Poliomyelitis	2–45	50–75
Pertussis	5–35	83–94
Measles[c]	7–16	83–94
Rubella	7–28	83–85
Mumps	8–32	75–86
Smallpox	9–45	80–85
Malaria	20	76–86
Tuberculosis	Months/years	Not well defined

[a] The serial interval is defined as the time between onset of symptoms in an index case and a secondary case directly infected by the index case. [b] The herd immunity threshold is defined as $1 - (1/R_0)$, where R_0 is the basic reproduction number for the disease in question. Sample estimates of R_0 for different diseases are given in Table 5.1 in Chapter 5. [c] See Figure 1.1.
Reproduced with permission from Vynnycky, E., White, R. (2010). *An Introduction to Infectious Disease Modelling*. Oxford: Oxford University Press.

1.2.2 Contagion: Separation and Space

In this subsection, we look at (i) the meaning of contagion, (ii) the scale and spatial structure of host populations, and (iii) the rules which govern the organization and evolution of these populations. Here our emphasis is on the host, the human population, rather than the infection.

Meaning of contagion

Contagion comes from two Latin words, the preposition *con* meaning 'together with' and the verb *tangere* meaning 'to touch'. The earliest use in English dates from the fourteenth century, coming from the Old French *contagious*, meaning 'contaminating', 'corrupting', or more generally 'communicating'. Usage over the centuries has tended to emphasize the bad sense of touching with an emphasis on its role in contamination. In medical use, there is some transatlantic divergence with the English usage retaining the original meaning and separating contact diseases from the broader class of infectious diseases. American usage tends increasingly to regard 'infectious' and 'contagious' almost interchangeably. Usage of the second word has become rarer, often replaced by the synonym 'communicable' as in the American Public Health Association's classic *Control of Communicable Diseases Manual* (Heymann, 2015).

One London School of Hygiene and Tropical Medicine epidemiologist has recently explored the much wider use of contagious concepts in a non-disease context (Kucharski, 2020). He shows how mathematical ideas common in disease studies can be used to explain 'why things spread, and why they stop'. His examples include rumours moving through social networks in the Trump Presidency back to the bursting of the 1720 South Sea bubble. See also Christakis and Fowler (2013) and Taylor and Eckles (2018).

Scale and spatial organization

In contagion, as opposed to infection, the emphasis is shifted from a concern with the microbial agent towards the human population itself—its numbers, its location, and its spatial organization.

Human geographers conceive a population as being organized into interlocking *nodal regions* at different spatial scales. Following Haggett et al. (1977), each is analysed in terms of:

1. *movements* or flows of people, information, and goods
2. *networks* which focus and constrain flows
3. *nodes* which grow up at critical points on the network
4. *hierarchies* which differentiate nodes into cities, villages, hamlets, etc.
5. density and potential *surfaces* which form around the hierarchies
6. diffusion *waves* which move through (1) to (5) at varying velocities.

Epidemic and pandemic waves are seen here as one class of diffusion wave (6).

One of the difficulties we face in trying to analyse a nodal regional system is that there is no obvious or single point of entry. Indeed, the more integrated the regional system, the harder it is to crack. In the words of one regional economist: 'The maze of interdependencies in reality is indeed formidable … Its tale is unending, its circularity unquestionable. Yet its dissection is imperative … At some point we must cut into its circumference' (Isard, 1960, p. 3). We choose to make that cut with spatial movements as it allows a logical progression towards the ultimate objective of understanding disease diffusion.

The spatial and hierarchical structure of populations (sometimes termed *metapopulations*) is attracting increasing interest in the epidemiological literature (Watts et al., 2005). A number of studies now rewrite models to build in the geographical structures of the population at risk (Sattenspiel and Herring, 1998; Sattenspiel, 2009, pp. 125–34).

Change in organization

The human population has just reached the 8 billion mark. On current United Nations forecasts, it is expected to stabilize later this century and demographers then expect it to begin a long decline. Table 1.3 shows the astonishing changes over the last four centuries during which our numbers have multiplied 16-fold. The table deliberately uses rounded figures since accuracy varies increasingly in earlier centuries.

The rest of Table 1.3 shows the way in which the human population has organized itself over the same four centuries. *Ceteris paribus*, population size will by itself be expected (through increasing size and density) to increase the likelihood of the spread of infections. But a second element, urbanization, compounds this by spatially concentrating that host population. Urbanization can be measured in many ways but we take a simple measure for which long historical records exist, the probable size of the world's largest cities. Even today, city size measurement is an art rather than a science, depending on an investigator's exact criteria. But, after looking at various measures, we are confident that the figures given are of the right order of magnitude. They show changes that substantially outpace the growth of the human population itself.

A third measure relates to transport. In 1492, Columbus crossed the Atlantic in 36 days while, today, one can travel from Western Europe to North America in less than a day. We have examined the impact of changes in travel times on epidemic disease 'jumps' for a number of times and locations—from Fiji in the late nineteenth

Table 1.3 Historical changes in the size, concentration, and flux in human populations

Year	World population		Urbanization		Travel	
	Total (billions)	Ratio	Largest city (millions)	Ratio	Days	Ratio (inverse)
2020	8.0	16	37.0	53	<1	50
1975	4.0	8	21.0	30	1–3	25
1925	2.0	4	7.7	11	3–5	13
1805	1.0	2	1.7	2	10	5
1600	0.5	1	0.7	1	50	1

Ratios for all indicators based on the year 1600 being set at 1.

century (Cliff and Haggett, 1985) to severe acute respiratory syndrome (SARS) in the twenty-first century (Cliff, Smallman-Raynor, Haggett, et al., 2009). There are many possible ways of measuring such changes but we choose in Table 1.3 a simple one as the time taken in days to cross the North Atlantic. Based on a sheaf of contraction charts drawn for intercontinental transport times, the conservative travel time figures show a 50-fold difference since 1600, with the switch from sail to steam within sea travel and, then, the switch from sea to air as the major discontinuities. Particularly significant is that the overall speed of change has been accelerating over the long historical period so that, in broad terms, half the change has occurred over the past few decades.

We expand upon the themes of population growth, urbanization, and transportation in our consideration of the disease implications of global change in section 3.3 in Chapter 3.

1.2.3 Disease: Definitions, Data, Burdens

We look here at the meaning of disease, the way contact between a disease agent and a host is recorded, and the role of infectious diseases within the overall pattern of mortality and morbidity—the so-called burden of disease.

Meaning and labelling

The word *disease* came into English usage by the fourteenth century from the two Old French words *dis* meaning 'without' and *aise* meaning 'comfort'. In a more general sense, it was used to indicate lack or want; distress; trouble, misfortune; and disease, sickness (Oxford English Dictionary). Its use in the restricted pathological sense of sickness or illness emerged by the start of the fifteenth century.

We all have labels for disease. The Bible spoke of plagues and scourges, Victorian novelists of early female deaths from maternal mortality, and our grandparents suffered from 'the screws'. A rich language has existed for centuries for medical conditions but the development of an internationally agreed labelling for disease came relatively late.

Infection impact: Evans's iceberg

The interactions between an invading agent and a host (the human body) are complex. Table 1.4 shows Evans's (1984) 'iceberg' concept of disease in which observable illness forms the upper part of a notional triangle (stage A) with death its vertex and subclinical illness (stage B), which is not overtly observable, the base. It has been modified to match the disease (measles) shown in Figure 1.1. Assault by a particular disease-causing organism may cause mild symptoms, severe symptoms, or even death. All three states are above the 'waterline' in the sense that they are felt by the patient.

Equally, the microbiological assault may be unnoticed by the human victim (below the 'waterline' or subclinical) and go either unnoticed or be picked up only in some investigative study. Each

Table 1.4 Iceberg concept of infectious disease as applied to measles

Stage	Human response	Population response	Types of epidemiological data
A. CLINICAL Level of disease needing clinical attention	Death of host **Tip of Evans's 'iceberg'**	Outbreaks; epidemics; pandemic	Death certificates, mortality statistics. Problems of disease identification when multiple causes of death. *MMWR* (USA)
	Severe illness with classic symptoms	Hospital admission if facilities available	Morbidity statistics (if reportable disease). *MMWR* (USA). Hospital statistics
	Illness needing GP attention Absence from work/school	Probable absence from work/school	GP records (including reports from sample of 'sentinel' practices)
B. SUBCLINICAL Level of disease not needing clinical attention	Mild illness not needing medical attention	Possible absence from work/school	Indication from non-clinical sources (e.g. absentee records). Inferred rise in related disease record (e.g. pneumonia/influenza link)
	Asymptomatic **Base of Evans's iceberg**		
C. NOT INFECTED	No clinical response but sheltering or lockdown behaviour at individual, group, and state levels during severe epidemics and pandemics		Normal range of demographic and economic statistics. Estimates of 'at-risk' populations. May be measured in special health surveys

MMWR, *Morbidity and Mortality Weekly Report.*

Source: Data from Evans, A.S. (ed.) (1984). *Viral Infections of Humans: Epidemiology and Control* (second edition). New York: Plenum.

infectious disease will have a different typical iceberg profile. In poliomyelitis, a large proportion of the invasions are below the waterline, with poliovirus only rarely causing the classical symptoms of paralysis. In rabies, severe 'above the waterline' effects, often leading to death, are a usual consequence.

Disease recording

The recording of disease is discussed in some detail in section 6.6 in Chapter 6. Here we note simply that the encounter between a disease agent and a host may result in the death of the host, in which case a *mortality* record in the form of a death certificate will typically be generated. This may or may not name a disease depending upon its role in causing death among the other contributing causes. Collection in a *morbidity* record will depend on hospital admission and/or diagnostic ability in general practice. Serious conditions may be legally reportable in some jurisdictions but not in others. And, in yet other jurisdictions, a patient may or may not have the resources to call on clinical help. It is also the case that the routine reporting of some diseases is supplemented by specific surveillance procedures. This is illustrated by occasional screening campaigns in which surveys of a population reveal the presence of conditions (e.g. tuberculosis, HIV/AIDS) which may not have been noted by the individual.

An extensive system of disease surveillance and data collection has been developed over the last 175 years, spanning all geographical scales from the local to the global. It is the output from such recording systems that enables us to estimate the global burden of disease. Some idea of the wide range of communicable diseases currently recognized by medical science can be obtained by turning the pages of a single week's report by any epidemiological agency. Thus, Australia's *Communicable Diseases Intelligence*, chosen for a random week in the last decade of the twentieth century (that ending on 4 April 1994), records over 120 different diseases and agents. The associated events include a major mumps outbreak in Western Australia, 131 cases of hepatitis C, and an outbreak of Ross River virus infection in the Northern Territory. Its overseas section records an outbreak of Japanese B encephalitis in Sri Lanka and a severe malaria outbreak on the Trobriand Islands off Papua New Guinea. Meanwhile, influenza A was sweeping through 21 Russian cities and cholera was continuing to invade northern Mozambique.

Disease records over time

Availability of disease data varies greatly over time. There is little consistent archival material until the second half of the nineteenth century. In the United States, Scandinavia, and Great Britain, legislation was passed at this time that ensured disease records were kept for afflictions considered to be of special risk to national populations. It is important not to see disease recording over time as progressing ever more accurately. In recent decades, the recording of some common diseases has been downgraded as their incidence and their perceived threat has fallen. In some countries, disease recording has moved from statutory reporting of all recognized cases to one of sampling and surveillance using devices such as 'sentinel' medical practices.

Disease records over space: mapping

Countries vary in what they can afford to spend on their medical services and the priority they give to recording particular diseases. In general, the richer the country, the better the disease data but the relationship is a complex one and there are many examples of small countries with excellent records (e.g. Iceland, Fiji) and vice versa.

Even where records are maintained, a significant mapping problem is the changing infrastructure of local boundary areas. We discuss in section 2.5.2, in Chapter 2, an 80-year sequence of maps of the medical districts in a country with outstanding medical records, Iceland. Here, the population over this period has been congregating around the major cities (notably the Icelandic capital, Reykjavík) and leaving the rural areas. This has led to a consequential relocation of physicians, so that some old urban areas may be split (as their populations grow) and some old rural areas may be amalgamated (as their populations dwindle). The fishing net by which diseases are caught and recorded is rarely stable, posing a continuing puzzle for map makers wishing to show local changes over time in a consistent manner.

The burden of infectious disease

Mortality

Death is, of course, the ultimate indicator of the importance of a disease. While death certificates (where they exist) give only a partial view of the cause of death, they represent the best evidence we have and the WHO goes to great lengths to collect and codify these data at the world level.

The first column in Table 1.5 lists the ten leading causes of death worldwide at the turn of the millennium. The table shows that infectious diseases occupied six of the top ten places as global killers. Taken together, communicable diseases (which include infectious and parasitic diseases, respiratory infections, maternal and perinatal conditions, and nutritional deficiencies) accounted for over 30% of the 56 million global deaths, a picture which had changed little by 2020.

Morbidity

Yet other ways of measuring the disease burden are in terms of illness (morbidity) rather than death and these are shown in the second two columns of Table 1.5. They show a very different pattern from that for deaths: where infectious diseases occur, they are often of a different kind and in a different order of priority.

Morbidity can be measured in different ways. We can (i) count the total number of new cases of a particular disease each year or during some other interval of time (the disease *incidence*). Or (ii) we can count the total number of people who continue to suffer with a particular disease, regardless of when they first contracted the disease (the disease *prevalence*). For example, when we state there were over 1 million new cases of leishmaniasis worldwide in 2000, we are describing its annual incidence. But when we state that in 2020 there were 10 million people worldwide permanently disabled by paralytic poliomyelitis, then we are talking about its prevalence.

Weighted measures

Although counting deaths from a particular cause in a particular year might seem a simple and unambiguous way of measuring the burden of disease, it avoids a central question. Are all deaths equal? Although this may depend upon one's personal viewpoint, the theological view might be exactly that—all lives, and therefore all deaths, are indeed equal. Let us think about this a little more.

Table 1.5 Different definitions of the global disease burden

Criterion I Deaths		Criterion II Morbidity (new cases)		Criterion III Permanent and long-term activity limitation	
1	Coronary heart disease (100)	1	**Diarrhoea (100)**	1	Mood disorders (100)
2	Cerebrovascular disease (64)	2	**Malaria (13)**	2	Hearing loss (84)
3	**ALRI (51)**	3	**ALRI (10)**	3	**Schistosomiasis (82)**
4	**HIV/AIDS (40)**	4	Occupational injuries (6)	4	**Lymphatic filariasis (82)**
5	COPD (39)	5	Occupational disorders (5)	5	Cretinoids (34)
6	**Diarrhoea (30)**	6	**Trichomoniasis (4)**	6	Mental retardation (25)
7	**Tuberculosis (25)**	7	Mood disorders (3)	7	Schizophrenic disorders (18)
8	**Malaria (18)**	8	**Chlamydial infections (2)**	8	Occupational injuries (17)
9	Prematurity (16)	9	**Hepatitis B (2)**	9	Occupational diseases (14)
10	**Measles (12)**	10	**Gonococcal infection (2)**	10	Cataract-related blindness (13)

Infectious diseases marked in bold. The leading cause in each of the three categories is set to 100 and other causes expressed in relative terms. Thus, in category I, the annual toll of deaths from tuberculosis (1.8 million) is 25 per cent of the deaths from the leading cause, coronary heart disease (7.2 million). ALRI, acute lower respiratory infections; COPD, chronic obstructive pulmonary disease. Diarrhoea includes dysentery.
Source: Data from the World Health Organization's *World Health Report*, 2000 edition.

We all have to die at some time, and while the death of a child might be seen as a tragedy (Christopher Marlowe's 'cut is the branch that might have grown full straight'; *Doctor Faustus*, Act V, scene 3), that of someone who is very old and perhaps very sick might sometimes be seen as a blessing. In other words, an argument exists that deaths of the young may cut off more potential years of living than deaths of the old. Clearly this is a huge simplification and leaves many moral questions unanswered.

Agencies such as the WHO and the United States Centers for Disease Control and Prevention (CDC) have been experimenting with statistics which measure *years of potential life lost* (YPLL). This takes into account the year at which a death occurs. For example, if we take the 'life tables' published by most national population agencies, we can look up life expectancy. In England in 2000, a 20-year-old male could expect on average to live for another 55 years (60 for a female) whereas an 80-year-old male could expect to live on average for another 7 years. So, under YPLL, the two deaths would be weighted differently, the younger death having a weight much higher than the older.

The effect of measures of this kind is to change the order of some leading causes of death, giving greater weight to the infectious diseases (which especially affect children) and to injuries (which especially affect young people). They also reduce the relative importance of heart disease and cancers (which tend to affect the old). With illness and disability, similar arguments may be used, giving special weight to diseases which cause a lifetime of disability (so-called *disability-adjusted life years* (DALYs)) rather than a brief illness. An introduction to the problem is given in Murray and Lopez's (1996) *The Global Burden of Disease*.

The WHO estimates that some 56 million deaths occurred worldwide in 2000. Using the WHO's main disease groups (infectious and parasitic diseases; cancers; diseases of the respiratory system; perinatal, neonatal, and maternal causes; diseases of the circulatory system; other and unknown causes), the leading group was infectious and parasitic diseases (such as tuberculosis, diarrhoea, malaria, and AIDS) which accounted for one-third of the total. Almost as many (29 per cent) were due to diseases of the circulatory system (e.g. coronary heart disease) and a further 12 per cent were due to cancers. Together, these three causes account for three-quarters of all deaths. There is a striking contrast in causes of death between the developing and the developed worlds. In the former, 43 per cent of deaths are due to infectious and parasitic diseases whereas these shrink to only 1 per cent in the latter. Diarrhoea in children aged under 5 years accounts for 1.8 billion episodes a year (and claims the lives of 3 million children). Acute lower respiratory conditions (especially in children), sexually transmitted diseases, measles, and whooping cough remain major problems in the developing world.

Disease impacts: national level

The contrasts outlined at the global level are echoed at the national level which means that each country is likely to have a different disease profile. Taking historical data for the purposes of illustration, **Figure 1.2** plots on a logarithmic proportional scale the number of deaths and number of cases for the main infectious diseases in the United States in the mid-1980s. Only those diseases which caused more than ten deaths or more than 1,000 cases per year are shown. The largest number of deaths (32,000) was caused by pneumococcal bacteria, followed by nosocomial deaths in acute (26,400) and chronic (24,700) care. In terms of morbidity, by far the largest number of cases was generated by the common cold viruses (rhinoviruses; 125 million) followed by another group of viruses, influenza (20 million). The diagram shows only the leading 50 specific infections, to which COVID-19 in the 12 months from March 2020 has been added. Although those not plotted had fewer than ten deaths per year or fewer than 1,000 cases, they include many diseases which rank highly on the 'dread' factor. For example, amoebic meningoencephalitis was recorded only four times in the United States in the period studied but each resulted in death; rabies killed all ten of those infected; and half of the 100 cases infected with the cryptosporidiosis parasite died. The diagonal lines in **Figure 1.2** show the case-fatality rates for the more frequently occurring diseases. Those which are on or above the 1:10 diagonal include HIV, Legionnaires' disease, and meningococcal meningitis.

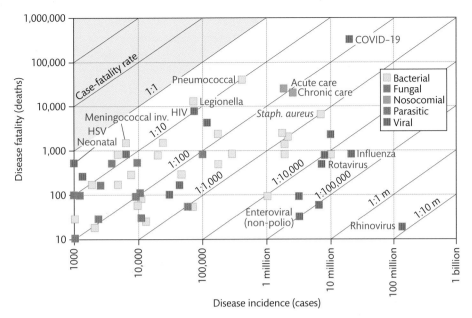

Figure 1.2 United States national mortality and morbidity framework for infectious diseases, 1980s. Annual mortality and morbidity from major infectious and parasitic diseases in the United States in the mid-1980s. Note that both disease fatality and disease incidence are plotted on logarithmic scales. The diagonal lines represent the case-fatality rate so that the most severe diseases are upper left, the mildest lower right. HSV, herpes simplex virus.

Source: Data from Bennett, J.V., Holmberg, J.D., Rogers, M.K., Solomon, S.L. (1987). 'Infectious and parasitic diseases.' In: R.W. Amler and H.B. Dull (eds.), *Closing the Gap: The Burden of Unnecessary Diseases.* Oxford: Oxford University Press, 100–20, supplemented with WHO COVID-19 data.

1.3 Nature of Epidemics

In this section, we focus on epidemics, looking at their definition, measurement, magnitude, and associated demographic impact.

1.3.1 Epidemic Concepts

Epidemic

The term *epidemic* comes from two Greek words, *demos* meaning 'people' and *epi* meaning 'upon' or 'close to'. It was used around 500 BC as a title for one major part of the Hippocratic corpus, but the section concerned was mainly a day-to-day account of certain patients and not an application of the word in its modern sense. In addition to its wider usage in terms of public attitudes (e.g. Burke's 'epidemick of despair'), the word has been used in the English language in a medical sense since at least 1603 to mean an unusually high incidence of a disease. Here, 'unusually high' is fixed in time, in space, and in the persons afflicted as compared with previous experience. The *Oxford English Dictionary* defines an epidemic as 'a disease prevalent among a people or community at a special time, and produced by some special causes generally not present in the affected locality'. The parallel term, epizootic, is used to specify a disease present under similar conditions in a non-human animal community.

Epidemicity is thus relative to the usual frequency of disease in the same area, among the specified population, at the same season of the year. It denotes the occurrence in a community or region of cases of an illness (or an outbreak) clearly in excess of expectation. The number of cases indicating the presence of an epidemic will vary according to the infectious agent, the size and type of the population's previous experience, or lack of exposure to the disease, and the time and place of occurrence. So, what constitutes an epidemic does not necessarily depend on large numbers of cases or deaths. A single case of a communicable disease long absent from a population, or the first invasion by a disease not previously recognized in that area, requires immediate reporting and epidemiological investigation. Two cases of such a disease associated in time and place are taken to be sufficient evidence of transmission for an epidemic to be declared.

Epidemiology, the scientific study of epidemics, has its own extensive vocabulary. The terms chosen here, from a very long and growing list, are based on those given in Halloran (1998), Vynnycky and White (2010), and Heymann (2015), but the language, like epidemics themselves, continues to grow and diversify.

1.3.2 Epidemic Models

The modelling of epidemics began in the laboratory with the study of mice populations. Mechanical analogues (coloured beads on a tray) were briefly in vogue, but from the time of P.D. En'ko's work in 1889 (Dietz, 1988), these were replaced by mathematical models which make statements based on increasingly complex equations. Solving such equations has been revolutionized by advances in computing, and mathematical epidemiology is now a well-established branch of applied mathematics. Bailey (1957, 1975), Anderson and May (1991), Vynnycky and White (2010), and Martcheva (2016) are classics in the field, while Sattenspiel (2009) is particularly relevant here since this work stresses the spatial and geographical aspects of model building. Such models are of two basic types: *deterministic*, which describe what happens on average in a population and do not incorporate the effects of chance; and *stochastic*, which make probability statements about the processes being modelled.

SIR compartment models

Most models are made up of boxes between which the population of interest is divided. The three basic divisions in a closed model are between *susceptible* (*S*), *infective* (*I*), and *recovered* (*R*) segments of a population, the so-called *SIR* family. The boxes may be then subdivided by factors of interest such as age, sex, ethnicity, or geographical location.

A distinction is drawn between models which are *closed* (restricted to the *SIR* segments and subsegments) and those which are *open* to the outside world (adding in births, deaths, in-migration, and out-migration, etc). Another difference is drawn between models which are *static* in that the parameters used are fixed in value and *dynamic* with parameter values which vary over the course of time (e.g. between the growth and decline phases of an epidemic wave).

Contact ratio

This is defined as a measure of contact sufficient to lead to transmission of the disease agent if it occurs between an infectious and a susceptible person. Technically, it is the per capita rate at which two specific individuals come into effective contact per unit time, and is commonly denoted by the Greek letter, β. It is also sometimes given other names, such as the transmission coefficient, transmission rate, or contact parameter.

Reproduction number

The basic reproduction number or ratio measures the average number of secondary infectives caused by one infectious person following their introduction into a totally susceptible population. It is denoted by R_0. There are at least a dozen ways of calculating this important aspect of epidemic growth ($R_0 > 1$) or contraction ($R_0 < 1$). In general terms, it is given as the ratio between an infection rate (β) and a recovery rate (γ), that is, $R_0 = \beta/\gamma$. R_0 is a number rather than a rate since there are no time units in the definition. Estimates of R_0 for sample diseases are given in Table 5.1 in Chapter 5.

Threshold

An epidemic threshold is the minimum proportion of the population that needs to be susceptible for the infection incidence to increase, calculated as $1/R_0$. The *herd immunity threshold* is the proportion of the population which needs to be immune for the infection incidence to be stable, calculated as $1 - (1/R_0)$. It is also referred to as the critical immunization threshold. To eliminate an infection from an area, the proportion of the population that is immunized must exceed this threshold. Threshold estimates are given for sample diseases in Table 1.2.

1.3.3 Types of Epidemics

Epidemics of communicable disease are of two main types. A *propagated epidemic* is one that results from the chain transmission of some infectious agent. This may be directly from person to person as in a measles outbreak, or indirectly via some intermediate vector (malaria) or a microparasite. The second type of epidemic is a *common-vehicle epidemic*. This type of epidemic results from the exposure of a group of people to a common medium (typically water, milk, or food) that has been contaminated by a disease-causing organism. Cholera and typhoid provide classic examples of diseases that are commonly transmitted in this manner.

1.3.4 A Simple Stage Model

We put forward here a simple description of the main stages through which an infectious disease event may evolve into an epidemic and, possibly, a pandemic. Only very few events progress through all of the stages described.

Stage 1: endemic reservoir

Natural disease reservoirs are commonly a population of animals or plant species within which an infectious disease agent may persist for the greater part of its life, often not appearing to harm that natural host. Natural reservoirs fall into three broad categories: human (e.g. measles, mumps, and smallpox), animal non-human (e.g. Ebola virus disease, plague, and rabies), and environmental (e.g. various forms of fungal agent). Essentially, reservoirs provide a long-term base where an organism can survive in an endemic state and reproduce in such manner that it can be transmitted from time to time to a susceptible host and invade the human population.

Stage 2: index cases

As we saw in section 1.2.1, the infection process by which an outbreak begins is immensely complex. An index case is the first documented patient within an outbreak or epidemic. Thus, a 2-year-old boy in a village in Guinea was established as the source of the large Ebola virus epidemic in West Africa in 2014 (see section 3.4.3 in Chapter 3). 'Patient 0', a sexually active flight attendant, was implicated in the early and rapid spread of the HIV/AIDS epidemic in the United States (see Figure 3.11 in Chapter 3). Other examples include a baby at 40 Broad Street, London, implicated in the 1854 cholera outbreak there, while Mary Malone (the superspreader 'Typhoid Mary') was a cook who infected 47 people in New England in the early 1900s. Even one of the authors of this book gained brief notoriety, aged seven, in bringing scarlet fever to all his older siblings, cousins, and Sunday School classmates in a Somerset village in 1939. Equally, the index cases in some outbreaks are never found or are wrongly attributed.

Stage 3: outbreak

A small but unusual cluster of cases defines an outbreak. If one child in a preschool class gets diarrhoea, that is an isolated case; if eight children get diarrhoea in the same week that is an outbreak and would be investigated by public health authorities to find its cause and attempt to prevent its further spread. As with so many epidemiological terms, the label relates to an event that is above some normal reference level. As we shall see in Chapter 5, the cluster of severe pneumonia cases among market-goers in Wuhan, China, presaged the start of the COVID-19 pandemic.

Stage 4: epidemic

If 'small, but unusual' characterizes an outbreak, then 'bigger and spreading' sums up an epidemic. As noted in section 1.3.1, there is no numerical size measure but large in relation to normal levels is again the key. Epidemics represent the second rung on the outbreak → epidemic → pandemic ladder, and monitoring the data to try and predict the likely outcome is a central concern of most epidemic modellers.

One general characteristic that separates an epidemic from an outbreak is the formation of a characteristic wave. **Figure 1.3** shows 25-year time series of reported measles cases (between 1945 and

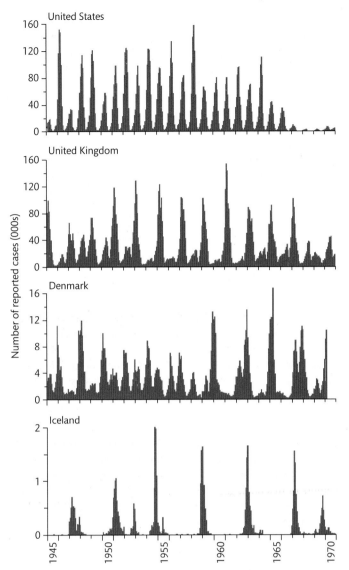

Figure 1.3 National measles cycles and host population size, 1945–70. The graphs plot the monthly count of reported measles cases in each of four countries (United States, United Kingdom, Denmark, and Iceland), arranged in descending order of national population size. Note the characteristic cyclicity in all instances, the dramatic reduction in amplitude for the United States after 1964 (because of vaccination programmes), and the fact that only Iceland has clear breaks indicating its non-endemicity.

Reproduced from Cliff, A.D., Haggett, P., Ord, J.K., Versey, G.R. (1981). *Spatial Diffusion: An Historical Geography of Epidemics in an Island Community.* Cambridge: Cambridge University Press. Reprinted with permission.

1970) for four countries, arranged in decreasing order of population size. In the United States, with a 1970 population of 205 million, and in the United Kingdom (56 million), epidemic peaks occur every 1 or 2 years. Denmark (5 million) has a more complex pattern, with a tendency for a 3-year cycle in the latter half of the period. Iceland (only 0.2 million) stands in contrast to the other countries in that only eight waves occurred over the period; several years are without cases.

Stage 5: pandemic

As outlined in section 4.1, the term *pandemic* describes a very large epidemic that is international, intercontinental, or even global in its extent. Global pandemics of such diseases as cholera, COVID-19, HIV/AIDS, influenza, and plague are treated at length in Chapters 4 and 5. Here, we note that—if pandemics deserve an epithet—then 'international and out of control' would serve. The WHO is careful about declaring an epidemic as a pandemic as this has political, legal, and financial implications.

Stage 6: dual outcome

At the end of each outbreak, epidemic, or pandemic, the biological clock is generally reset and a disease agent reverts to its natural reservoir. An exception is the smallpox virus which was finally eradicated at the end of a long international campaign (see section 6.5 in Chapter 6).

1.3.5 The Magnitude of Epidemic Events

The first paragraph of Norman Bailey's classic 1957 edition of *The Mathematical Theory of Epidemics* reads as follows:

> The fearful toll of human life and happiness exacted through the ages by widespread disease and pestilence affords a spectacle that is both fascinating and repellent. A recital of the astronomical numbers of casualties suffered in this way by the human race is almost stupefying in its effect, and makes the consequences of all past wars seem almost trivial in comparison. Thus in Europe in the 14th century there were some 25 million deaths out of a population of perhaps 100 million from the Black Death alone. In 1520 the Aztecs lost about half their population of 3 million from smallpox. The downfall of their empire in 1521 was due more to smallpox than to Cortes. It has been estimated that Russia suffered about 25 million cases of typhus in the years from 1918 to 1921 with a death-rate of approximately 10 per cent. In the world pandemic of influenza in 1919 the total number of deaths is thought to have been in the region of 20 million over twelve months. Examples such as these could be multiplied *ad nauseam.* (Bailey, 1957, p. 1)

Shortly after, Bailey was to leave the groves of Cambridge to take over the headship of the WHO Epidemiological Research Unit in Geneva and be involved in the new epidemics that the later decades of the twentieth century would throw at the global population.

In Table 4.1, in Chapter 4, we list sample pandemic events in history. This table began life with the optimistic hope that reasonable estimates of deaths and death rates caused by each event globally, or at least in England and Wales, could be straightforwardly compiled. That hope was rapidly dashed; inspection of Table 4.1 shows that, even for the numbers we have gathered, there is a high frequency with which numbers are 'estimated' (est.). There are two compelling reasons. 'Largest' implies the need both for some precision and that one can confidently sift out and apply numbers to events, some of which occurred at distant times or in distant places far removed from precise medical measurers. As we noted in section 1.2.3, accurate diagnosis and reliable international records are matters for the last century at best.

Two examples serve to show how historical estimates permit these gaps to be filled. For the Black Death in England, one indicator lies in the parish records of incumbents. We know that a ship docked at the Dorset port of Melcombe in June 1348 and correspondence tells that deaths from a new plague were being recorded in surrounding places within a few weeks. In a study of the adjacent county of Somerset, Haggett (2012, pp. 94–6) calculated the rate of replacement for priests serving in each parish. When plotted on a time chart, a peak in new appointments soars in 1348–50 above the

Table 1.6 Spectrum of pandemic and epidemic events

Size	Time period	Location	Disease	Estimated number of deaths	Estimated ratio of deaths to population
>10 million deaths	2018	Worldwide	Disease X[a]	90,000,000	1:90
	1346–52	Western Europe	Black Death Bubonic plague	20,000,000	1:4
	1918–19	Worldwide	Influenza A	>20,000,000	1:25 (India)
>1 million deaths	2020–?	Worldwide	COVID-19	2,759,000[b]	
>100,000 deaths	1741	Ireland	Famine, typhus, dysentery	300,000	1:6
	1098–99	Palestine (First Crusade)	Epidemic diseases, famine	240,000	1:1.25
	1781–2	Europe	Influenza	>100,000	?
>10,000 deaths	c.1438	Paris	Smallpox	50,000	1:4
	1870–71	Paris (siege)	Smallpox	75,162	1:29
	1870	England & Wales	Whooping cough	c.36,000	1:650
	1875 (Jan–June)	Fiji	Measles and sequelae	30,000	1:4
	1801–03	Haiti (French troops)	Yellow fever	22,000	1:1.13

[a] The number of deaths for Disease X (see section 3.5 in Chapter 3) is based on a simulation at Johns Hopkins University using a set of mid-range estimates. [b] Cumulative reported total to 27 March 2021.
Source: Data from Cliff, A.D., Haggett, P., Smallman-Raynor, M.R. (1998). *Deciphering Global Epidemics: Analytical Approaches to the Disease Records of World Cities, 1888–1912.* The original extensive table gives, for each epidemic cited, a list of sources on which the table is based.

'normal replacement' rate. On this basis we can roughly estimate that a quarter to a third of incumbents (and probably their flocks, too) lost their lives to an epidemic in this period.

A second example is the great Fiji measles epidemic in 1875 (Cliff and Haggett, 1985). At the time, the archipelago of hundreds of volcanic islands and atolls stretching over a sea area the size of France had one medical officer to oversee a native population that was uncounted but was certainly in excess of 100,000. Here, the loss from measles was estimated from church records. Western missionaries from the Methodist Church in England had established a large network of chapels throughout Fiji with pastors and church leaders making an annual return of worshippers to the main church. That this dipped by a quarter to a third on average gives a rough estimate of the impact of the epidemic.

Any list of epidemic events has to be taken with a pinch of salt. It is critically dependent on the various assumptions made and on which any number estimates are based and the time period in months or years to which it refers. With this caveat, Table 1.6 gives some idea of the mortality, geographical and temporal scope, and the size of a tiny sample of the pandemics, epidemics, and local outbreaks of infectious and contagious diseases which have occurred in human history.

1.4 Epidemics in the Time Domain

The second half of this opening chapter is concerned with the ways in which the progress of epidemics has been studied, giving special weight to those capable of geographical application. We look first at the analysis of epidemics over the single dimension of time using epidemic matrices (section 1.4.1). We then turn to modelling the data, first as waves of increasing complexity (sections 1.4.2–1.4.3) and then as branching networks (section 1.4.4).

1.4.1 The Epidemic Data Matrix

Much epidemiological investigation starts with a simple data matrix. Typical are those assembled over decades of practice by a Yorkshire general practitioner, William Pickles, whose work is analysed in detail in Chapter 2. As illustrated there (see Figure 2.2), Pickles's data include both hand-drawn coloured graphs and detailed epidemic data pages assembled by Pickles, his wife, and the practice's dispenser, from surgery records and daily home visits. Time was made to record and chart each day's record of infectious disease for every village and hamlet in the practice. Six diseases (each plotted in a different colour) were carefully recorded and plotted day by day in the fashion of a school register. This simple process of counting diseases, by time and by place, has proved to be a cornerstone of epidemiological investigation. It stretches back to John Snow's counts and maps of cholera in the Soho district of London, through to today's 'track and trace' of COVID-19 as used in a myriad of countries. The difference is only one of scale. Pickles's modest 6 diseases × 8 parishes over 91 days each quarter year (4,368 cells in all) is replaced by today's massive matrices with millions of space–time cells. By way of example, the Johns Hopkins website in the United States keeps a daily electronic world data log for COVID-19, of which each of the United States' 50 states and over 3,000 counties comprise but a tithe of the areas reporting.

From chart to matrix

One way of looking at Pickles's chart is as an *epidemic data matrix* (EDM), a cube with disease, time, and space forming its three dimensions (**Figure 1.4**). The epidemic data on one plane can thus be analysed in terms of the other two, either separately, as in this section, or taken together in a space–time framework as in sections 1.5 and 1.6.

The geometry of the page keeps the dimensions to three but tracking epidemics in reality is conducted in a k-dimensional hypercube. Each disease will be measured in several ways—cases

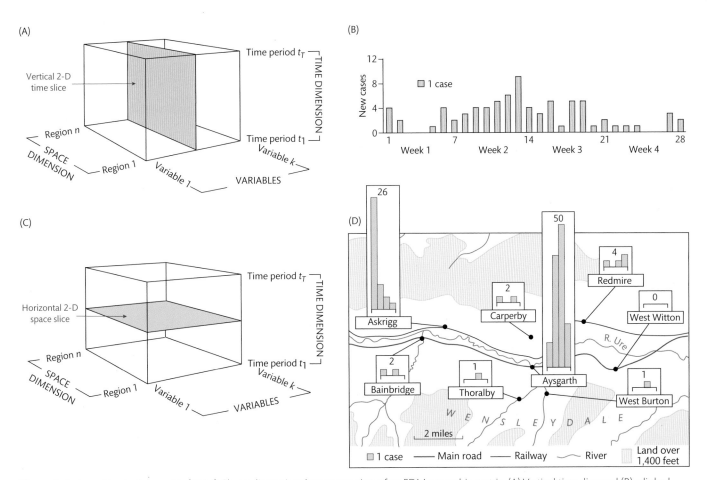

Figure 1.4 An epidemic data matrix (EDM). Three-dimensional representation of an EDM as a cubic matrix. (A) Vertical *time* slice and (B) a linked histogram. (C) EDM with a horizontal *space* slice and linked map (D). Both show newly diagnosed cases of Sonne dysentery by a country doctor in a Yorkshire practice in February 1932 (see section 2.2 in Chapter 2). Cases are plotted on the same scale on both the histogram and the map. 2-D, two dimensional.

Reproduced from Cliff, A.D., Ord, J.K. (1975). 'Space-time modelling with an application to regional forecasting.' *Transactions of the Institute of British Geographers*, 64, 119–28. Reprinted with permission. Source: Data from Pickles (1939, chart pp. 24–5).

diagnosed, strains identified, hospital admissions, deaths, and so on. Analysis of charts and trends will draw on contextual data—age, sex, occupation, household size, and so on. Equally, epidemic analysis will draw on demographic and economic data to describe the background populations through which a disease is spreading. The potential EDM grows, especially if dyadic data is added (see section 1.6.4).

1.4.2 The Single Epidemic Wave

Much thought was given by early observers to the nature of the curves that might best match histograms like **Figure 1.4B**. The argument ran that if we could find a 'natural' epidemic curve then this might provide clues to epidemic behaviour and allow some foresight into how a growing epidemic might shape itself into the future in the remainder of the curve. Thus, William Farr (1840) smoothed quarterly data on deaths from smallpox in England and Wales over the period 1837–39, suggesting that the pattern might follow the Gaussian normal curve of error. This empirical curve-fitting approach was further developed by Brownlee (1907) who considered in detail the 'geometry' of epidemic curves.

Statistical distributions

One method of curve recognition that we have used in the past (Cliff et al., 2000) relates to the various moments of a statistical distribution. As **Figure 1.5** shows, we have followed the Farr–Brownlee

approach in our own studies of Icelandic measles epidemics (Cliff and Haggett, 1983; Cliff et al., 1993). The three upper curves follow the S-shaped curves identified in Hägerstrand's diffusion work (see following subsections) and are well described by the logistic model. In Figures 1.5A–C, the cumulative share of the epidemic is plotted against time, where $\hat{b}$ is the rate of build-up. The lower seven waves plot the number of cases over time and show the mean times (D, H); s, the standard deviations (E, G, I); and b_2, a measure of kurtosis or peakedness (F, J). These measures are discussed further on p. 52. The upper left wave is the fastest of the seven, and shows (i) strong peaking and (ii) is sharply skewed to the left; most cases occur early. Slower moving epidemic waves lie in the right-hand column. For the Icelandic measles epidemic waves examined in section 2.5.4, for example, the five between 1916 and 1944 were faster and deadlier than the nine between 1946 and 1974. The post-war waves were on average more frequent but half the size and slower moving around the island.

Empirical evidence

A separate strand of empirical evidence has come from diffusion studies within the social sciences. Swedish human geographer, Torsten Hägerstrand, in his *Innovation Diffusion as a Spatial Process* (1953, 1967a) was concerned with the acceptance by farmers of several agricultural innovations in an area of central Sweden. These

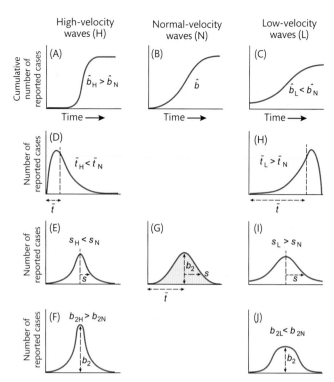

Figure 1.5 Characteristic case distributions for Normal, high, and low velocity epidemic waves. (A–C) Sinusoidal curves (above) and (D–J) bell-shaped curves below. Individual variants described in text.

Reproduced from Cliff, A.D., Haggett, P., Smallman-Raynor, M.R. (1993). Measles: An Historical Geography of a Major Human Viral Disease from Global Expansion to Local Retreat, 1840–1990. Oxford: Wiley.

innovations ranged from farmers taking up the control of bovine tuberculosis (through vaccination) to adopting government subsidies for the improvement of grazing. Here the object was to speed up the adoption of good practice and mirrored similar practical studies of innovation on farms in the United States.

These studies of the progress of a contagious wave through a population suggested to Hägerstrand and his colleagues a four-stage process for the passage of what he termed 'innovation waves' ('innovationsförloppet'). The *primary stage* marks the beginning of the diffusion process. A centre of adoption is established at the origin. There is a strong contrast in the level of adoption between this centre (high) and remote areas (low) which is reflected in the steep decline of the level of the adoption curve beyond the origin. The *diffusion stage* signals the start of the actual spread process. There is a powerful centrifugal effect, resulting in the rapid growth of acceptance in areas distant from the origin and by a reduction in the strong regional contrasts typical of the primary stage. This results in a flattening of the slope of the proportion of adopters curve. In the *condensing stage*, the relative increase in the numbers adopting an innovation is equal in all locations, regardless of their distance from the original innovation centre; the acceptance curve moves in a parallel fashion. The final *saturation stage* is marked by a slowing and eventual cessation of the diffusion process, which produces a further flattening of the acceptance curve. In this stage, the innovation being diffused has been adopted throughout the country, so that there is very little regional variation.

Other Swedish geographers carried out similar studies to test the validity of this four-stage process. For instance, Tornqvist (1967)

traced the spread of television ownership in Sweden using information obtained from 4,000 Swedish post office districts. His findings again followed the four-stage model.

The logistic model

The shape of the diffusion profile in time and space has been formally modelled. We consider first the build-up in the number of adopters of an innovation over time t. If the total susceptible population at the start ($t = 0$) of the process is known, then the cumulative number of that total who will have become adopters at $t = 1, 2, \ldots$ commonly follows an S-shaped curve when plotted against t (**Figure 1.5A–C**).

The model most commonly fitted to profiles of the form of **Figure 1.5B** is either the logistic or the Gompertz distribution. The logistic model is given by:

$$p_t = \left(1 + e^{a-bt}\right)^{-1} \tag{1.1}$$

or:

$$y_t = k\left(1 + e^{a-bt}\right)^{-1} \tag{1.2}$$

where p_t is the proportion of adopters (or infectives in the case of an epidemic) in the population at t, y_t is the number of adopters, and a, b, and k are parameters. The parameter k is usually interpreted as the saturation level (everyone has adopted or has become infected), a is the intercept, and b is the slope coefficient. Since p_t is the proportion of the population which has actually adopted by time t, $(1 - p_t)$ is the proportion still to adopt; $p_t (1 - p_t)$ then represents the probability that a random meeting between two individuals is between an adopter and a potential adopter, while the parameter b represents the rate at which meetings take place (the rate of mixing). Note that b is the same *whatever the distance between the adopter and the potential adopter*; that is, equation 1.1 implies spatially homogeneous mixing between adopters and potential adopters. This assumption is in conflict with the idea of compartment models discussed in section 1.3.2, so that Cliff and Ord (1975) have suggested an extension of the logistic model that allows homogeneous mixing within regions, but less mixing between regions.

Kendall waves

The relationship between the input and output components in existing wave-generating models was explored by Cambridge statistician, David Kendall (1957). He demonstrated that if we measure the magnitude of the input by a diffusion coefficient, β say, and the output by a recovery coefficient, γ, then the ratio of the two, γ/β, defines a threshold, ρ, in terms of population size. For example, where γ is 0.5 and β is 0.0001, then ρ would be estimated as 5,000.

Figure 1.6A illustrates a sequence of outbreaks in a community where the threshold has a constant value and is plotted as a horizontal line. Given a constant birth rate, the susceptible population increases and forms a diagonal line rising over time. Three examples of virus introductions are shown. In the first two, the susceptible population is smaller than the threshold ($S < \rho$) and there are a few secondary cases but no general epidemic. In the third example of virus introduction, the susceptible population has grown well beyond the threshold ($S > \rho$); the primary case is followed by many secondaries and a substantial outbreak follows. The effect of the outbreak is to reduce the susceptible population as shown by the offset curve in the diagram.

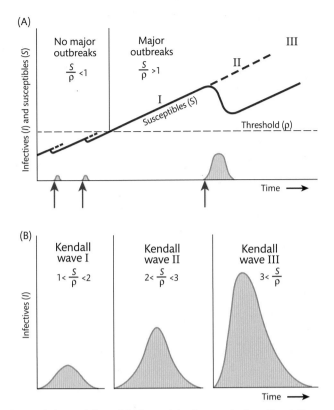

Figure 1.6 Kendall model of an epidemic wave in time. Kendall's (1957) model of the relationship between the shape of an epidemic wave and the susceptible population/threshold ratio. (A) Growth of a susceptible population over time showing the effect of infections introduced at the red arrows. (B) Three typical Kendall waves for the locations I, II, and III on (A).

Reproduced from Haggett, P. (2000). *The Geographical Structure of Epidemics.* Oxford: Clarendon Press.

Kendall investigated the effect of the S/ρ ratio on the incidence and nature of epidemic waves. With a ratio of less than one, a major outbreak cannot be generated; above one, both the probability of an outbreak and its shape changes with increasing S/ρ ratio values. To simplify Kendall's arguments, **Figure 1.6B** illustrates the waves generated at positions I, II, and III in **Figure 1.6A**. In wave I, the susceptible population is only slightly above the threshold value. If an outbreak should occur in this zone, then it will have a low incidence, and will be symmetrical in shape with only a modest concentration of cases in the peak period; as **Figure 1.6B** shows, a Kendall wave I approximates a Normal curve. In contrast, wave III is generated when the susceptible population is well above the threshold value. The consequent epidemic wave has a higher incidence, is strongly skewed towards the start, and is extremely peaked in shape with many cases concentrated into the peak period. Wave II occupies an intermediate position and is included to emphasize that the changing waveforms are examples from a continuum.

The spatial search for the kinds of waves predicted by the Kendall model has revealed some unexpected results. A geographer, Andrew Gilg (1973), analysed the shape of epizootic waves generated by an outbreak of Newcastle disease (fowlpest) in poultry populations in England and Wales in 1970–71. Study of Gilg's maps suggest that Kendall type III waves were characteristic of the central areas near the start of an outbreak. As the epizootic spread outwards, so the

waveform evolved towards type II and eventually, on the far edge of the outbreak, to type I.

A generalization of Gilg's findings is given in **Figure 1.7**. This shows, in panel (A), in an idealized form, the relationship of the wave shape to the map of the overall outbreak and, in panel (B), the waveform plotted in a space–time framework. In both diagrams, there is an overlap between relative time as measured from the start of the outbreak and relative space as measured from the geographical origin of the outbreak; in essence, the energy of the wave becomes dissipated as it moves through time and over space.

If we relate the pattern to Kendall's original arguments in **Figure 1.6**, then we must assume that the S/ρ ratio was itself changing over space and time. This could occur in three ways, either by a reduction in the value of S, or by an increase in ρ, or by both acting in combination. A reduction in the susceptible population is plausible in terms of both the distribution of poultry farming in England and Wales, and by the awareness of the outbreak stimulating farmers to take counter-measures in the form of both temporary isolation or, where available, by vaccination. Increases in ρ could theoretically occur either from an increase in the recovery coefficient (γ) or a decrease in the diffusion coefficient (β). The efforts of veterinarians to protect flocks would have been likely to force a reduced diffusion competence for the virus.

1.4.3 Complex Wave Trains

In this section, we move from the study of the single wave towards those created by a series of epidemics (cf. **Figure 1.3**) which we term *wave trains*. Modelling interest in these multiple events is of some antiquity. Among the first applications of mathematics to the study of infectious disease was that of Daniel Bernoulli (1760) when he used a mathematical method to evaluate the effectiveness of the techniques of variolation against smallpox. Names in mathematical epidemiology such as En'ko, Hamer, Ross, Soper, Reed, Frost, and Kermack and McKendrick are linked to the conversion of ideas about disease spread into simple, but precise, mathematical statements. A summary of their work is given in the definitive accounts by Bailey (1975) and Anderson and May (1991). We look at two models that illustrate deterministic and stochastic approaches (see section 1.3.2).

Deterministic *SIR* model

The simplest form of an epidemic model, the Hamer–Soper model, is shown in **Figure 1.8**. It was originally developed by Hamer in 1906 to describe the recurring sequences of measles waves affecting large English cities in the late Victorian period and has been greatly modified over the last 50 years to incorporate probabilistic, spatial, and public health features.

At any time t, we assume that the total population in a region can be divided into three classes: namely the population at risk or susceptible population of size S_t at time t, the infected population of size I_t, and the removed population of size R_t. The removed population is taken to be composed of people who have had the disease, but who can no longer pass it on to others because of recovery, isolation on the appearance of overt symptoms of the disease, or death. Four types of transition, i, are allowed:

1. A susceptible being infected by contact with an infective.
2. An infective being removed. We assume that infection confers life-long immunity to further attack after recovery, which

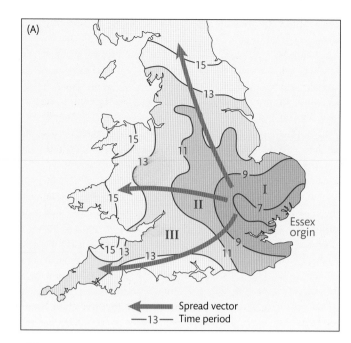

(A)

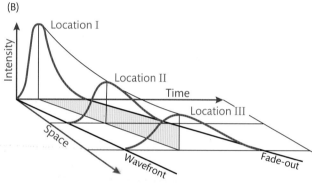

(B)

Figure 1.7 Changes in the shape of an epidemic wave with distance from the origin of an outbreak. (A) Gilg's findings on the spread of a Newcastle disease epizootic in England and Wales. The epizootic started in Essex and the contours of spread are in 15-day steps (i.e. contour 11 = 165 days after the start). (B) Generalized wave model set in time and space: locations I, II, and III refer to the positions on the map in (A).
Reproduced from Cliff, A.D., Haggett, P. (1988). *Atlas of Disease Distributions: Analytical Approaches to Epidemiological Data*. Oxford: Wiley. Source: Data from Gilg (1973, Figure 6, p.89).

is reasonable for many infectious diseases like measles and whooping cough.

3. A susceptible 'birth'. This can come about either through a child growing up into the critical age range (i.e. reaching about 6 months of age when mother-conferred immunity wanes), or through a susceptible entering the population by migration into the region from outside.

4. An infective entering the *I* population by migration into the region from outside. For simplicity, we assume that there is no migration out of the region.

Suppose that transition *i* occurs at the rate r_i (*i* = 1, 2, 3, 4); that is, in a small time interval $(t, t + \delta t)$ the probability of transition *i* occurring is $r_i \delta t + o(\delta t)$ where $o(\delta t)$ means a term of smaller order (i.e. considerably smaller) than δt. All events are assumed to be independent and to depend only on the present state of the population.

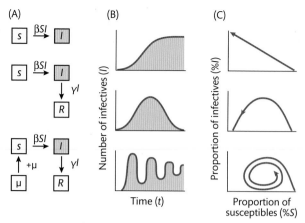

Figure 1.8 The Hamer–Soper model. Basic elements in the three simplest Hamer–Soper models of wave generation. (A) Model elements: *S*, susceptibles; *I*, infectives; *R*, recovereds; μ, births; β, infection (diffusion) rate; γ, recovery rate. (B) Typical time profiles for the model with number of infectives shown by the red shading. (C) Trajectory of typical waves in infective–susceptible space. The basic wave-generating mechanism is a simple one. The infected element in a population is augmented by the random mixing of susceptibles with infectives ($S \times I$) at a rate determined by a diffusion coefficient (β) appropriate to the disease. The infected element is depleted by recovery of individuals after a time period at a rate controlled by the recovery coefficient (γ). As Figure 1.8A shows, the addition of parameters to the model, such as the birth rate (μ), allows successively more complex models to be generated.
Reproduced from Haggett, P. (2000). *The Geographical Structure of Epidemics*. Oxford: Clarendon Press.

The probability density of the time between any pair of successive transitions is:

$$r \, exp(-rt) \tag{1.3}$$

where:

$$r = \sum_{i=1}^{4} r_i \tag{1.4}$$

and the probability that the next transition is of type *i* is $\frac{r_i}{r}$, *i* = 1, 2, 3, 4.

We assume, in the transitions 1–4, that the infection rate is proportional to the product *SI*, that the removal rate is proportional to *I*, and that the birth and immigration rates are constant.

Bartlett threshold models

Empirical validation of the mass action models for measles was provided by the work of statistician Maurice Bartlett (1957). He investigated the relationship between the periodicity of measles epidemics and population size for a series of urban centres on both sides of the Atlantic. His findings for British cities are summarized in **Figure 1.9**. The largest cities have an endemic pattern with periodic eruptions (type I), whereas cities below a certain size threshold have an epidemic pattern with fade-outs. Bartlett found the size threshold to be of the order of 250,000 inhabitants.

The critical community size for measles (the size for which measles is as likely as not to fade out after a major epidemic until reintroduced from outside) is found for the United States to be about 250,000–300,000 in terms of total population (Bartlett, 1960, p. 37). These figures agree broadly with the English statistics, provided notifications are corrected as far as possible for unreported cases. Subsequent

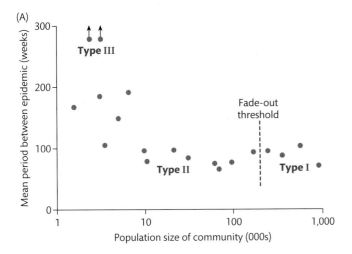

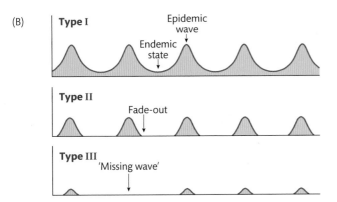

Figure 1.9 British towns' thresholds. Bartlett's findings on city size and epidemic recurrence. (A) The impact of population size on the spacing of measles epidemics for 19 English towns. (B) Characteristic epidemic profiles for the three types indicated in (A).

Reproduced from Cliff, A.D., Haggett, P., Ord, J.K., Versey, G.R. (1981). *Spatial Diffusion: An Historical Geography of Epidemics in an Island Community.* Cambridge: Cambridge University Press. Reprinted with permission.

research has shown that the threshold for measles, or indeed any other infectious disease, is likely to be somewhat variable with the level influenced by population densities and vaccination levels. However, the threshold principle demonstrated by Bartlett remains intact.

If the population size of an area is below the threshold, when the disease concerned is eventually extinguished, it can only recur by reintroduction from other reservoir areas. Thus, the generalized persistence of disease implies geographical transmission between communities as shown in **Figure 1.10**. We can see that in large cities above the size threshold, like community A, a continuous trickle of cases is reported. These provide the reservoir of infection which sparks a major epidemic when the susceptible population, S, builds up to a critical level. This build-up occurs only as children are born, lose their mother-conferred immunity, and escape vaccination or contact with the disease. Eventually the S population will increase sufficiently for an epidemic to occur. When this happens, the S population is diminished and the stock of infectives, I, increases as individuals are transferred by infection from the S to the I population. This generates the characteristic D-shaped relationship over time between the sizes of the S and I populations shown on the end plane of the block diagram.

1.4.4 Epidemics as Branching Networks

We noted earlier that in spatial epidemiology, as in physics, phenomena may be viewed differently at different levels of resolution. At one level of resolution, an epidemic is simply an aggregation of infected individuals and its passage is seen as a wave. But at a higher level of resolution, the same process can be seen as individuals passing infection on in a chain-like structure (**Figure 1.1C**). In **Figure 1.1C**, an individual implies a single human being. But, with some loss of generality, the same arguments can be used for spatial districts (villages, parishes, counties, etc.) as appropriate. A range of chain models is reviewed by Vynnycky and White (2010, pp. 151–69), while an overview of geographical applications is provided by Sattenspiel (2009, pp. 151–60).

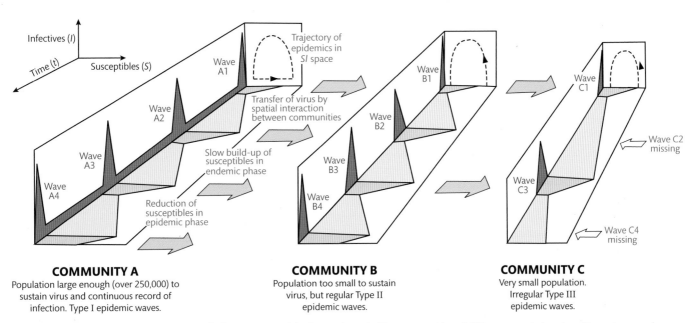

COMMUNITY A
Population large enough (over 250,000) to sustain virus and continuous record of infection. Type I epidemic waves.

COMMUNITY B
Population too small to sustain virus, but regular Type II epidemic waves.

COMMUNITY C
Very small population. Irregular Type III epidemic waves.

Figure 1.10 Conceptual view of the spread of a communicable disease (measles) in communities of different population sizes. Stages in spread correspond to the Bartlett model.

Reproduced with permission from Cliff, A.D., Haggett, P. (1988). *Atlas of Disease Distributions: Analytical Approaches to Epidemiological Data.* Oxford: Wiley.

The Reed–Frost model

The Reed–Frost model is the name usually given to this class of models to mark its development by two American epidemiologists in the 1920s. The approach is based on chain frequencies that are analysed using the binomial distribution—hence the class name of chain binomial models. They were developed to run in parallel rather than in competition with mass action models. The latter were constructed for use with aggregated data, and can be readily adapted to deal with spatial units at the regional, national, and international level. Although the chain binomial was originally developed for the micro-scale analysis of intra-family chains of transmission of infectious diseases, they have been adapted to provide forecasts based on aggregated data at a regional scale (Bailey, 1975; Cliff et al., 1981).

The basic model for a single district supposes that it is possible to record the state of the system at times $t = 1, 2, \ldots$. Ideally, the time interval between recording points should correspond in length to the serial interval of the disease. This ensures that we do not witness multiple epidemic cycles in a single time period, provided that each infected individual is isolated after the appearance of symptoms. The total population in a given recording district at the beginning of time period t, which we denote by N_t, will contain S_t susceptibles, I_t infectives who can transmit the disease to susceptibles, and R_t removals. During the t-th time period, N_t may be modified by the addition of A_t arrivals (births and/or immigrants) and the loss of D_t departures (deaths and/or emigrants). Finally, let X_t denote the number of new cases which occur in time period t.

The following accounting identities may then be written down for each recording district:

$$N_{t+1} = N_t + A_t - D_t,$$
$$N_t = S_t + I_t + R_t \tag{1.5}$$

If $\alpha_t A_t$ denotes the number of individuals among the new arrivals who are infectives, while $\delta_t D_t$ denotes the number of infectives among the departures, then:

$$I_{t+1} = I_t + X_t - \left[R_{t+1} - R_t \right] + \alpha_t A_t - \delta_t D_t \tag{1.6}$$

The arrivals term in equation 1.5 is vital in cases where we are considering a disease that has to be re-imported into an area after *local* fade-out; these arrivals are the individuals who, if they are infected, can trigger a recurrence of the disease when the number of susceptibles is high.

Postscript: chain geometry

One aspect of chain models that deserves further exploration is their link to graph theory. We explored the applications of graph theory to geographical structures in one volume (Haggett and Chorley, 1969) and a series of papers (Cliff and Haggett, 1981; Cliff et al., 1979) several decades ago, but these have only recently seen an avenue opening into epidemiological applications for chain models.

1.5 Epidemics in the Space Domain, I: Mapping

The history of epidemiology is closely entwined with maps. John Snow's famous sketch of cholera deaths in 1854, arranged like coffins along the streets of London's crowded Soho, remains iconic. Maps pose two separate sets of challenges. For the map maker, the task is one of design, of *encoding* data onto a map (section 1.5.1). For the map user, the parallel task is one of interpretation, of *decoding* the map (section 1.5.2). Both stages of the map cycle are subject to error.

1.5.1 Encoding Epidemic Maps

Maps are one of the key ways for portraying information about how a disease varies across the earth's surface. An example of an early epidemic map appears in Figure 6.4 in Chapter 6. Four centuries later we can turn to our laptop and dial up from a Johns Hopkins University website a screen map of the latest world distribution of COVID-19 cases, dipping down through the spatial scales from continent to country to cities and subdivisions. Interpretation is enhanced by 'on-call' graphs, statistics, and analytic tools of ever-increasing speed and sophistication.

There is a wealth of beautifully illustrated surveys of sample maps from the archive, of which Koch's *Cartographies of Disease* (2005) is a good example. Our *World Atlas of Epidemic Diseases* (2004) is primarily concerned with the existing distribution of 38 infectious diseases, and it includes a sample of many historical reproductions. Here, we limit our attention to maps of the worldwide distribution of diseases.

World mapping

By the very late eighteenth century, the idea of mapping diseases at the global scale seems to have been developing. Leonard Finke (Finke, 1792–95) may have been the first to have written about this notion in his *Attempt at a General Medical-Practical Geography*. In three volumes, this work maps out medical descriptions of the world. It contains anthropological descriptions of its peoples and their possible diseases. However, as Finke's work implies, the actual mapping of disease at the world scale was costly and needed agreements on both disease definitions and adequate disease data collection. It was the 1840s before such conditions were in place.

Filling in the world map was to await the critical work of the German physician, August Hirsch, who avoided cartography himself but pioneered the global study of diseases. His two-volume *Handbuch der Historisch-Geographischen Pathologie*, the first edition of which was published between 1859 and 1864, was a monumental attempt to describe the world distribution of disease, drawing upon more than 10,000 sources. Hirsch had close links with England and dedicated his book to the London Epidemiological Society. Twenty years later, a much revised version was translated by Charles Creighton as *Handbook of Geographical and Historical Pathology* (Hirsch, 1883–86) but again with no maps.

Clemow's *Geography of Disease* (1903) was the first world survey to include a small number of maps. A physician with experience in Russia and the Ottoman empires, Clemow set out to record (i) the recent geographical distribution of a disease in text, tables, and maps (only nine in all); and (ii) the factors governing that geographical distribution.

It was to be the middle of the twentieth century before the publication of two pioneering atlases of disease: the *Seuchen Atlas* and the atlas of the American Geographical Society.

1. *Seuchen Atlas*. The *Seuchen Atlas* (Zeiss, 1942–45; Anderson, 1947) was conceived by the German High Command as an adjunct to war, enhancing that country's ability to mount military campaigns in Europe and adjacent areas. Its circulation was confined to military institutes and to those German university institutes involved in

training medical students. The scope of the atlas was largely limited to those areas where the German High Command expected to be fighting. This was revised at Heidelberg at the end of World War II as a bilingual, three-volume *World Atlas of Epidemic Diseases* (Rodenwaldt, 1952–61) which included 120 maps of disease and background maps of climate and population.

2. *American Geographical Society*. In 1948, the New York-based American Geographical Society began a programme in medical geography under the direction of a French surgeon, Jacques May.

A series of 17 world maps were published as supplements to the Society's quarterly journal, the *Geographical Review* (May, 1950–54). The large foldout sheets included poliomyelitis, cholera, malaria, dengue, and yellow fever, as well as a wide variety of tropical diseases. The meticulous drafting set new standards in detail and accuracy as shown in the fragment for the leishmaniasis map in **Figure 1.11**.

The American Geographical Society cartographer responsible for the maps (William Briesemeister) developed an innovative

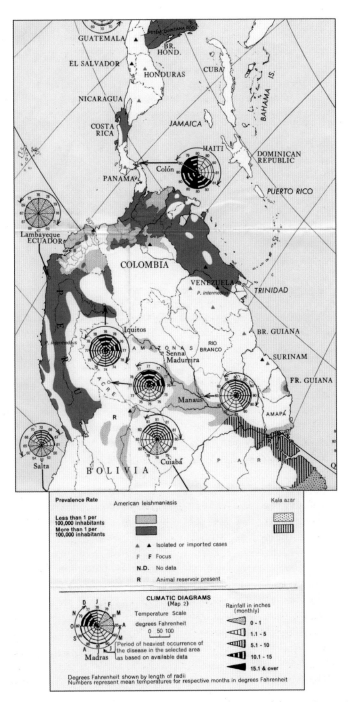

Figure 1.11 Central America: fragment from a global map of the world distribution of a tropical disease. Drawn in 1954 it shows the varying prevalence (two shades of green) for the American form of leishmaniasis. The circular climatic diagrams plot the seasonal distribution of the disease at contrasting locations. Original scale: 1:25,000,000.

Reproduced from May, J. (1954). 'Map of the world distribution of leishmaniasis.' *Geographical Review*, 44, 583–4.

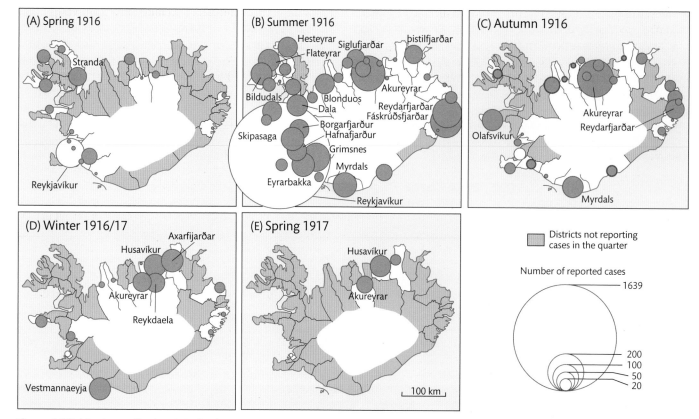

Figure 1.12 Measles notifications in Iceland, wave III. Quarterly distribution from spring 1916 to spring 1917, with circles drawn proportional to the number of cases in each medical district.

Reprinted by permission from Springer Nature, *Journal of Geographical Systems*, 'A swash-backwash model of the single epidemic wave', 8: 227–252. A.D. Cliff, P. Haggett, © 2006.

equal-area projection for the world base map (Briesemeister, 1953),[2] adroitly nesting enlarged higher-resolution insert maps into the vacant ocean areas. The reverse of each map sheet provides a dense thicket of detail on the multiple sources from which the drawings had been made.

1.5.2 Decoding of Disease Maps

The obverse of map making is map analysis. What does a map mean? What clues, if any, does mapping provide for disease aetiology?

A regional example

We start by considering a typical epidemic map of an area (Iceland) that we have used frequently in our earlier studies (Cliff et al., 1981); see Figure 1.12 and section 2.5 in Chapter 2. The epidemic in question is that of measles which spread across Iceland in 1916–17. Underpinning the distribution is the base map of reporting areas (63 medical districts) that, given the essentially empty interior of the island, are arranged around the coast. The most populous medical district was the capital (Reykjavík) in the south west making up a quarter of the island's (then) 80,000 population. This dominance is reflected in the map where the capital and nearby large towns have to be shown as open circles to allow the many smaller settlements to appear as proportional solid orange circles.

The epidemic wave shown in **Figure 1.12** was large. There were 4,900 notified cases with 1,600 in the capital alone. The epidemic occurred 8 years after the last wave of measles, indicating that the measles virus had died out locally and needed to be reintroduced from northwest Europe or North America. The five maps indicate that the infection started in the western part of the island in the first quarter and reached its peak that summer. Thereafter, cases dwindled through the autumn and winter, with the spring of 1917 marking the last gasps of the epidemic. Measles was not to return to Iceland for another 11 years by which time the number of unexposed children had grown large enough to sustain another major wave (5,300 cases). A more formal analysis of this Iceland map is discussed in the next section.

Themes

Probability mapping

Comparisons of the spatial distribution of different diseases, at different time periods, and in different parts of the world, calls for some common standard. Learmonth (1954) was one of the earliest to make use of standard statistical measures. His maps of changing cholera prevalence in pre-partition India between 1921 and 1940 include a histogram of all 212 districts over all 20 years. The distribution allowed him to measure the standard deviation of prevalence over both time and by district to create a nine-fold cross classification.

In a similar fashion, Michael and Bundy (1997) investigated the distribution across Africa for case prevalences of bancroftian filariasis. Here proportional circles were used to indicate the observed

---

[2] This lenticular equal-area projection is an oblique Hammer projection, centred at 45°N, 10°E, and scaled to different proportions with an axis ratio of 1.75 to 1, instead of 2 to 1.

raw prevalences in each country. Three bands of shading indicated the probability that these prevalences were significantly different from the mean regional value for Africa of 10.3 per cent. For example, the darkest shading indicated countries where there was a 'high probability' that a country was significantly higher than the African mean.

Use of such statistical measures for area-based data depends critically on the nature of the distribution being modelled. More recent contributions have proposed more stable and effective measures for probability mapping (Ord and Getis, 1995).

Regional trends

It is frequently useful with geocoded data to establish broad regional trends as an aid to map interpretation. One of the commonest ways of doing so is to fit a generalizing surface of some kind. There are many ways of doing this (Haggett and Chorley, 1969; Angulo et al., 1977; Carrat and Valleron, 1992). **Figure 1.13A** illustrates one such approach by fitting a quartic kernel estimator to the spatial distribution of acute poliomyelitis notifications in England and Wales in the 26-week epidemic period, 14 June–6 December 1947. Estimation was undertaken using a grid cell size of 10 km^2 and a bandwidth of 144 km. The choice of bandwidth was based on an exploratory examination of intensity surfaces using different degrees of smoothing and reflected the desire to capture national trends rather than local variations in the geographical distribution of poliomyelitis notifications. The surface was based on 8,123 notified cases from 1,471 local authority districts of varying order (metropolitan, county, and municipal boroughs; urban and rural districts). The reported cases were treated as a spatial point pattern, with the first-order properties of a spatial point process used to describe how case intensity (defined as the mean number of notifications per unit area) varied across space. The surface depicts a bipolar distribution of disease activity that broadly follows the (then) underpinning distribution of the population of England and Wales; there is a primary 'southern' focus of high intensity centred on London and the southeast and a secondary 'northern' focus centred on the adjoining counties of Cheshire, Derbyshire, Lancashire, Staffordshire, and the West Riding of Yorkshire. Levels of intensity fall with distance from these two centres.

Base-map standardization

A different approach has been pioneered by Dorling (1995) as illustrated in **Figure 1.13B**. This shows a measure of mortality for England and Wales, 1981–89, based on average years of expected life lost (YLL). Each of the 4,000 individual wards is drawn as a circle with its size proportional to the size of the population and colour shaded from dark grey (low YLL) to dark red (high YLL). County boundaries are shown. The effect is to enlarge on the map those areas with large populations (e.g. London swells to fetal proportions with closely packed wards). Conversely, lightly peopled counties such as in southwest England have few dots. Creating these maps is a mammoth piece of computing equivalent to trying to lay (i) many thousands of tiles, (ii) each of different size, but (iii) with common flexibility. The side conditions are (iv) to maintain contiguity with surrounding wards, and (v) to optimize the resulting pattern so as to retain the closest match with the familiar geographic shape. The spatial solution that emerges is fascinating. For example, the contrast

between the inner, poorer areas of London (with high average YLL) and the affluent suburbs (with lower average YLL) is evident.

Spatial standardization can also be approached via multidimensional scaling (MDS). Again, this moves away from the conventional map by substituting for geographical distance some measure of separation relevant to the disease under study. For example, infection flow between two areas may be a function of the numbers of people moving been two areas rather than raw distance itself. A physical model might be to have a set of billiard balls (settlements) connected by springs whose length is inversely proportional to population flow. MDS is equivalent to forcing out a flat 'map' (in two dimensions) which best represents the separation values between the settlements. An example of MDS appears in section 2.2.2 in Chapter 2, while the potential of MDS methods in spatial epidemiology is set out in Cliff et al. (1995).

Regional trends and local anomalies

If we look at the Dorling map (**Figure 1.13B**) from a distance, the detail disappears and we see a gradual colour change as the grey become less marked and red starts to dominate as we move from south to north. A side benefit of trend recognition is to identify local anomalies or residuals which may prompt further research questions. For example, on the Dorling map, *positive anomalies* (an unhealthy Yarmouth within a lower trending East Anglia) or negative anomalies (a lower Harrogate within a higher trending Yorkshire) stand out on **Figure 1.13B**.

1.6 Epidemics in the Space Domain, II: Models

In this section we return to the EDM of **Figure 1.4** but dissect it along the spatial rather than the temporal plane. We can do this in two ways: (i) by modifying existing time-series models to add a suitable spatial component or (ii) inventing models for the kinds of map data surveyed in section 1.5. We have already written at length on (i) in Cliff et al., (1981, pp. 132–58) so here we follow the second path. A sketch of an evolving epidemic (section 1.6.1) is followed by a consideration of an edge model (1.6.2), a simulation model (1.6.3), and two groups of dyadic models (1.6.4).

1.6.1 An Epidemic Cycle in Space

In section 1.4, we asked whether epidemics in the time dimension could be thought of as waves and, if so, did they approximate to any standard shape or model? Here we ask the same question for waves moving across a two-dimensional map.

Maps of thousands of outbreaks of infectious diseases are now extant in the epidemiological literature. We reproduce a broad sample of these in our *World Atlas of Epidemic Diseases* (Cliff et al., 2004). The many we have interrogated suggests that there may well be a characteristic, even a dominant, pattern and we outline our suggested spatial structure of a typical epidemic as a three-dimensional sketch in **Figure 1.14**. The model assumes an idealized epidemic wave in the spatial domain (u, v) with infection being introduced into an island (green). It suggests that a wave's evolution over time may go through several distinctive spatial morphologies irrespective of the geographical scale of the event. We show this as five phases: onset, youth, maturity, decay, and extinction.

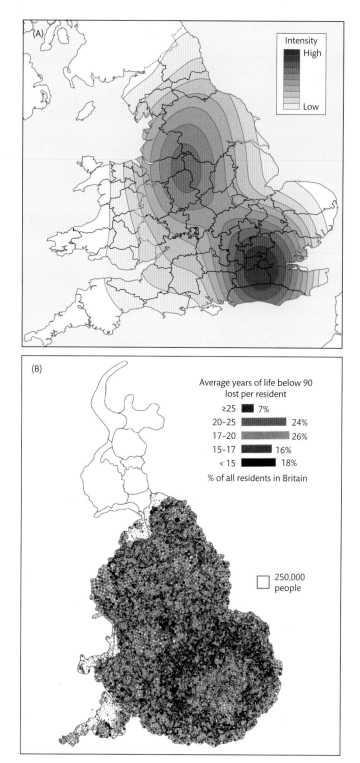

Figure 1.13 Regional trends and population proportional map. (A) Generalized surface map fitted to poliomyelitis notifications in local authorities in England and Wales, June–December 1947. (B) Map of mortality in England and Wales using years of life lost, 1981–89. See text.

(A) Reprinted from *Journal of Historical Geography*, Vol. 40, Smallman-Raynor, M.R., Cliff, A.D., 'The geographical spread of the 1947 poliomyelitis epidemic in England and Wales: Spatial wave propagation of an enigmatic epidemiological event', p. 43, © 2013, with permission from Elsevier. (B) Adapted from Dorling, D. (1995). *A New Social Atlas of Britain*. Chichester: Wiley.

1. *Onset.* This is marked by the introduction of an infectious agent (virus, bacterium, etc.) into a new area with a susceptible population that is open to infection. Typically, this initial invasion occurs either in one or in a small number of locations. Cases are reported locally and, with notifiable diseases, passed on up the reporting hierarchy to national and international health agencies.

2. *Youth.* A very active, aggressive, stage marked by the rapid spread of infection from the original point of introduction to

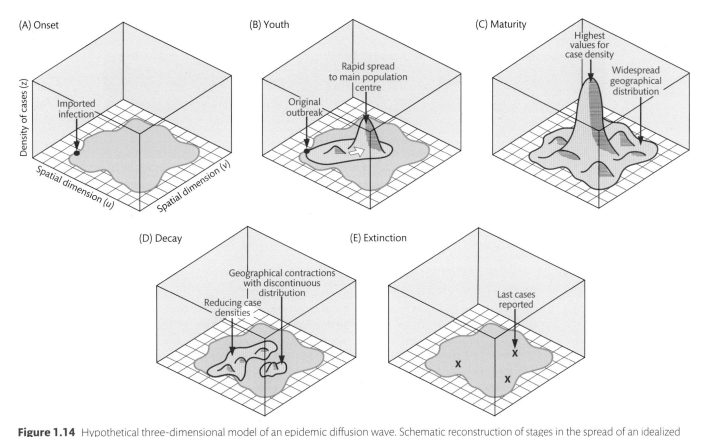

Figure 1.14 Hypothetical three-dimensional model of an epidemic diffusion wave. Schematic reconstruction of stages in the spread of an idealized epidemic wave. Cases are given in the vertical (z) direction and the spatial extent of the infection is given by the horizontal plane (u, v).
Reprinted by permission from Springer Nature, *Journal of Geographical Systems*, 'A swash-backwash model of the single epidemic wave', 8: 227–252. A.D. Cliff, P. Haggett, © 2006.

the main population centres. Historical studies indicate that this may occur through a mix of both local (neighbourhood) diffusion and by long-range (cascade) diffusion following the settlement hierarchy.

3. *Maturity*. In this central stage, the epidemic peaks at its highest intensity with strong clusters of cases widely spread through the susceptible population. In **Figure 1.14C** this is shown as affecting the whole island. Here the epidemic is at its maximum intensity with strong contrasts in infection density between the various sub-areas. In this phase, the map of infection may well mirror the urban hierarchy of the island.

4. *Decay*. This phase is marked by a lengthy period of declining intensity with fewer reported cases and a rather chaotic and disorderly spatial pattern. Typically, the spatial structure tends to be less coherent than in earlier stages with a scatter of low-intensity infected areas whose location may be hard to explain other than by random or local factors.

5. *Extinction phase*. This represents the last throws of the epidemic wave with a final scatter of cases. Spatially, such cases often tend to be found in the less accessible areas. Extinction may be achieved through natural cessation as the potential cases are protected by herd immunity and/or by active reduction and elimination measures of the type discussed in Chapter 6.

The sequence in **Figure 1.14** is not intended as a sufficient summary of spatial epidemic behaviour. Rather it serves as a visual spatial marker against which the outputs from quantitative spatial models can be checked and refined.

1.6.2 A Swash–Backwash Spatial Model

The edges of epidemics

In a study of measles outbreaks in South West England in the late 1960s, we inspected the 222 weekly maps from 1967–70 for the 179 General Register Office (GRO) recording areas which comprise the six counties of Cornwall, Devon, Somerset, Dorset, Gloucestershire, and Wiltshire (Cliff et al., 1975, pp. 83–106). In addition to case numbers, we identified each area in terms of whether it was (i) reporting cases for the first time (*newly infected*), (ii) continuing to report cases (*infected*), (iii) not reporting cases (*inactive*), or (iv) had stopped reporting cases less than 2 weeks ago (*fade-out*). An outbreak was assumed to have ended when a GRO failed to report new cases for three consecutive weeks. As Table 1.7 shows, there was strong evidence of geographical contagion when we looked at the spatial pattern of newly infected areas in a sample period of 1969–70. Thus, of 416 newly infected areas, 316 were located adjacent to an existing infected area.

Cliff and Haggett (2006) followed up this study by exploring the stages by which given areas move the through inactive → active → recovered sequence. These terms map directly onto those used in the Hamer–Soper ($S \rightarrow I \rightarrow R$) models *but refer to areas or recording units rather than individuals*. The method was demonstrated by operations on a simplified case of 12 areas × 10 time

Table 1.7 Measles in South West England, 1969–70. Location of newly infected General Register Office districts with reported measles cases

Distance from existing outbreak[a]	GRO areas outside existing outbreaks		Location of new outbreak areas		Risk ratio (B):(A)
	Number (A)	%	Number (B)	%	
Contiguous to existing measles-infected GRO (= 1 link apart)	2,603	52.7	316	76.0	1:8
Two links	1,749	35.4	83	19.9	1:21
Three links	529	10.7	17	4.1	1:31
Four links	55	1.1	0		
Total	4,936	100.0	416	100.0	1:12

[a] Two links = one intervening area between the GROs; three links = two intervening areas between the GROs; four links = three intervening areas between the GROs.

Reproduced with permission from Cliff, A.D., Haggett, P., Ord, J.K., Bassett, K., Davies, R.B. (1975). *Elements of Spatial Structure: A Quantitative Approach*. Cambridge: Cambridge University Press.

periods EDM (**Figure 1.15**), with areas coloured in terms of the three *SIR* classes.

In a topological move (analogous to twisting a Rubik's cube to align colours), cells are moved in the EDM array so that all the starting dates for an outbreak or epidemic are aligned from earliest to latest (**Figure 1.15C**, left). This diagram arranges all areas in terms of their *leading edge* (*LE*). This matrix twisting operation is then repeated (**Figure 1.15C**, centre) to realign all the *following* or *trailing edges* (*FE*) of the epidemic in a similar manner.

Plotting both *LE* and *FE* together (**Figure 1.15C**, right) yields a phase transition diagram of susceptible (*S*), infected (*I*), and recovered (*R*) areas to show the transitions $S \to I$ and $I \to R$ between them. If we scale both axes to the form $0 \to 1$, they yield integrals with dimensionless numbers that provide a useful summary of the shape of epidemic events. Such numbers apply regardless of the true size of the event. This integral method has been borrowed from Strahler (1952) who used it to describe the distributions of heights within a watershed in flood susceptibility studies.

The swash–backwash analogue

The two edges, *LE* and *FE*, can also be used to throw light on the changing spatial structure of an epidemic wave over time. **Figure 1.15D** uses the data in the 12×10 example in (B) and (C) to plot the changing position of the *LE* cells and *FE* cells over time. In the early stages, newly infected sub-areas are being added and in the later stages sub-areas are subtracted as their local outbreaks come to an end and no further cases are recorded. The shaded areas show the number of cells added and subtracted, while the heavy line traces show the net balance of areas; this is positive in the earlier time period and negative in the later period. The positions of the two means are shown on this graph. The median position between them, λ_t, say, broadly separates the early-positive from the later-negative stages.

Using the results, we define in **Figure 1.15E** a two-stage swash–backwash model of the spatial spread of a single epidemic wave. The terms, 'swash' and 'backwash', are taken from coastal geomorphology (Chorley et al., 1984) where the dynamics of waves breaking on a shoreline are described as going through two distinctive stages. In the *swash* (or onset) stage, the wave rushes up the beach occupying a larger area of sand; the direction of the wave

front is determined by the direction of the approaching wave trains with respect to the shoreline. In the *backwash* (or withdrawal) stage the wave retreats down the beach relinquishing the area formerly occupied but with the direction of retreat determined by the slope of the beach. In epidemiology, the context is clearly different but the analogy of a wave occupying and then retreating from an infected area remains useful.

Phase transition in a hypothetical wave

Assuming that both the sub-areas and the time periods are discrete, we use the following notation:

A Area covered by an epidemic wave in terms of the number of sub-areas infected, where a_i is a sub-area in the sequence $1, 2, \ldots, a_i, \ldots, A$.

T Duration of an epidemic wave, defined in terms of a number of discrete time periods, t_j, in the sequence $1, 2, \ldots, t_j, \ldots, T$.

N Total cases of a disease recorded in a single epidemic wave measured over all sub-areas and all time periods; n_{ij} is the number of cases recorded in the cell formed by the *i*-th sub-area and the *j*-th time period of the $A \times T$ data matrix.

Note that, whereas this overall wave is continuous (no time periods with zero cases), for individual sub-areas the record may be discontinuous with one or more time periods with zero cases. The overall wave is given by the marginal summation of cases for each time period.

Estimation of phase transitions

The method followed in our simple 12×10 example was essentially geometrical and it was used largely for a pedagogic purpose. In practice, and when studying large epidemic waves, standard statistical analysis of the distribution of cases (*N*), areas (*A*), and the two edges (*LE* and *FE*) can be substituted to yield the same results more economically. The arithmetic mean $\bar{t}$ of all four characteristics can be computed as a time-weighted mean. For example, for cases *N*, the equation is:

$$\bar{t}_N = \frac{1}{N}\sum_{t=1}^{T} t n_t \tag{1.7}$$

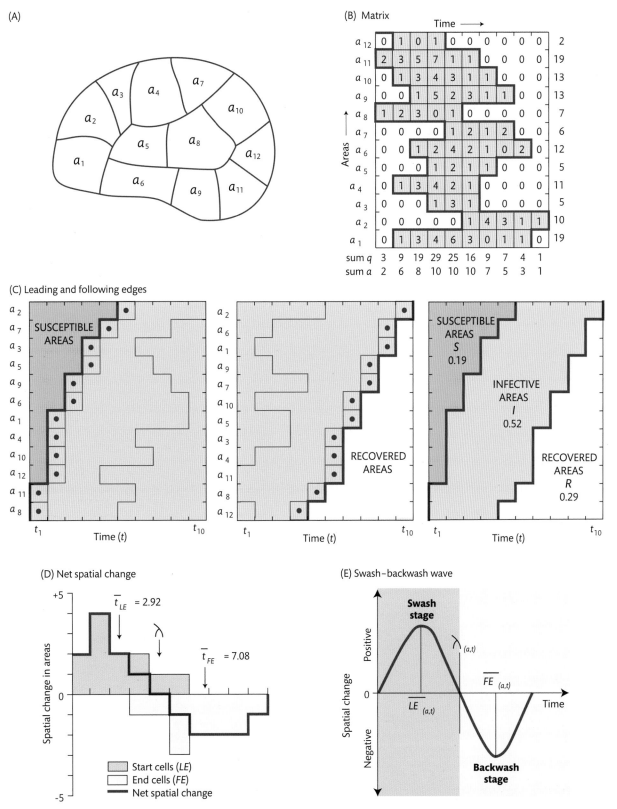

Figure 1.15 Swash–backwash model: exemplar of hypothetical epidemic spread within a 12 (areas) × 10 (time periods) matrix. (A) Hypothetical 12-area map. (B) Reported cases by area ($a_1 \ldots a_{12}$) and time period ($t_1 \ldots t_{10}$). (C) Space–time data matrix rearranged to order leading edges by start date (left matrix) and following or trailing edges (centre matrix). In the right-hand matrix, the leading and following edges are plotted as a phase-transition diagram with susceptible (S), infected (I), and recovered (R) integrals. (D) Distribution of leading and following edges by time, with the average times to infection and recovery of areas given ($\bar{t}$). λ is the switch-over point from swash to backwash. (E) Concept of a swash–backwash wave.

where n_t is the number of cases notified at time t and $N = \sum n_t$ over all t. The first time period, say month, of an epidemic is coded as $t = 1$. The subsequent months of the epidemic may then be coded serially as $t = 2$, $t = 3$, ..., $t = T$, where T is the number of monthly periods from the beginning to the end of the epidemic (i.e. $T = 10$ in our example). The time-weighted means yield not only a useful measure of central tendency but of the velocity of the wave in terms of time to infection. Similar measures can be made for areas, leading edges, and following edges. The values for $\bar{t}_N$ and $\bar{t}_A$ are 4.75 and 5.71 respectively; those for $\bar{t}_{LE}$ and $\bar{t}_{FE}$ are plotted in **Figure 1.15D**. They show that the epidemic wave for cases was faster than that for areas; this implies a relatively spatially concentrated epidemic. Higher moments about the mean can also be computed to yield valuable measures of epidemiological behaviour. The r-th central moment about $\bar{t}$ for cases may be written as:

$$m_r = \frac{1}{N}\sum_{t=1}^{T}\left(t - \bar{t}\right)^r n_t. \tag{1.8}$$

Using equation 1.8, we may then define further measures of velocity as:

$$s = \sqrt{m_2} \tag{1.9}$$

and:

$$b_1 = \frac{m_3^2}{m_2^3} \quad \text{and} \quad b_2 = \frac{m_4}{m_2^2} \tag{1.10}$$

The quantity s defined in equation 1.9 is the familiar standard deviation of the frequency of cases against time, while b_1 and b_2 in equation 1.10 are the Pearson measures of skewness and kurtosis respectively. Skewness indicates the tendency of the distribution to

peak before or after the mean, and kurtosis is a gauge for whether the distribution clusters more closely or less closely than would be expected under the Normal curve. See the discussion of **Figure 1.5** for further details.

S, I, R integrals

The means of the two wave edges can be used to generate estimates of the susceptible, infected, and recovered integrals within the phase diagram of **Figure 1.15C** (right). The susceptible areas integral in the spatial domain can be measured as:

$$S_A = \frac{\left(\bar{t}_{LE} - 1\right)}{T} \tag{1.11}$$

while the infected areas integral in the spatial domain is measured as:

$$I_A = \frac{\bar{t}_{FE}}{T} - S_A \tag{1.12}$$

and the recovered areas integral as:

$$R_A = 1 - \left(S_A + I_A\right) \tag{1.13}$$

All three integrals are dimensionless numbers with values in the range [0, 1]. The parameters of the swash–backwash model, and their interpretation, are summarized in **Table 1.8**.

Spatial basic reproduction number

As discussed in section 1.3.2, in conventional *SIR* epidemic models, the basic reproduction number, R_0, is one of the most useful parameters for the mathematical characterization of infectious disease processes. Its equivalent in the spatial domain, the *spatial reproduction number*, denoted by R_{0A}, is the average number of secondary

Table 1.8 Summary descriptions of the parameters of the swash–backwash model

Model parameter	Equation	Description
$\bar{t}_{LE}$	$\bar{t}_{LE} = \frac{1}{N}\sum_{t=1}^{T} tn_t,$	For the leading edge, gives the average time of arrival of the epidemic wave across the set of areas, where n_t is the number of units whose leading edge occurred in epidemic week t and $N = \sum n_t$. A similar equation can be written for $\bar{t}_{FE}$
$\bar{t}_{FE} - \bar{t}_{LE}$		Average duration of infectivity. Relatively low (high) values denote infection waves of relatively short (long) duration
V_{LE}	$V_{LE} = 1 - \frac{\bar{t}_{LE}}{T}$	Dimensionless velocity ratio in the range [0, 1], measuring the average time from the onset of an outbreak to the first notified case of a disease in a given area. Relatively low (high) values denote relatively slow (fast) spreading infection waves. A similar equation can be written for V_{FE}; relatively low (high) values denote relatively slow (fast) retreating infection waves
S_A	$S_A = \frac{\left(\bar{t}_{LE} - 1\right)}{T}$	Susceptible integral. Defines the proportion of geographical units in the study area A which are at risk of infection. Relatively low (high) values denote relatively fast (slow) spreading infection waves
I_A	$I_A = \frac{\bar{t}_{FE}}{T} - S_A$	Infected integral. Defines the proportion of geographical units in the study area A which are infected with a disease. The integral forms a measure of the *relative* rate of spatial advance and retreat of an infection wave. Relatively low (high) values denote infection waves in which the rate of spatial retreat is relatively fast (slow) compared with the rate of spatial advance
R_A	$R_A = 1 - \left(S_A + I_A\right)$	Recovered integral. Defines the proportion of geographical units in the study area A which have recovered from infection. Relatively low (high) values denote relatively slow (fast) retreating infection waves
R_{0A}	$R_{0A} = \frac{1 - S_A}{1 - R_A};$ $R_{0A} = \frac{V_{FE} + (1/T)}{V_{LE}}$	Spatial basic reproduction number, measures the propensity of an infected geographical unit to spawn other infected units in later time periods. Values of R_{0A} calibrate the spatial velocity of disease spread, with relatively low (high) values denoting relatively slow (fast) spatial propagation

infected geographical units produced from one infected unit in a virgin area *A* and is given by:

$$R_{0A} = \frac{1 - S_A}{1 - R_A} \qquad (1.14)$$

Other specifications of R_{0A} are also possible (**Table 1.8**).

Regional application

So far, our study of the swash model has been conducted in terms of a small, idealized epidemic wave and methods have been put forward to allow its measurement and analysis. But how far do the methods work when applied to actual epidemic waves of infectious diseases? These may be several orders of magnitude larger and considerably more complex in their spread. To conduct a more realistic test, we use outbreaks of the highly contagious human virus disease, measles, for our epidemic modelling. The specific example chosen is taken from the extensive work we have done on the Icelandic records (Cliff et al., 1981). We take wave III which we already encountered in section 1.5.2 (see **Figure 1.12**, and also section 2.5 where wave III is set in the context of the other Icelandic measles waves).

Swash edge analysis was conducted for this wave, and the results are given in the series of graphs drawn in **Figure 1.16**. Wave III impacted heavily on Iceland after a long interval without the virus. In a 14-month period from April 1916, the island experienced almost 5,000 recorded measles cases, of which over 100 proved fatal. **Figure 1.16** consists of five graphs. Graph (A) shows the monthly time series of both reported cases and the number of districts in which cases occurred. Inset (B) shows the average of cases per district over time and identifies two surge peaks. Graph (C) plots the number of newly infected districts and compares it with the trace of newly terminated districts each month. Inset (D) is small but critical since it posts the differences between the two preceding curves which allows the *S* and *R* phases of the wave to be defined. The last graph, (E), shows the cumulative curves for the number of newly infected and newly terminated districts. This is used to define the susceptible (*S*), infective (*I*), and recovered (*R*) districts as conceived in the early Hamer–Soper *SIR* type of models.

1.6.3 Simulating Waves on Spatial Lattices

Simulation using numerical rather than mechanical models is well developed in epidemiology. Rochester, Minnesota, home of the Mayo Clinic, was the scene for many experiments with influenza described in *Simulation of Infectious Disease Epidemics* (Ackerman et al., 1984). Simulation has the benefit of allowing experiments to be conducted without putting real people (or indeed real reputations) at risk. Schools, playgroups, and shops may be closed, borders shut, vaccinations given or refused, all within the safety of rule changes built within a traditional *SIR* model. The Rochester 'city' had 1,000 persons structured into 254 families and five age-groups with 'preschool' given a choice of 30 playgroups. The exponential growth of computer power means today's equivalents such as ONCHOSIM, SCHISTOSIM, or SIMULAIDS can be much more fine grained (Vynnycky and White, 2010, pp. 149–76).

Geographical work on simulation

Geographical work on simulation followed a different route. Torsten Hägerstrand at Lund University published the first of his

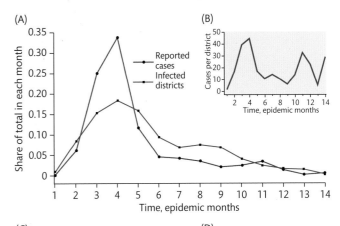

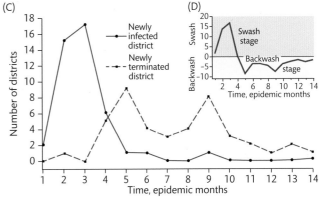

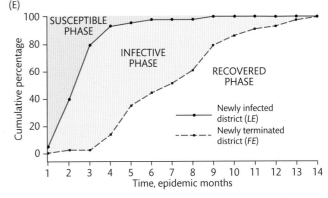

Figure 1.16 Swash–backwash model: some wave parameters for Icelandic measles wave III. The data analysed here refer to the outbreak mapped in Figure 1.12. (A) Monthly time series for the number of cases reported and for the number of districts infected. (B) Monthly time series of density of reported cases per infected district. (C) Monthly time series of the number of districts newly infected (i.e. measles cases first recorded) and of the number of districts where infection terminated (i.e. measles cases last recorded). (D) Differences between the series plotted in (C) used to define swash and backwash stages of the epidemic. (E) Cumulative curves for the number of newly infected and newly terminated districts used to define susceptible, infective, and recovered districts.

Reprinted by permission from Springer Nature, *Journal of Geographical Systems*, 'A swash-backwash model of the single epidemic wave', 8: 227–252. A.D. Cliff, P. Haggett, © 2006.

papers on diffusion in 1952. His initial simulations were done without computer aid, substituting random number tables (an essential constituent) and family members/students (equally essential) to produce a limited number of trials by hand. Hägerstrand's approach to maps had three steps (**Figure 1.17**). The best analogy is weather forecasting—looking at past weather patterns on maps,

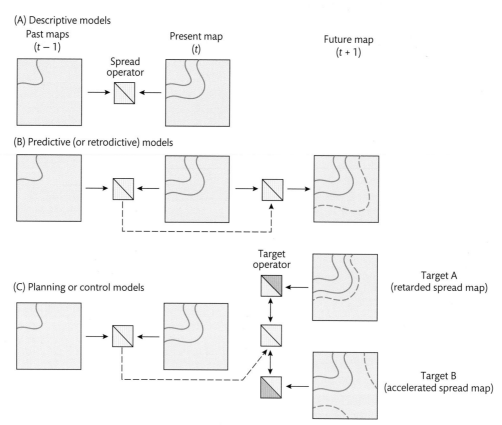

Figure 1.17 Map sequences as a predictive device. Descriptive, predictive, and interdictive models of a spatial diffusion process. The creation of operators (e.g. mean information fields, MIFs) from a sequence allows the forward projection of the map to a future time period. Reproduced from Haggett, P. (1990). *The Geographer's Art*. Oxford: Blackwell.

projecting them forward to the present, and then on further to estimate likely future weather maps. At step 1, Hägerstrand assumed that, if a map shows numerical data, then there must be a spread operator which converts the first number field in map $t - 1$ (the past) into the second map (the present) at time t. From an accurate observation of a sequence of maps, we may be able to identify the change mechanism and summarize our findings in terms of a *descriptive model* (Figure 1.17A). What we are doing is searching for the operator which appears—in terms of our model—to convert early maps of the past into later maps of the past and then into the present.

The second step looks to the future. If we can find such an operator, and if we can assume some continuity in this process (the heroic assumption that lies behind so much forecasting), then we can sketch a future map at time $t + 1$ (a *predictive* or *retrodictive* map; Figure 1.17B). The error bands associated with each 'contour' will be given by the width of the lines on the map; the further forward in time, the wider these bands are likely to be.

But planners and decision-makers may want to alter the future, say, to accelerate or stop a diffusion wave. So our third step asks: what will happen in the future, if we intervene in some specified way? Models that try to accommodate this third order of complexity are termed *interdictive models* (Figure 1.17C).

Articulation of Hägerstrand's models was achieved through Monte Carlo simulation of spatial processes, that is, by providing a well-defined copy or mimic of an observed historical sequence and projecting this into the future. In the years following its publication in 1953, his model was adapted and applied to a wide range of regional cases, from the spread of ghetto housing in American cities to the early settlement of Polynesian islands.

Deriving a mean information field

Values for any spatial operator may be calculated in two different ways. An *external* operator may be deduced from existing knowledge of the spread process. Thus, Hägerstrand knew that adoption by one Swedish farmer of a particular innovation depended on seeing its beneficial effects on a neighbour's farm rather than on government advertising. So any operator was likely to be both local in reach and to drop off in an exponential way from the location of the adopting farmer. His 5 km × 5 km *mean information field* (MIF) therefore had its highest contact probabilities (CP) = 0.443 over the central cell, falling exponentially away towards the four most distant corner cells each with very low values (CP = 0.009).

An *internal* operator uses sets of maps over time in the estimation process (best-fit values have been computed by regression, linear programming, and maximum entropy methods). A study by Tinline (1972) of foot-and-mouth disease (FMD) among a population of cattle herds in northwest England produced operators that had an asymmetric pattern of CP values, reflecting the role of wind (coming dominantly from the west-southwest direction) in the spread of the FMD virus.

Rules of the Hägerstrand model

Hägerstrand's model was stochastic and was based upon the following rules (the language of which can readily be adapted to

Table 1.9 Spatial structure of Monte Carlo simulation of diffusion waves

Type of model	Spatial operator (MIF) floating grid	Source of spatial process values	Geographical area, elements, source
Diffusion waves: model determined from external evidence	001 014 017 014 001 014 030 055 030 014 017 055 443 055 017 014 030 055 030 014 001 014 017 014 001 Symmetric operator (numbers × 10³)	Values determined from examination of exponential distance decay functions	Central Sweden farms Innovations *Source:* Hägerstrand (1953)
Diffusion waves: internal evidence	Asymmetric MIF operators determined from pattern of spread data	Examination of disease records and prevailing wind vectors. Statistical fits	Cheshire Plain farms FMD *Source:* Tinline (1972)
Individual vectors used to build up probability maps of a diffusion field	Each day's movement determined by combination of wind and wave probabilities which vary by season	Examination of wind/wave direction, strength, frequency. Length of voyage distributions	South Pacific Ocean voyages Inter-island migrations *Source:* Levison et al. (1973)

cover epidemics such that an adopter = 'infective' and a potential adopter = 'susceptible'):

1. The input numbers and spatial locations of potential adopters in the model were the actual configurations at the start of the diffusion process.
2. The study area was divided up by a lattice composed of 5 km × 5 km squares.
3. A potential adopter was assumed to adopt the innovation when contacted by an adopter.
4. In each iteration of the model, every adopter was allowed to contact one other person, either an adopter or a potential adopter. The probability, p_i, that an adopter would contact an individual located in the i-th cell of the study lattice was determined by the probabilities in the MIF as described previously.

The MIF can be conceived of as a floating grid. Each cell in the MIF was a 5 km × 5 km square to match the cell size in the study area lattice; outside the floating grid, $p_i = 0$ (Table 1.9, row 1). These probabilities were estimated from an analysis of migration and telephone traffic data. The floating grid was placed over each existing adopter in turn, so that the adopter was located in the central cell of the MIF. What Table 1.9 tells us is that an adopter located in the centre of the central cell of the MIF has approximately a 44 per cent chance of contacting someone within (about) 0–2.5 km of themselves, and that this contact probability decays over space to 1 per cent at a distance of about 14 km (along diagonals) from the adopter, and to zero beyond 14–18 km. Since the probability is taken as zero beyond 18 km, it is clear that the MIF is exponentially bounded.

The location of each adopter's contact was determined in two steps. First, a random number, $r, 0 \le r \le 1$, from a rectangular distribution, located the cell i according to the rule:

$$\sum_{m=1}^{i-1} Q_m < r \le \sum_{m=1}^{i} Q_m \tag{1.15}$$

where Q_m, the probability of a contact in cell m with population n_m, is:

$$Q_m = \frac{P_m n_m}{\sum_{m=1}^{25} P_m n_m} \tag{1.16}$$

Here P_m is the probability that an adopter would contact an individual in the m-th cell of the MIF. A second random number from a rectangular distribution on $[l, n_m]$ was drawn to locate the receiver in the cell. If the receiver was a potential adopter, he immediately became an adopter by rule (3); if the receiver was an existing adopter, the message was lost; if the receiver was identical with the carrier, a new address was sampled. To take into account the reduction in interpersonal communication likely to be caused by physical features such as rivers and forests, two simplified types of barrier were introduced into the model plane, namely zero- and half-contact barriers. When an address crossed a half-contact barrier, the telling was cancelled with probability 0.5. However, two half-contact barriers in combination were considered equal to one zero-contact barrier. Using this model, Hägerstrand performed a series of computer runs to simulate the spatial pattern of acceptance of a subsidy for the improvement of pasture on small farms in the Asby district of central Sweden (Figure 1.18).

1.6.4 Dyadic Models

So far in our treatment of both temporal and spatial modelling we have concentrated on analysis of the EDM introduced in section 1.4.1. Here we consider studies that go beyond the *primal* matrix to analyse its dual, the *dyadic* matrix (dyad coming from the Greek for 'pair' or 'two'). We look at two examples: (i) lag correlation models, and (iii) spatial interaction models.

Lag correlation models

Consider the map of the English county of Cornwall illustrated in **Figure 1.19**. It shows in part (A) the pattern of the 27 areas (GROs) which provide weekly information on notifiable diseases. The primal EDM is therefore a cube made up of diseases along one axis and time (weeks) and areas (GROs) along the others. The spread of an epidemic involves movements of infectives *across* spatial boundaries as well as within them. If we label the GRO areas as N, then the duals are N^2 if the link data are *directional* and $(N^2 - N)/2$ if the links are symmetric.

Varying contact patterns

Figure 1.19B and **Table 1.10** show the contiguity between each area and the immediately adjoining areas. The map is now reduced to a graph with an associated contact matrix (1, 0) based on contiguity (1). Matrix algebra can be used to determine the number

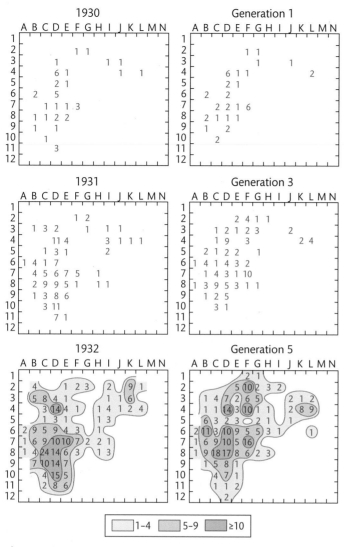

Figure 1.18 Central Sweden: historical and simulated spatial diffusion patterns for an improved pasture subsidy, 1930–32. The observed distributions of adopters appear in the left-hand column of maps; the corresponding simulated distributions from the Monte Carlo model are mapped in the right-hand column.

Reproduced with permission from Hägerstrand, T. (1967). 'On Monte Carlo simulation of diffusion.' In: W.L. Garrison and D.F. Marble (eds.), *Quantitative Geography* (Volume 1). Evanston, Illinois: Northwestern University Studies in Geography, 13, 1–33. Reprinted by permission, Northwestern University Press.

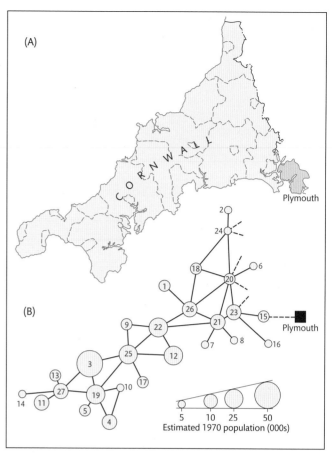

Figure 1.19 Cornwall: conversion of primal matrix to dyadic form. (A) General Register Office (GRO) areas in Cornwall. (B) Areas reduced to a graph based on contiguity between GRO areas. Pecked lines show links to adjacent Devon GRO areas.

Reproduced from Cliff, A.D., Ord, J.K. (1975). 'Space-time modelling with an application to regional forecasting.' *Transactions of the Institute of British Geographers*, 64, 119–28. Reprinted with permission.

of links or steps between areas. More importantly, the areas may be connected up in different ways (rather like plugging in cables in a telephone connection board) to allow different spatial spread patterns to be explored. For example, if an epidemic wave were to move in a hierarchic fashion infecting the larger centres first, then this could be tested.

Haggett (1976) explored measles cases over a 222-week period against graphs representing seven different spread hypotheses (some 6,216 cells in all). Each GRO area was recorded as reporting cases (black, B) or clear (white, W). A standard BW spatial autocorrelation test (the Moran test; Cliff and Ord, 1973) was used to measure the strength of spatial clustering on each of the seven graphs for each week. A hybrid model for epidemic spread was proposed based on the findings. Journey to work links proved the most significant

factor, plausible since it reflected school journeys for what was mainly a disease of children. GRO population size came in second place, reflecting the urban–rural hierarchy.

The Cornwall study was part of a much wider project (Cliff et al., 1975) looking at measles records over the whole of South West England for the same 222-week period. Here we were dealing with a geographically much larger six-county area, a little larger than Massachusetts, and with over 2.7 million population in 1970. Statistical analysis of the primal matrix (222 weeks × 179 areas = 39,738 cells) was first performed using spectral analysis to determine temporal patterns. More rewarding results were generated from interrogating the associated dual matrix (222 weeks × 31,506 dyads = 6,994,332 cells). Figure 1.20 shows the result achieved by lag correlation analysis. At first glance, the diagram seems to be like a Himalayan mountain range seen from the south, low plains and foothills rising to majestic towering peaks in the background. Here, time is measured in a conventional metric along the horizontal axis in weeks, going in 222 steps from January 1967 to January 1971. Space is measured in dyadic terms as a contagion factor, the nearness of one GRO to another. This can be measured in several ways but here we chose the simplest, the shortest number

Table 1.10 Cornwall: order of spatial lags separating the 27 General Register Offices in the county

GRO name		1	2	3	4	5	6	7	8	9	10	11	12	13	14	15	16	17	18	19	20	21	22	23	24	25	26	27
		Order of spatial lag																										
Bodmin MB	1	0	4	4	5	5	4	3	3	3	4	6	3	6	6	4	4	4	2	4	3	2	2	3	3	3	1	5
Bude–Stratton UD	2		0	6	7	7	3	4	4	5	6	8	5	8	8	4	4	6	2	6	2	3	4	3	1	5	3	7
Camborne–Redruth UD	3			0	2	2	5	4	4	2	2	2	3	2	2	5	5	2	4	1	4	3	2	4	5	1	3	1
Falmouth MB	4				0	2	6	5	5	3	1	3	4	3	3	6	6	3	5	1	5	4	3	5	6	2	4	2
Helston MB	5					0	6	5	5	3	2	3	4	3	3	6	6	3	5	1	5	4	3	5	6	2	4	2
Launceston MB	6						0	3	3	4	5	7	4	7	7	3	3	5	2	5	1	2	3	2	2	4	3	6
Liskeard MB	7							0	2	3	4	6	3	6	6	3	3	4	3	4	2	1	2	2	3	3	2	5
Looe UD	8								0	3	4	6	3	6	6	3	3	4	3	4	2	1	2	2	3	3	2	5
Newquay UD	9									0	2	4	2	4	4	4	4	2	3	2	3	2	1	3	4	1	2	3
Penryn MB	10										0	3	3	3	3	5	5	2	4	1	4	3	2	4	5	1	3	2
Penzance MB	11											0	5	2	2	7	7	4	6	2	6	5	4	6	7	3	5	1
St Austell/Fowey UD/MB	12												0	5	5	4	4	3	3	3	3	2	1	3	4	2	2	4
St Ives MB	13													0	2	7	7	4	6	2	6	5	4	6	7	3	5	1
St Just UD	14														0	7	7	4	6	2	6	5	4	6	7	3	5	1
Saltash MB	15															0	2	5	3	5	2	2	3	1	3	4	3	6
Torpoint UD	16																0	5	3	5	2	2	3	1	3	4	3	6
Truro MB	17																	0	4	2	4	3	2	4	5	1	3	3
Camelford RD	18																		0	4	1	2	2	2	1	3	1	5
Kerrier RD	19																			0	4	3	2	4	5	1	3	1
Launceston RD	20																				0	1	2	1	1	3	2	5
Liskeard RD	21																					0	1	1	2	2	1	4
St Austell RD	22																						0	2	3	1	1	3
St Germans RD	23																							0	2	3	2	5
Stratton RD	24																								0	4	2	6
Truro RD	25																									0	2	2
Wadebridge/Padstow RD/UD	26																										0	4
West Penwith RD	27																											0

[1] Identity numbers correspond with areas mapped in Figure 1.19B.

of steps moving only through contiguous spread. So the minimum lag (1) on the scale is for immediately connected neighbours, while the maximum (15) is for a very distant neighbour 15 steps away. Such a measure is clearly unique to each geographical area studied. The vertical axis is a measure of association between the measles time series using the correlation coefficient. Only positive values are shown so the scale runs from zero up to 0.4. As expected, the values at spatial lag 1, which forms the back wall of the diagram (shaded orange), are consistently positive and large, reflecting the high spatial autocorrelation between adjacent GROs—a local neighbourhood effect. Correlations generally fall away as areas become more distant from each other.

Across the generally irregular terrain we have highlighted lags at 5 and 12 steps. These show consistently positive correlation values and probably reflect the urban hierarchy within the South West with (i) Plymouth–Exeter–Bristol–Gloucester/Cheltenham as an upper tier and (ii) smaller market towns being linked to the spatial interaction of people. Other ripples in the peaks probably reflect a scatter of random cases and small outbreaks over the 4 years.

Further analysis of epidemic links on the lines of Figure 1.20 may be justified for diseases like COVID-19. But it is important not to confuse precision with accuracy. Given the colossal computing power now available, we can readily increase the precision of our findings. More difficult is to remember the fragile base on which the original data may be collected. Non-parametric analyses may well be more accurate since they make fewer assumptions about the distribution of epidemic data.

Spatial interaction models

This second group of dyadic models has deep historic roots. Over a century ago, Ravenstein (1885, 1889) put forward his laws of migration, suggesting that movements might make use of Newton's Second

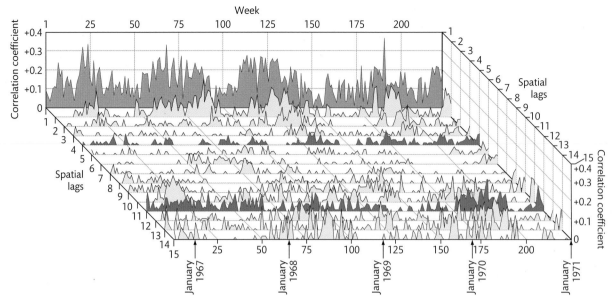

Figure 1.20 South West England measles activity, 1967–71. Lag correlation plot of 222 weeks of measles activity in 179 GRO areas. The correlation for each week between all pairs of GROs at each spatial lag is plotted. Only positive correlations are shown. The local maxima at spatial lags 5 and 12 are shaded green. Lag 1 is plotted in orange and illustrates the strong correlations among adjacent GROs—a contiguity effect.

Reproduced from Cliff, A.D., Ord, J.K. (1975). 'Space-time modelling with an application to regional forecasting.' *Transactions of the Institute of British Geographers*, 64, 119–28. Reprinted with permission.

Law of Motion—namely that migration might be directly related to the populations of the sending and receiving areas and inversely related to the square of the distance separating them. More generally, this law can be restated as an entropy maximizing problem. Again, the idea arose in physics, but it is not dependent on this and it seems to work very well in traffic flow problems for 'it turns out the most probable state is very much the *most* probable—which no doubt accounts for the success and robustness of the model's performance' (Wilson, 2000, p. 63). In addition to entropy maximizing gravity models, both linear and non-linear programming, originally developed to solve economic flow problems, can be used in the study of infection flows.

Given the potential of spatial interaction models, it is surprising that only a few examples of epidemiological applications exist. A Russian group at Leningrad (Baroyan et al., 1969) pioneered the use of gravity models in modelling Hong Kong influenza flows between Russian cities, 1968–69, as have Chen et al. (2021) in modelling COVID-19 movements among cities in China's Hubei province in 2020. Cliff and Haggett (1988, pp. 105–7) used maximum entropy gravity models to study flows of measles cases from Mexico, Canada, Japan, and 12 European countries into each state of the United States. The Lagrangian multipliers which are a by-product of the computations have a potential role in identifying levels of risk both for exporting and importing units. Finally, Tinline (1972) used linear programming methods to identify MIF values for his FMD outbreak studies.

1.7   Conclusion

In this first chapter, we have reviewed the key role of contagion in the spread of infectious diseases through the process of spatial diffusion.

Our emphasis has been on the impact of population distribution and movement in shaping both the emergence and the phasing of epidemics and pandemics. We have deliberately chosen to stress the role of geographical space in epidemiology and to expand on models developed in that field of research. Understanding epidemic behaviour is, in our view, enriched by drawing on the insights provided by a wide range of university disciplines that already stretch from molecular biology through applied mathematics to archaeology and anthropology.

A second bias in this chapter has been to emphasize the role of scale in epidemic studies. Using the conventional metric scale (Brillouin, 1964) we note that the light and electron microscopes allow the study of epidemic disease agents down to the near-atomic level at 10^{-10} metres. But by using the 'macroscopes' provided by maps and geographical information systems, geographical research moves over a similar magnitude range out to 10^{10} metres at the global level. Our *World Atlas of Epidemic Diseases* (Cliff et al., 2004) includes hundreds of maps which span spatial scales from street to world level.

1.7.1   Book Structure

This first chapter has aimed to set the subject of geographical contagion in a very broad-brush context. The chapters that follow are more specific in purpose, use finer brushes, and a more selective palette of diseases. In Chapter 2, we study epidemic outbreaks which are smaller in the numbers infected and are typically confined to a smaller geographical area. We look at outbreaks meticulously recorded within two GP practices, one in Yorkshire (Wensleydale) and the other in Gloucestershire (Cirencester) where two pioneering doctors threw crucial light on how their patients contracted illnesses. In Iceland, we also look at practice data in the northwest where excellent records have survived.

In Chapter 3, our spatial scale changes from the local to the international, and the palette of diseases we consider is wider. At this broader level of resolution, the focus moves from individual cases and outbreaks to full-blown epidemic waves. Where on Earth did the classic crowd diseases originate, and what are the factors that have facilitated the emergence of a raft of so-called new infectious diseases in recent decades? Our examination covers factors that, inter alia, have tended to increase the geographical scale of disease cycles: the revolution in population growth, the fall in transport costs, and the mass movements of people for the purposes of trade, migration, and tourism. The Brownian motion of the human population, its population flux, has increased exponentially since the industrial revolution and, with that, the opportunities for the spread of diseases over large distances has never been higher.

Chapter 4 moves to the outcomes of the forces unleashed in the previous chapters. It tracks the great pandemics in world history, seeking to find order and rationales for their spatial form. It contrasts the movements of past plague, cholera, and influenza pandemics, and the ongoing HIV/AIDS pandemic. Where do these pandemics come from? Why do they travel so fast and jump from continent to continent ever more easily?

Given the current crisis of the global COVID-19 pandemic, it would have been easy for a preoccupation with this to have drowned out consideration of the other pandemic-causing diseases described in Chapter 4. And so, COVID-19 is treated in a separate Chapter 5. Although we describe the temporal and spatial patterns that COVID-19 has created, we also try to place this pandemic within the longer historical perspective provided by Chapter 4. Our discussion of COVID-19 covers the period from its putative beginning in late 2019 to the turn of 2021. At that point, mass vaccination—at least in the economically more advanced countries of the world—began to take hold, thereby offering a glimmer of light at the end of the pandemic tunnel.

The last key chapter, Chapter 6, is different in both spirit and purpose to the others. It moves from a concern with understanding epidemic diffusion to exploring how that knowledge can be applied to infectious disease prevention and control.

2 Epidemics in Small Communities

CONTENTS

2.1 Introduction

An implication of the Bartlett model, described in section 1.4.3 in Chapter 1, is that diseases which ultimately burgeon into epidemics and pandemics must begin initially with just a handful of infectives. The personal contact or mean information field (MIF; see section 1.6.3 in Chapter 1) of these infectives enables them to pass on the disease agent to other susceptible individuals with whom they come into contact. Over time, the continual repetition of this simple process will, if unhindered, enable an infection to enter general circulation in a population. Eventually the disease agent will become dispersed through villages, towns, and cities, and up the geographical scale hierarchy into global diffusion. As we saw in section 1.3.2, in Chapter 1, epidemiologists and statisticians capture the speed of this growth process through the quantity R_0, the so-called *basic reproduction number*, which we defined as the number of secondary cases that, unchecked, one infected individual would produce in a completely susceptible population.

In this chapter, we develop our understanding of the way infection achieves community circulation by looking at epidemic outbreaks which are small in the numbers infected and which are initially confined to a small geographical area. At this local geographical scale, the history of medicine is rich with examples of how individual doctors, sometimes in small communities in remote locations, gained insights into the ways in which epidemic diseases spread. Perhaps Jenner (1798), in his study of cowpox and smallpox in his practice at Berkeley in Gloucestershire, represents the supreme example.

In the twentieth century, two doctors in general practice in the United Kingdom dominated observational epidemiology at the microscale. In the first half, there was William Pickles, who worked in Wensleydale in North Yorkshire from 1912 until the early 1960s and meticulously recorded the patterns of epidemic diseases in eight villages and a series of isolated farmsteads. His *Epidemiology in Country Practice* (1939) remains a model of careful observation and insight into disease transmission between farm, family, school, and village. Pickles's classic book begins:

> A gipsy woman driving a caravan into a village in the summer twilight, a sick husband in the caravan, a faulty pump at which she proceeded to wash her dirty linen, and my first and only serious epidemic of typhoid, left me with a lasting impression of the unique opportunities of the country doctor for the investigation of infectious disease. This incident showed me clearly the ease with which the *fons et origo* [source and origin] of an epidemic could be traced in the country and the simple steps that were sufficient to bring it to an end. (Pickles, 1939, p. 1)

Quoting from William Budd's *Typhoid Fever* (1873), Pickles (1939, pp. 1–3) goes on to elaborate the features of rural general practices which make them ideal epidemiological laboratories in which to study the origin, spread, and behaviour of epidemic diseases:

1. They have a simple geographical structure of small communities spaced on well-defined lines of communication like beads on a necklace. 'It is equally obvious that where the question at issue is that of the propagation of disease by human intercourse, rural districts where the population is thin, and the lines of intercourse are few and always easily traced, offer opportunities for its settlement which are not to be met with in the crowded haunts of large towns' (pp. 1–2).

2. Detailed knowledge of the social structure of the susceptible and infective populations facilitates contact tracing. 'Having been born and brought up in the village, I was personally acquainted with every inhabitant of it; and being, as a medical practitioner, in almost exclusive possession of the field, nearly every one who fell ill, not only in the village itself, but over a large area around it, came immediately under my care. For tracing the part of personal intercourse in the propagation of disease, better outlook could not possibly be had' (p. 2).

3. Country doctors tend to remain in one practice and so see epidemics come and go. Inter alia, this permits epidemic return times to be investigated. 'The daily, even hourly, exposure to infection so easy to ascertain gives us the opportunity of fixing the incubation period and the infectivity period [of a disease] in a way which is withheld from our town brother' (p. 2).

4. Knowledge of the social engines of spread. 'He [the village doctor] knows the relationships, friendships and love affairs of all his patients, because he is interested in the people and they are a major part of his life. He knows the markets they frequent, the schools which their children attend, and the memorable trips to the seaside or the pantomime. The annual feast is not quite a thing of the past, although in most of our villages it is now merely a memory of what it has been. Every year the inhabitants of one of the villages, with due solemnity and ritual, burn the effigy of their patron saint—St. Bartholomew being thinly disguised as "Old Bartle"—and a large gathering from all the districts around assists in the process. Something like a revival of the old carefree gaiety of pre-war [1914–18] was seen in the Silver Jubilee [1935] and Coronation celebrations [1937], but it is a melancholy reflection how often these and similar festivities have been responsible for the spread of infectious disease. A short time ago, isolated cases of diphtheria were occurring in young people who seldom left their homes. Every one of these had gone joyfully to a dance or fair about three days before he or she was stricken, and that joyful occasion provided the only possible source of infection' (pp. 2–3).

After a 15-year overlap, but then following on from Pickles in the second half of the twentieth century, Edgar Hope-Simpson in general practice in Cirencester, Gloucestershire, from 1947 until the mid-1970s, made detailed records of infectious diseases, especially influenza, by geographical location and virus type. These influenza records enabled him to propose radical ideas about the transmission of epidemic influenza A. Pickles drew inspiration from the great Scottish doctor, James Mackenzie, who worked in general practice in Burnley from 1879 to 1907 and established the Institute for Clinical Research at St Andrews University in 1919; Hope-Simpson saw himself as following in the footsteps of Pickles, and he remained active in retirement until the early 1990s.

Parallel arguments to those of Pickles have been adduced in Cliff et al. (2000, pp. 41–83) for the use of islands as sites for the study of epidemiological processes. And so, to complement the United Kingdom examples, our other case studies in this chapter stay at the individual scale but switch the geographical setting from the United Kingdom to the sub-Arctic island of Iceland. In the northwest of the country, around the fishing town of Ísafjörður, excellent medical practice and Lutheran church records have survived which enable the microscale geographical spread of epidemics

among the dispersed rural population to be tracked and mapped. Equivalent data spanning 100 years also exist for the rest of Iceland. We use these to treat Iceland as an epidemiological laboratory in which we study the spread of communicable diseases as chains and waves. We look especially at measles but also analyse Iceland's waves of diphtheria, influenza, pertussis, poliomyelitis, rubella, and scarlet fever.

And so, in this chapter, we look at the contribution of doctors and community paramedics who used their general practices and observational skills, alongside church demographic records, to study the behaviour of epidemic diseases at the microscale. Ultimately their work helped to specify the processes whereby single infected individuals can seed community-wide epidemics. In more recent years, the trend of local observational epidemiology has been away from individual practices towards samples of practices as the framework for epidemiological study. In England, the decennial surveys of disease morbidity in sentinel practices undertaken by the Royal College of General Practitioners (RCGP) represent one such example. G.I. Watson, a GP working near Guildford in the mid-twentieth century, played a central role in setting research in general practice on a sound footing at the RCGP, serving both on RCGP committees and heading up the RCGP Epidemic Observation Unit at Peaslake from 1954. This was the first of a number of RCGP research units established in the 1960s and 1970s around the country.

2.2 William Pickles of Wensleydale, 1913–63

William Pickles was born on 6 March 1885. Educated at Leeds Grammar School and the medical school of the (then) Yorkshire College (later Leeds University) and in London, he became an MD in 1918. His first visit to Aysgarth (Figure 2.1) was as a locum for Dr Hime in 1912 and he joined the practice in 1913. Internal isolation of settlements from each other and external isolation (out of Wensleydale) was high for much of the period. As a consequence, contact tracing was straightforward:

> In my early days of practice in Wensleydale, twenty-five years ago, there were people in the district who had never been in a train, and even today many, especially women, seldom leave their homes; it is therefore possible for me to state definitely that such a one suffering from an infectious disorder could only have been infected on a certain date. (Pickles, 1939, p. 7)

The main external line of communication was the Wensleydale railway from Northallerton on the east coast mainline from London to Edinburgh, to Hawes Junction/Garsdale Head on the Leeds–Settle–Carlisle line in the west. Infection commonly arrived in the dale via this route since none of the settlements in Wensleydale had a large enough population to sustain endemically the common infectious diseases (see Figures 1.9 and 1.10 in Chapter 1). As a consequence, epidemics occurred discretely in time and space, first imported into the area and then spreading from one village to another. Pickles (1939, pp. 20–1) comments:

> The only epidemics that I have myself encountered have been those spread by personal contact … the great majority of our people rarely leave their homes, but there are annual visits to the pantomime and school trips to the seaside, and on many occasions these expeditions have resulted in the importation of infection. Living as we do between

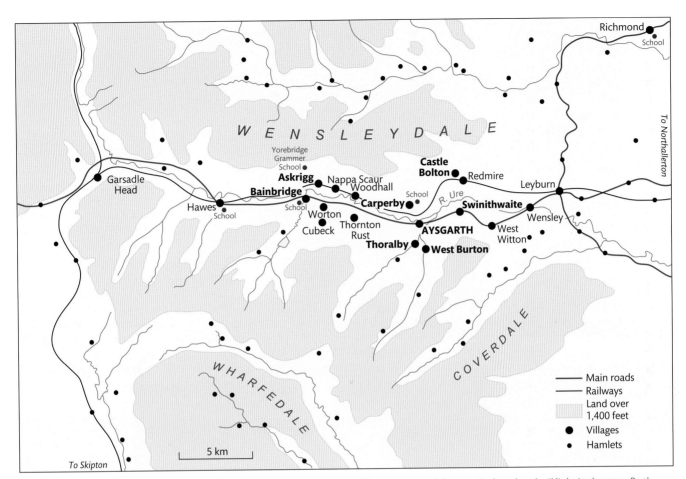

Figure 2.1 Geography of the Aysgarth practice in the 1930s. The map shows Wensleydale and the principal road and rail links in the area. By the time Pickles arrived permanently in the practice in 1913, it exclusively served an area of the dale from West Witton in the east to Bainbridge in the west (21 km); the practice population was about 4500 in 1930. The River Ure flows down the dale, and north and south tributaries flow into it from the surrounding fells. Large solid circles mark the chief villages and market centres in the practice. Dispersed settlements and isolated farmsteads, many scattered along the north–south tributaries of the Ure, and other small communities, are marked by small circles. The rail links were available throughout Pickles's time in the practice. Public road transport took off in the 1930s. Prior to that, train, horse, motorcycle, cycle, and foot were the main means of getting about.

two small market towns [Hawes and Leyburn], which our farmers and others visit weekly, we find that many of our instances of epidemic disease take their origin from these weekly visits, and in the case of the farmers I suspect the covered auction marts as the chief source of infection, especially influenza infection. There are also more direct means by which these infections reach this particular neighbourhood. … a few years ago, a particularly worthy schoolmistress returned to her home after a Christmas holiday spent with her relatives. On the morning of the school opening, knowing she was ill [with influenza], with commendable if mistaken zeal, she attended her school. In the afternoon she was utterly unable to return, but from that brief morning session a crop of 78 cases resulted.

Having reached the district, it is easy to understand the method of spread of these infections. There are now cinemas, … concerts, whist-drives, and dances, which are available to the inhabitants over a wide area owing to the increase of transport facilities, of which a recent development is an excellent bus service. All these channels have provided opportunities for infection …, but the school remains and will remain the largest factor in disseminating the infective agent of an epidemic.

And so we see the role of people travelling to places outside the dale importing infection on their return and then the part played by markets, schools, and social events in spreading infection within the dale.

On control, Pickles was alert to the issue of school closures to prevent the spread of infection:

> School closure is a vexed question. … There are occasions early in an epidemic when a temporary closure might be completely effective, but my policy is to exclude children from outlying farms and hamlets. … What would also be satisfactory would be to close all the churches and chapels and cinemas, and to issue an order against public meetings, dances and whist drives … I find this does not appeal to the very people who clamour for school closure. (Pickles, 1939, p. 22)

Analysis of Pickles's epidemic records (Figure 2.2) enables the geographical spread of disease between individuals to be specified, and it is to this that we now turn.

2.2.1 Epidemic Records

From 1931 to 1963, Pickles's wife and daughter, Gertrude and Patience, along with Madge Blades, the practice dispenser, recorded the primary data from which Pickles drew his conclusions on the

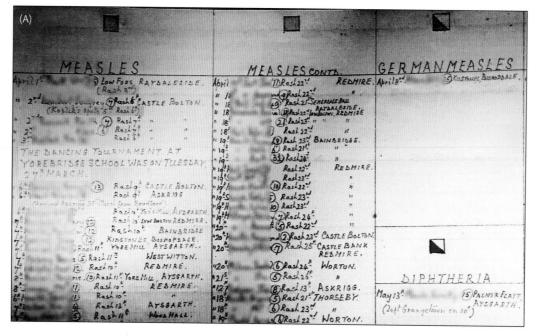

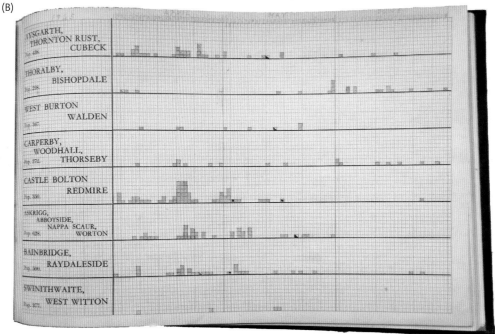

Figure 2.2 Recording epidemic diseases in Wensleydale. (A) Part of a page during a measles epidemic, April–June 1945, from Pickles's records preserved in two volumes at the Royal College of General Practitioners. Pickles's wife Gerty maintained the records on a daily basis for ten common infectious diseases—influenza, measles, scarlet fever, whooping cough, mumps, chickenpox, and shingles, Sonne dysentery, 'epidemic catarrhal jaundice' (hepatitis A), and Bornholm disease—as well as many less-commonly occurring infections. Each entry gives the patient's name, age, village, disease, and any additional information such as where and by whom infected. Family names have been redacted to ensure patient anonymity. The contact information (highlighted in yellow) links the early April cases to attendance at a dancing tournament held at (the former) Yorebridge Grammar School near the market town of Hawes in late March. The contact information also records a measles infective arriving in the dales at Askrigg from Bradford, and a diphtheria case from Grangetown near Middlesbrough appearing in Aysgarth. Disease diagnostic information (for measles, date of rash, date of infection, and Koplik's spots) is also noted and is highlighted in blue. (B) The textual information was then displayed as a simple bar graph, with one square per case. The chart reproduced here plots the 1945 measles epidemic using green squares. Other diseases are plotted in different colours.

Source: images from Pickles's data books held by the Royal College of General Practitioners. Reproduced with the permission of the Royal College of General Practitioners (UK), 1939.

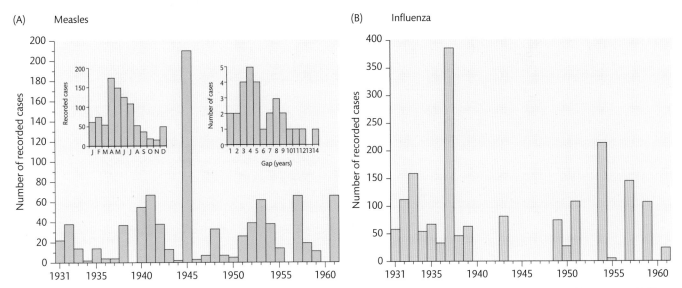

Figure 2.3 Measles and influenza in Wensleydale. Annual time series of (A) measles and (B) influenza cases recorded in the Pickles practice, 1931–61. Pickles recorded a total of 916 measles cases and 1764 influenza cases over the 31-year period. The inset graphs in (A) show (left) the monthly distribution of cases and (right) the frequency of return times for measles epidemics; see text for details.

mode of spread, incubation, and infectivity periods of various epidemic diseases in Wensleydale. As **Figure 2.2** shows, the recording took two forms. **Figure 2.2A** illustrates one of the sample tables giving the date a patient was diagnosed by Pickles as infected, their name, age, village of residence, the disease involved, and, crucially, any additional information on the infection. The additional information includes, where known, how and from whom the infection was acquired. **Figure 2.2B** charts the daily time series numbers of each disease as a bar graph.

Pickles's epidemiological writings suggest his recording was particularly directed at four issues—the incubation and infectious periods of different epidemic diseases, their varying degrees of infectiousness, and epidemic return times which produce the repeating cycles of infections. Contact tracing is essential to an understanding of all of these, and we sample from Pickles's observations on two classic epidemic diseases, measles and influenza, to illustrate his contribution.

2.2.2 Measles

Figure 2.3A shows the annual time series of measles cases recorded by Pickles in his Wensleydale practice. Pickles notes (1939, p. 33) that the return time for measles epidemics in Wensleydale is about 9 years and that they last around 6 months. All the dales villages are well below the critical community size for endemic measles (~250,000 in the pre-vaccination era) and, as noted by Pickles as previously mentioned, all epidemics would have been started by importation from outside the immediate dale. In terms of the Bartlett model of measles waves, the villages are type III communities (see Figure 1.9 in Chapter 1).

In the light of Pickles's remark that major measles epidemics in Wensleydale have a return time of about 9 years, we applied time series methods, best subsets regression, and fitted sine/cosine waves to (i) the measles total cases time series of **Figure 2.3A** and to (ii) each of the annual case time series of the eight principal villages (Askrigg, Aysgarth, Bainbridge, Carperby, Castle Bolton, Swinithwaite, Thoralby, and West Burton; **Figure 2.1** shows

locations). No statistically significant regular period of recurrence was found. As Pickles noted (see previously), this suggests that, once the susceptible population, S, is large enough, measles epidemics can be seeded anywhere in the dales system of settlements by a chance introduction of the measles virus from outside the area.

We then focused on the time gap between major epidemic peaks in each village. We declared any given year in a village time series as a peak year (coded 1) if the cases that year were more than double the village's average annual case load over the 31 years of the time series. All years which failed to meet this test were coded 0. The inset histogram (right) in **Figure 2.3A** shows the frequency distribution of gap lengths. While the average gap or return time for measles peaks was 5.76 and the median 5.0 years, as **Figure 2.3A** (inset) shows, there is a secondary peak in the gap lengths at 7–9 years, consistent with Pickles's estimate of a 9-year cycle. The 9-year return time for measles epidemics in Wensleydale suggested by Pickles reflects the small populations of the villages in the practice and the commensurately long time required for the susceptible population to build up to a critical level again after an epidemic. It provides an explanation for something which puzzled Pickles (p. 35): 'I cannot say why we do not have the biennial epidemics which admittedly recur in the large towns.'

The degree of epidemiological cohesiveness of the dales villages can be assessed using correlation and multidimensional scaling (MDS). We define cohesiveness of a village as the average correlation between its annual measles time series and the seven other villages in the system. The values for Pickles's villages were as follows: Askrigg 0.41, Aysgarth 0.44, Bainbridge 0.32, Carperby 0.16, Castle Bolton 0.49, Swinithwaite –0.01, Thoralby 0.40, and West Burton 0.22. These cohesiveness values were then used as the response variable in a multiple regression with the village populations shown in **Figure 2.2B** and the length in kilometres of the minimum spanning tree (MST; Graham and Hell, 1985) on the road network as the explanatory variables. The MST is one measure of the connectedness of each village to the transport network; a small MST distance characterizes a well-connected village whereas a large MST distance characterizes villages

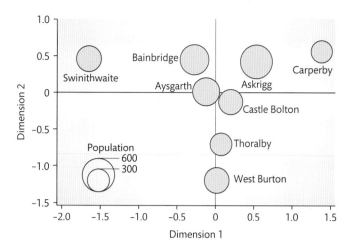

Figure 2.4 MDS measles map for eight villages in Wensleydale, 1931–61. Minimum stress two-dimensional map based on correlations between the time series of the villages. See text for details. Circle sizes are proportional to populations of the villages shown in Figure 2.2B. The stress of the final configuration is 0.08 and $R^2 = 0.97$.

whose location is remote from other villages in the network. Neither explanatory variable was significant although their regression coefficients had the expected sign; cohesiveness and MST were inversely related (i.e. cohesiveness increased for better connected villages in the road network) while cohesiveness and population size were positively related (larger places were more cohesive). Population size was more important than distance as an explanatory variable. This would be expected from the Bartlett model, and it is reinforced by the MDS 'map' (Cliff et al., 1995) computed from the correlation matrix between the annual time series of the eight practice villages as the measure of similarity between the villages. An MDS map is constructed so that the locations of points on the map correspond not to their (scaled) geographical locations as on a conventional map, but to their degree of similarity on some variable measured for them. For example, we might map points into a time space; locations separated by short travel times will appear central and close together in such a space, while centres linked by long travel times will be widely separated and peripheral.

This basic idea can be extended to the mapping of points from geographical space into a disease space. Points with, say, similar attack rates for an infectious disease will be located close to each other on the MDS map even though they may be far removed geographically. The greater the degree of similarity between places on the variable measured, the closer together the places will be in the MDS space. Conversely, points which are dissimilar on the variable will be widely separated in the MDS space, irrespective of their geographical location on the globe. Thus, broadly stated, the problem of MDS is to find a configuration of n points in m-dimensional space such that the inter-point distances in the configuration in some sense match the experimental dissimilarities of the n objects. This may be viewed as a problem of statistical fitting.

Figure 2.4 is the MDS measles map for the villages in the Pickles practice, 1931–61. Circle sizes are proportional to the village populations for 1931 as given in **Figure 2.2B**. The configuration shows that the four largest settlements cluster together in the centre of the map, with the other villages scattered around this core. Such a pattern illustrates again the importance of population size in determining the shape of the measles time series in the dale.

Pickles's comments on Wensleydale's measles epidemics show how careful observational epidemiology can help to flesh out our understanding of the processes whereby epidemics of infectious disease begin with a handful of cases in a small geographical area, develop through the social contact network, pass into general circulation, and cause a significant epidemic. Just as Peter Panum (1847) had done nearly 200 years ago in the Faroe Islands, when he recognized the epidemiological significance of social gatherings associated with the whaling year, so Pickles identified the role of schools, markets, dances, and, as shown later, other social gatherings in driving the early stages of an epidemic.

2.2.3 Influenza

Pickles's interest in influenza focused upon the seemingly erratic behaviour of the disease in Wensleydale (Pickles, 1939, pp. 30–3; Pickles et al., 1947). The massive pandemic of 1918 had high mortality in Wensleydale as elsewhere:

> Since that dread time, in 1924, 1927, 1929, and 1931, we have had extensive epidemics of this complaint, but with this difference, that there was hardly a patient in any of these epidemics who gave us a moment's anxiety, and the death rate was providentially negligible. The next epidemic, in 1937, … spread more rapidly than in previous visitations, due probably to the improved methods of transport. (Pickles, 1939, p. 31)

The nature of the influenza virus is discussed later in section 4.4.1 in Chapter 4. Here we simply note that the pandemics and repeated epidemics of influenza experienced across the globe are usually caused by the A strain of the virus. In 1973, E.D. Kilbourne proposed the simple model illustrated in **Figure 2.5A** to explain the temporal pattern of repeating influenza waves. This model helps to account for the cycles and varying sizes of influenza outbreaks observed by Pickles in Wensleydale. If a new strain of the A virus (A_2, say, in **Figure 2.5A**) is introduced into a population, population antibody levels to it will be low and a large epidemic/pandemic will result. As more and more individuals become infected, population antibody levels and, therefore, resistance to the virus strain in circulation will build and subsequent epidemics will be smaller and smaller. As a result of natural selection pressure on the virus, mutations will occur as described in section 4.4.1 in Chapter 4, and a new strain (A_3 in **Figure 2.5A**) will emerge which has not been encountered previously by individuals and to which population antibody levels are low. Such a strain will have the potential to cause a major epidemic or pandemic; the cycle will then repeat itself.

In Wensleydale, in addition to the influenza epidemics noted previously, there had also been small outbreaks in 1933 and 1935. 'One of these [1933] … originating in a schoolmistress, raises a notable point. The area which suffered in this epidemic of 78 cases practically escaped in 1937, a circumstance which may indicate some degree of partial immunity in the inhabitants of the area' (Pickles, 1939, pp. 32–3). Since it is likely that the same virus strain was involved, this is entirely consistent with the Kilbourne model. Pickles investigated the point further in his 1947 paper. Data from the three influenza epidemics of 1933, 1937, and 1943 showed that, except for West Burton, the villages in the practice exhibited an alternating series for case rates, in which a large epidemic one year was followed by a small one the next, and vice versa (**Figure 2.5B**). The causative virus would have been influenza A (H1N1) in all three epidemics

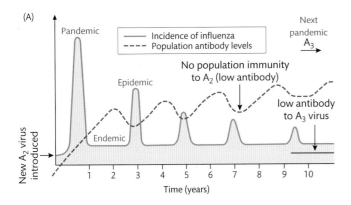

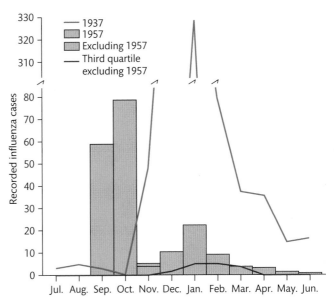

Figure 2.6 Seasonal influenza case distribution in the Pickles practice, 1931–61. The graph shows the monthly case distribution averaged over all years, 1931–61 but excluding 1957 (blue columns; third quartile red line trace), for 1957 as orange columns, and for the 1937 epidemic (green line trace).

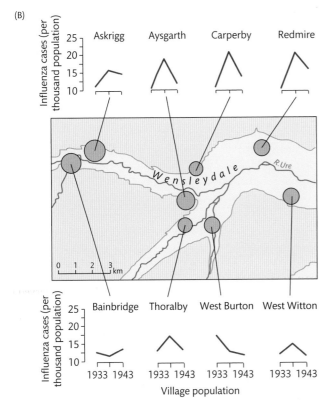

Figure 2.5 Influenza in Wensleydale. (A) Kilbourne's 1973 model of repeating influenza epidemic waves. (B) Attack rates from three successive influenza A epidemics (1933, 1937, 1943) in eight villages of a country practice in Wensleydale, North Yorkshire. A statistical analysis appears in Cliff et al. (1986, pp. 27–8). The causative virus would have been influenza A (H1N1) in all three epidemics, so a high attack rate in a village in the first epidemic would have significantly reduced the susceptible population in the second, leading to lower attack rates, and vice versa.

(A) Reproduced from Kilbourne, E. D. Influenza in perspective: 1967–1968. *Sandoz Panorama*, 6:7–11, 1968. (B) Source data from Pickles (1939, pp. 24–5) and Pickles et al. (1947).

(cf. A₂ in **Figure 2.5A**), so a high attack rate in a village in the first epidemic would have significantly reduced the susceptible population in the second, leading to lower attack rates, and vice versa. The negative correlation between attack rates in successive epidemics broke down in the 1945–46 outbreak which was caused by influenza B. The larger than expected case load would be expected under the Kilbourne model since the population was exposed to a different virus strain.

For much of Pickles's working lifetime, the type A influenza virus in circulation was H1N1. But, as described in section 4.4 in Chapter 4, in 1957 there was a major shift of both surface antigens from H1N1 to H2N2, so-called Asian influenza. As a result, the population in the dales and worldwide became susceptible. The impact upon the 1957–58 influenza season in Wensleydale was immediate. As **Figure 2.6** shows, the season began in September and had ended in November as opposed to all other seasons which, on average, ran from November to March/April. Not only was the season earlier but much sharper than any other influenza season except the epidemic of 1937. We shall see this tendency for virus shift years to generate more cases and to peak earlier than a normal influenza season when we turn to Hope-Simpson's work in section 2.3.

2.2.4 Contact Tracing

As we noted earlier, Pickles's writings stressed the key role of personal contact fields in facilitating the growth of individual cases into community-wide transmission of infectious disease agents. The 1938 measles epidemic in the dales makes the point:

> Two children, a brother and a sister, attended one of our schools feeling out of sorts. … The rash of measles commenced in each on March 3. There were no other sufferers from measles in the whole district, but these children had been to a pantomime in Leeds, where measles was rife, on Feb. 15 and no doubt were infected with the disease during this excursion. … the boy's symptoms definitely began on the 27th giving an incubation period of twelve days. The whole of the susceptible population of the school with two possible exceptions then contracted the disease. (Pickles, 1939, p. 4)

In the same vein:

> A boy in a farm 'place' arrived at the surgery and announced he had 'gitten measles' (contracted measles). This was certainly the case, and he was told to go to his mother's home, and shout to her the same

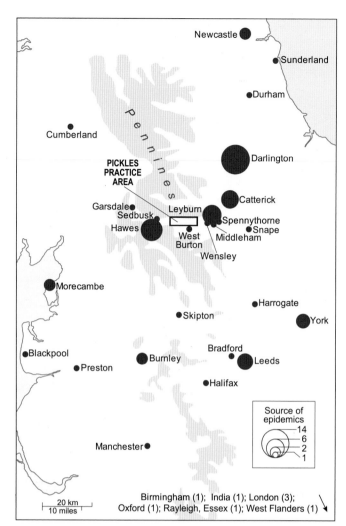

Figure 2.7 Geographical sources of measles and influenza epidemics in Wensleydale. The map shows the settlements outside the Pickles practice area from which measles and influenza infections were transferred into Wensleydale.

As already noted, measles and influenza epidemics in Wensleydale were generally seeded by infectives coming into the dale from the surrounding regions or by Wensleydale residents visiting places outside the dale in which epidemics were ongoing. **Figure 2.7** maps the locations, as recorded by Pickles, from which measles and influenza infection was transferred into Wensleydale between 1931 and 1961. Most were close to the dale with a preponderance from adjacent areas of Yorkshire.

2.3 Edgar Hope-Simpson and Peter Higgins in Cirencester, 1947–73: A Study of Influenza

Hope-Simpson joined the Cirencester practice (**Figure 2.8**) in 1945, after some years in a rural practice in West Dorset. For the next quarter of a century, Hope-Simpson was a working physician in a practice which varied between 3,000 and 4,000 patients. He was fascinated by the epidemiology of the common infectious diseases of the children and adults he attended, and he kept very detailed day-by-day records of the incidence of these diseases for each patient. Like Pickles, he and his wife spent every evening producing Pickles-style charts in their living room.

Uniquely at the time, the practice had associated with it an Epidemiological Research Unit which, from 1946, was a constituent laboratory of the United Kingdom's Public Health Laboratory

tidings outside the door in order that she might have the living-room cleared of his small brothers and sisters. He then repaired to his bedroom, where he remained a fortnight. On the twelfth day after his arrival, his aunt, and only his aunt, became a victim of the disease, although she had never seen the boy, and left the house the day after his arrival. It was found that the boy's bedroom and the living room directly below, by an unusual and capricious arrangement of the builder, were lighted by one long window, giving direct aerial access from one room to another. The meal table was below this gap, and the aunt, who sat directly underneath at meals, was apparently thus infected. (Pickles, 1939, p. 36)

Over the period 1931–61, Pickles recorded a total of 2,855 cases of measles and influenza. For 73 of these, Pickles explicitly noted the setting in which the infection was acquired: 41 (56 per cent) in school (Richmond, Bainbridge, Carperby, Yorebridge, and Hawes); six at a party; four at a dance; eight socially (concert, wedding, fair, circus, or pantomime); seven at market in Hawes or Leyburn; and seven were visitors. In addition to social events and school, we can deduce from the name and address information of patients that about 55 per cent of infections in the dataset occurred between members of the same family.

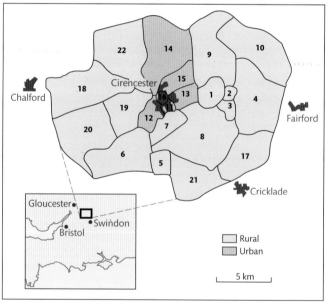

Figure 2.8 Location of the Cirencester practice. The map shows the geographical location and extent of Hope-Simpson's practice including the boundaries of the 22 units into which he divided the practice for data collection purposes. Cirencester is a market town, with a population of around 12,000 in 1957, lying between Swindon and Gloucester in the middle part of the English Cotswolds. The practice covered an area of some 210 km². Patient records span the 30-year period, 1946–76. The demographic structure of the practice at the time was representative of geographical variations in the local population (Cliff et al., 1986, pp. 47–52). The panel size was stable over the period and showed a similar level of secular ageing as the Cirencester population more generally.

Reproduced with permission from Smallman-Raynor, M.R., Cliff, A.D. (2012). *Atlas of Epidemic Britain: A Twentieth Century Picture*. Oxford: Oxford University Press.

Service. It was also supported by a Medical Research Council grant from 1947 to 1973. In 1960, a small virological laboratory was established in the Unit until transferred to Gloucester in 1973. Hope-Simpson and the Unit continued their epidemiological studies until 1996. From 1960, the laboratory was run by Dr Peter Higgins. Higgins (b. 1926) was a member of the scientific staff of the Public Health Laboratory Service from 1955, seconded to the Common Cold Unit, which he joined in 1981 until its closure and his retirement in 1990 (Tansley et al., 1998, p. 254).

Although Hope-Simpson worked on a number of diseases, his consuming passion was understanding the epidemiology of influenza. At Dyer Street, individual patients were identified and influenza diagnosed by a single doctor and his partner over an approximate 30-year period. Links can be established between virologically and serologically confirmed cases of influenza and those recognized simply by clinical symptoms. From c.1945, a series of papers reported findings from this practice (e.g. Hope-Simpson, 1948, 1952, 1958, 1970, 1978, 1979; Hope-Simpson and Sutherland, 1954). As a result, the practice became internationally known as providing a special window into the operation of epidemiological processes at the micro level. The period from 1961 to 1973, when Higgins was in charge of the laboratory and Hope-Simpson was Director of the whole Unit, was particularly profitable; it was when much of the basic virological work was undertaken (see Tansley et al., 1998, pp. 108–10 and 254).

2.3.1 Epidemic Records

Records of clinical cases of influenza were kept in the Hope-Simpson practice for 28 years, 1946–74. More than 10,000 cases were recorded with the annual totals fluctuating between a minimum of 117 in the influenza season (defined as July to June of the following year) of 1946–47 (a non-epidemic year) to a maximum of 669 in 1957–58 (the first season of Asian influenza). About 60 per cent of all cases were recorded in years dominated by influenza A viruses.

2.3.2 Seasonality

In Figure 2.6, it was shown how the influenza A virus shift from H1N1 to the (then) new virus strain H2N2 (Asian flu) produced an influenza season in Wensleydale which occurred earlier in the year and yielded more cases than usual. The same effect can be seen in the Hope-Simpson data. Epidemic curves are usually bell-shaped and very commonly right-skewed—that is, in an epidemic, reported cases build up rapidly to a single peak and then fade out more slowly than they build, thus producing a right skew; see Figure 1.5. A symmetric bell-shaped case incidence over the duration of an epidemic implies that the build-up and fade-out phases occur at the same secular rate. For such a symmetric curve, a graph of the cumulative percentage of cases (y-axis) against time on the horizontal x-axis would assume a sigmoidal shape known as a *logistic* curve with the mid-curve turning point corresponding to the peak of the epidemic (see Cliff et al., 1986, pp. 85–6); see Figure 1.5B. As compared with a logistic, a right-skewed epidemic (faster build-up than fade-out) would have a cumulative case curve lying to the left of the logistic in the early stages (Figure 1.5A); a left-skewed epidemic (slower build-up than fade-out) would lie to the right (Figure 1.5C).

Figure 2.9A shows what happened in the Hope-Simpson practice around the influenza virus shift seasons of 1957–58 (from H1N1 to H2N2) and, in the lower row of graphs, 1968–70 (from H2N2 to H3N2). The virus shift seasons are characterized by a sharp build-up in cases as compared with seasons before and immediately after the shift. Figure 2.9B illustrates the effect in a different way by plotting as a block diagram the time series of weekly case counts of clinically confirmed cases for the period 1946–74. Under the Kilbourne model, elevated case incidence should occur in virus shift seasons and, because population immunity to the new strain will be very low, it might reasonably be expected that cases would occur earlier in the season than in non-shift years; we have already seen that case levels in Cirencester rose sharply in shift seasons as compared with non-shift years. Figure 2.9B shows the number of clinically diagnosed influenza A cases recorded in the Cirencester practice by influenza season from 1946–47 to 1973–74. In the shift seasons, 1957–58 and 1969–70, it is evident that the build-up and peak incidence of influenza occurred much earlier in the year than was usual in the practice. This is especially true in 1957–58 which peaked in October as compared with the practice norm of February–March.

2.3.3 Velocity of Epidemics

If influenza epidemics in A-virus shift years are more intense than usual and peak earlier in the season, do they also spread geographically more quickly? This question has been considered for the Hope-Simpson practice by Cliff, Smallman-Raynor, Haggett, et al. (2009, pp. 572–5) using the parameter R_{0A} of the swash model described in section 1.6.2 in Chapter 1. Figure 2.10 gives the results for serologically or virologically confirmed cases of type A influenza in the practice. These are available between 1963 and 1975. There was a sharp upturn in the rate of spread through the practice population in the second season of Hong Kong influenza (1969) when Europe was principally affected—Viboud's (2005) 'smouldering pandemic'. Thereafter, wave velocities fell slowly back to reach pre-1969 levels by 1973 as the population still susceptible to the new strain diminished.

Geographically, the spread of influenza in Cirencester was led through the urban areas of the practice into the less densely populated rural parts in five of the nine seasons in which influenza A epidemics occurred, on average by about a week. When influenza A epidemics occurred first in rural areas (four seasons), they did so by about 10 days before spreading into urban areas.

2.3.4 Within-Family Transmission

Multiple case data from households within the Hope-Simpson practice shows some evidence, through the small peak at 4 days, of the short serial interval generally associated with influenza A (Figure 2.11). This is consistent with the evidence in Table 1.2.

2.4 Summary

The first half of this chapter has highlighted the contributions of two general practitioners, William Pickles and Edgar Hope-Simpson, in enhancing our understanding of the temporal and spatial behaviour of epidemic diseases in the twentieth century through their epidemiological observations, and their assiduous collection and analysis of microscale data. We now move on to a different arena, Iceland, and look at similar data collected there.

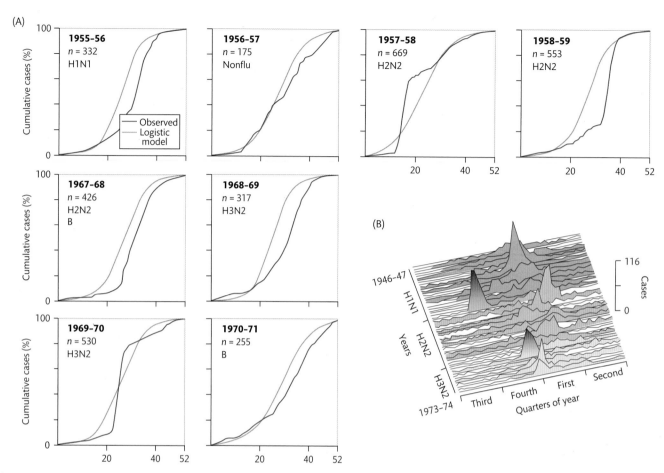

Figure 2.9 The shape of epidemics and influenza virus shift seasons, Cirencester, England. (A) The graphs plot, against time, the cumulative percentage of observed clinical cases (red line) and the cumulative percentage expected under the logistic model (grey line) for each week of the groups of influenza seasons, 1955–56 to 1958–59, and 1967–68 to 1970–71. The sample size (*n*) and virus strains in circulation are recorded. In both groups, the seasons prior to the virus shift are characterized by a slow build-up of cases, whereas the virus shift seasons of 1957–58 and 1969–70 are both characterized by a sharp build-up of cases after a slow start. As noted in Viboud et al. (2005), the 1968–69 shift primarily affected North America in its first season and Europe in its second. This is evidenced in Cirencester. (B) Clinically diagnosed influenza cases in the Hope-Simpson practice, weekly, for 28 influenza A seasons, 1946–47 to 1973–74. The two peaks of cases highlighted in red which correspond with the major virus shift seasons, 1957–58 and 1969–70, stand out to the left (i.e. earlier start) of the main range of peaks which represent the normal late winter seasonal maximum. This appearance of an early peak at times of antigenic shift in the influenza virus can be related to the larger stock of susceptibles available for infection on such occasions in the Kilbourne model (Figure 2.5A).

Reproduced with permission from Smallman-Raynor, M.R., Cliff, A.D. (2012). *Atlas of Epidemic Britain: A Twentieth Century Picture*. Oxford: Oxford University Press.

2.5 Iceland: Measles in the Twentieth Century

2.5.1 Introduction

Iceland's centuries-long history of epidemics and its unusually complete disease records have attracted study from many disciplines. The detailed spatial records of most interest to epidemic modellers date from 1895 and were consistently maintained for a century. For a shorter, 87-year long window, from 1902 to 1988, there exist unbroken, geo-coded, monthly time series of the incidence of several infectious diseases. Here we examine the unique nature of Iceland as an epidemic laboratory (section 2.5.2) and the history of the measles epidemics which struck the island over that historical period, tracing both (i) the chain of contacts that brought the virus into and around the island (section 2.5.3) and (ii) the waves of morbidity these index cases triggered (section 2.5.4). We have argued elsewhere (Cliff et al., 1993, pp. 4–8) that measles is a useful indicator disease widely used in early epidemic modelling. But the Iceland record is much richer

than measles alone, and we go on to compare it with six other infectious diseases (section 2.5.5). Finally, we draw together the broad themes which underlie the shape of both the measles and other disease epidemics over this study period (section 2.5.6) in the hope that the lessons learnt may throw light on the much larger epidemic canvas covered in the rest of this volume.

2.5.2 Iceland as an Epidemiological Laboratory

We look here at three aspects of Iceland: (i) its setting and context which separate it out from the complex and more difficult to trace continental areas; (ii) the uniquely rich data sources and collecting infrastructure which provide the data matrices for study; and (iii) the measles epidemics that have been isolated for special study.

Iceland: setting and context

Iceland is a large but sparsely peopled island located in the North Atlantic between Greenland and Norway on the edge of the Arctic Circle. It was settled from AD 870 by Norse peoples and its subsequent

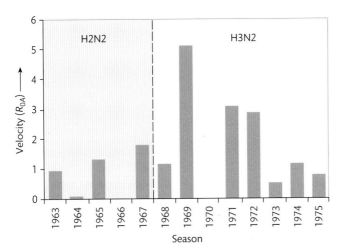

Figure 2.10 Velocity parameter values from a spread model of influenza epidemics in Cirencester, 1963–75. Time series of values of the velocity parameter (R_{0A}) for each type A influenza epidemic wave as it spread across the Hope-Simpson practice. The larger the value of R_{0A}, the greater the velocity of spread. In Cirencester, the 1968–70 pandemic associated with the shift from Asian (H2N2) to Hong Kong (H3N2) influenza moved more rapidly and struck earlier than epidemics in non-pandemic seasons. The gaps for 1966 and 1970 were non-influenza seasons in the practice.

demographic history has shown strong fluctuations, mainly related to epidemic mortality, famine, and waves of out-migration. Today (2021) it has a total population of nearly 350,000 (slightly more than that of Northumberland) but set in an area of 103,000 km² (half the size of England). It is Europe's most sparsely populated state. Much of Iceland's land surface is made up of high plateaus, a stubborn environment dominated by ice sheets, lava fields, or subarctic tundra. The harshness of the interior has largely restricted human settlement to the peripheral lowlands (see the blue area in **Figure 2.12A**).

Iceland's settlements are thus isolated at two geographical levels: (i) externally from Northern Europe and North America through a mid-Atlantic location, and (ii) internally from each other by being scattered along its deeply indented coast. Until the end of World War

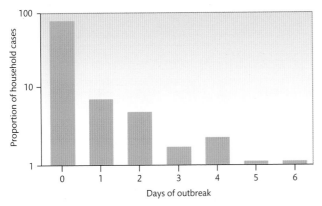

Figure 2.11 Within-household transmission of influenza A in Hope-Simpson's practice. Analysis of 134 household outbreaks of influenza A to show the proportion of cases occurring on each day of the household outbreak. The y-axis is on a logarithmic scale.

Source: data from Hope-Simpson, R.E. (1979). 'Epidemic mechanisms of type A influenza.' *Journal of Hygiene (London)*, 83, 11–26.

II, communication within the country was dominantly by coastal shipping around the perimeter. It is therefore more appropriate from an epidemiological point of view to think of Iceland as a ring-shaped archipelago of discrete population 'islands' rather than as a single cohesive unit.

Iceland's 1902 population was 79,000 but, over the course of the next nine decades (the period studied here), it grew to 252,000 by 1988. Growth reflected declining mortality, especially among infants, with deaths in the first year of life falling from 267 (133 per 1,000) to 29 (7 per 1,000) over the same period. Over the last half century this has been bolstered by high birth rates by European standards, so that today Iceland has one of the youngest populations in the industrialized world.

The Icelandic database

A major reason for selecting Iceland for epidemiological study is the quality of the country's demographic and disease data. Records in some detail go back to 1751 and through them it is possible to build up an outline picture of Iceland's twinned demographic and epidemiological history over the last 250 years. For the last century, the key source is *Heilbrigðisskýrslur* (*Public Health in Iceland*), first published in 1896; this provides for each medical district (i) a monthly record of cases of infectious diseases as observed and recorded by physicians, and (ii) an annual commentary by each physician on the course of the disease in their own district. These commentaries vary in quality from doctor to doctor and are generally richer in detail in the early decades.

At their best, they give useful insights into the microgeography of disease spread, with comments on the severity and spread of the various epidemic diseases in each community. They indicate (where known to the reporting doctor) the external source of the disease and how it diffused from village to village or even from farm to farm within the district. Not surprisingly, this information was easier to obtain when movements were few and mostly by local boats; with the coming of air transport, the motor car, and tourism, the quality of this case-tracking evidence deteriorates in the second half of the study period.

Reporting units

The basic geographical unit of reporting for health statistics in Iceland is the medical district. Each district is based on a parish or group of parishes. Names and boundaries of districts have been periodically reviewed during the century and a half from 1840 with the number of districts varying between 42 and 63. Major revisions were undertaken in 1875, 1899, 1907, 1932, and 1955 (**Figure 2.13**). At each major boundary revision, names of medical districts were often changed, and new districts were created by dividing or amalgamating old districts in response to population changes and the location of doctors' surgeries.

A critical figure in establishing the island-wide disease recording system was the appointment in 1895 of a new chief medical officer for the island, Jonas Jónsson. Having studied in the medical school at Copenhagen, where Dr Panum (the Danish physician who had studied the Faeroes measles epidemic of 1846) worked, he was seized with the importance of monitoring epidemics. He reorganized the medical districts in 1899 and ensured each district was allocated at least one of Iceland's 60 physicians or medical assistants. Each was required to maintain and report consistent and regular records of

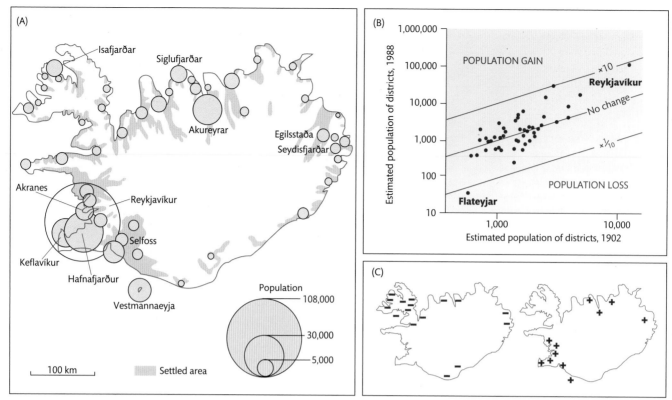

Figure 2.12 Iceland: the geographical setting. Population distribution in Iceland by medical district. (A) Population at the end of the study period (1988). Settled areas are shown in blue and circle areas are proportionate to the population size of each medical district. (B) Graph of 1902 district populations plotted against 1988 population. Note that both scales are logarithmic and areas of population gain and loss are labelled. (C) Distributions of population change 1902–88 showing (*left*) districts which have lost population [–] and (*right*) districts which more than doubled their population [+]. Data from Hagstofa Íslands.

Reproduced with permission from Cliff, A.D., Haggett, P., Smallman-Raynor, M.R. (2009). 'The changing shape of island epidemics: Historical trends in Icelandic infectious disease waves, 1902–1988.' *Journal of Historical Geography*, 35, 545–67.

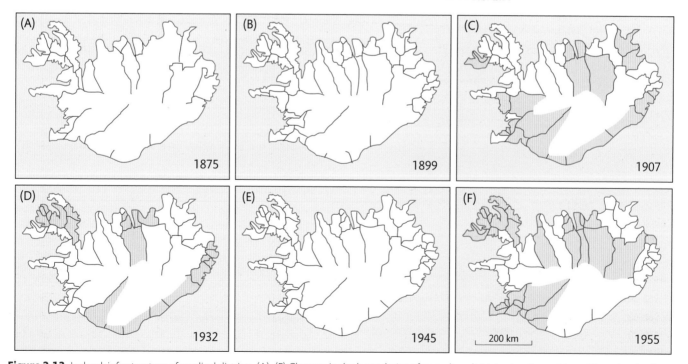

Figure 2.13 Iceland: infrastructure of medical districts. (A)–(F) Changes in the boundaries of recording districts at major revisions. These involved joining districts together in areas where population was falling, and splitting where population was growing. Orange tint indicates unchanged districts with red lines showing boundaries. Individual district boundaries shown for four revision dates in (A)–(D). (E) Consistent set of district boundaries to 1945. (F) All boundaries on earlier maps.

Reproduced from Cliff, A.D., Haggett, P., Ord, J.K., Versey, G.R. (1981). *Spatial Diffusion: An Historical Geography of Epidemics in an Island Community*. Cambridge: Cambridge University Press. Reprinted with permission.

infectious diseases within each district. The picture of the diffusion of epidemics in Iceland presented here rests on the records of a handful of qualified men. Even by 1900, there were only 60 qualified doctors practising in Iceland.

Jónsson (1940, p. 162) has provided a vivid account of the work of the rural doctor in such districts, where the distance from the doctor's residence to an outlying farm might be up to approximately 100 km:

> Over this the doctor must make his way, often across mountains and uninhabited areas, or over desert sands and unbridged rivers. At the best such journeys are made on horseback, but in winter when even this method of travelling is impossible the doctor has often to go on foot, or on skis; in other places the journeys are made by boat across fjords and bays and even round promontories which project right out into the open oceans. At such times it may take the doctor the whole of a long day or even days to reach his patient and cost him and those who have to come to fetch him.

But there were major differences between the towns and the sparsely settled districts. In the latter, the pressures were less and the annual reports correspondingly fuller.

Wave identification

Several criteria have been proposed in the literature for deciding when an outbreak is sufficiently large to be called an epidemic (Cliff et al., 1975, pp. 101–4). All involve monitoring two pieces of information, namely (i) *epidemic size*, as measured by the total number of cases reported in a given length of time; and (ii) *epidemic intensity*, as measured by the rate of attack (number of cases per head of population) in a given length of time. In general, we require outbreaks

to pass both. Criterion (i) prevents short, sharp bursts of infection being called epidemics, while criterion (ii) ensures that long strings of small numbers of cases are not called separate epidemics.

Given that Iceland lies well below Bartlett's endemicity threshold (see section 1.4.3, Chapter 1), individual epidemics are easily identifiable. The average number of measles cases recorded in a non-epidemic year was in single figures. The records for measles (and subsequently for the six other infectious diseases examined in this chapter) can be broken down into discrete waves as shown in Table 2.1. In the case of measles, the separation of the 16 different waves is straightforward with each discrete epidemic separated from the preceding and following wave by months or years with no recorded measles activity. In these long inter-epidemic periods, the island's population was effectively free from the virus.

2.5.3 Measles Epidemics as Chains

As we saw in Chapter 1, an epidemic may be studied in close-up by tracing the intricate tapestry of infected cases and at longer range as a wave of infected cases. We look first at the chains for (i) individual epidemics and then (ii) at the collective pattern for all 16 twentieth-century measles waves.

Individual measles chains

Wave I: April–November 1904

The first example (wave I) occurred during the summer of 1904. Iceland had been free of measles between 1788 and 1846 when it was affected by the same outbreak which ravaged the Faroe Islands. Another major epidemic hit the island after a further interval of

Table 2.1 Characteristics of the 16 Icelandic measles waves, 1904–74

Wave and date	Cases	Cases/1,000 population	Deaths	Deaths/1,000 cases	Months since previous epidemic	N of districts affected (%)	T	$\bar{t}$	s	$\sqrt{b_1}$	b_2
I 1904–05	822	10.4	23[a]	?		8 (19)	8	4.53	1.23	0.97	4.03
II 1907–08	7,398	89.2	354	47.9	29	38 (86)	16	7.05	1.52	0.45	5.84
III 1916–17	4,944	55.0	118	23.9	91	42 (88)	14	4.80	2.46	1.61	5.09
IV 1924–26	6,130	61.2	34	5.6	84	39 (80)	26	7.61	5.22	1.69	4.77
V 1928–29	5,317	50.8	16	3.0	23	42 (86)	17	6.15	2.45	0.86	3.71
VI 1936–37	8,408	71.9	60	7.1	73	47 (94)	14	5.41	2.14	1.58	5.54
VII 1943–44	7,155	56.8	18	2.5	70	44 (88)	16	5.74	2.67	1.71	5.50
VIII 1946–48	4,791	35.3	6	1.3	29	46 (90)	22	8.42	3.74	0.77	3.04
IX 1950–52	6,645	45.2	11	1.7	16	43 (84)	27	15.45	3.52	−0.28	4.86
X 1952–53	1,872	12.5	1	0.5	3	23 (45)	10	5.22	1.77	0.14	3.52
XI 1954–55	7,787	49.9	4	0.5	10	45 (88)	21	9.05	2.92	1.24	5.98
XII 1958–59	7,102	42.1	3	0.4	27	45 (79)	22	11.29	2.03	0.59	5.58
XIII 1962–64	7,405	40.4	6	0.8	27	41 (72)	26	10.54	3.54	1.86	7.58
XIV 1966–68	6,152	30.4	4	0.7	29	41 (72)	22	5.85	2.40	2.17	11.76
XV 1968–70	3,625	17.8	0	0.0	1	39 (68)	27	13.32	3.96	0.14	3.97
XVI 1972–74	3,953	18.2	0	0.0	21	39 (68)	16	6.46	2.33	1.42	5.19
TOTALS	89,506		658			622					

[a] Ísafjörður only. T = number of months in the epidemic, $\bar{t}$ = mean, s = standard deviation, $\sqrt{b_1}$ = skewness, b_2 = kurtosis of the histogram of the number of cases reported in each month of the epidemic.

Reproduced with permission from Cliff, A.D. Haggett, P., Ord, J.K., Versey, G.R. (1981). *Spatial Diffusion: An Historical Geography of Epidemics in an Island Community*. Cambridge: Cambridge University Press.

36 years, in 1882. The 1904 epidemic was the shortest and most spatially confined of the whole sequence of Icelandic measles waves. In its 8 months' duration, it spread only to the fishing villages and isolated farmsteads of northwest Iceland, and at no time were the two leading towns of Reykjavík and Akureyri affected.

The general course of the epidemic in northwest Iceland, from its commencement in April 1904 until its demise in November of that year, is outlined in **Figure 2.14A**. Some 2,000 cases of the disease were recorded in a population of less than 11,000, an attack rate of nearly 20 per cent. As the inset graph of number of cases against month of reporting shows, more than two-thirds of the cases occurred in the months of July and August, when the three doctors in the region were overwhelmed and noted in their journal that the epidemic was 'out of control'. The number of reported cases of measles by medical district is given using proportional circles. These indicate that the disease was focused upon the main town in the region, Ísafjörður. Of the 2,000 cases of measles which occurred in the region as a whole, about 1500 were reported in Ísafjörður alone where new cases occurred at the rate of some 20 a day for 2 months and involved half the population of the area.

The doctors' accounts relate how measles arrived in the northwest fjords in late April when a Norwegian whaling ship visited the whaling station in Hesteyrar. It brought the disease from its home port near Bergen in Norway where an epidemic was in progress. Despite attempts to contain the disease by quarantine, the crew members came into contact with the crew of a local shark-fishing vessel and both subsequently set sail for the town of Ísafjörður and the whaling stations near the local farm and church of Eyri, taking the disease with them. Quarantine succeeded in eliminating secondary cases in the main town but failed to snuff out the disease at the whaling stations near Eyri.

Using local parish records, we have reconstructed the details of the course of the epidemic in the two contiguous parishes of Eyri and Ögur that lie on the southern side of the main fjord. A brief lull in the spread of the epidemic was sustained until 21 May when a Whitsuntide confirmation ceremony occurred at the church in Eyri (**Figure 2.14B**). Most of the confirmed children were about 14 years old. The church was packed with the families and friends of the confirmees. Many of the adults had been in contact with the crew members of the infected whaler and some of the crew members of

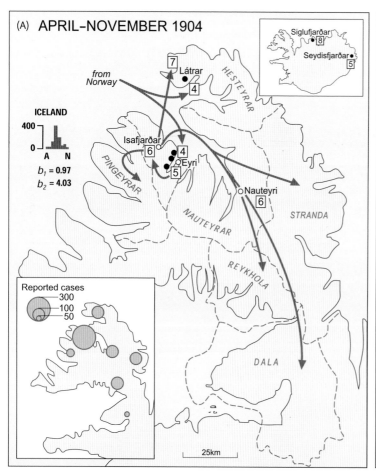

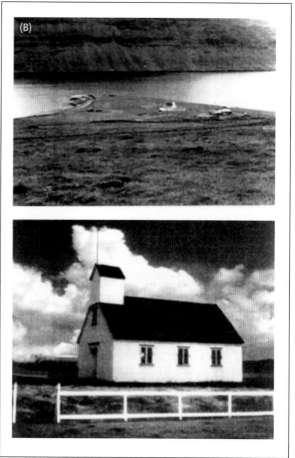

Figure 2.14 Measles in northwest Iceland. (A) Spread of wave I in northwest Iceland, 1904. Black circles indicate whaling stations and vectors the inferred lines of epidemic spread based on reports by medical practitioners in each parish. The histogram shows the reported number of measles cases in each month and numbers on the map (4, 5, 6) indicate the month of the year (April, May, June) in which measles cases were first recorded. The number of reported cases in each of the seven affected medical districts is shown (inset map) using proportional circles. (B) Eyri church: focus of the 1904 measles epidemic. Located on a remote fjord in northwest Iceland (upper photograph), it was here that a confirmation service on 21 May 1904 brought children together and accelerated the spread of the epidemic.

Reproduced from Cliff, A.D., Haggett, P., Ord, J.K., Versey, G.R. (1981). *Spatial Diffusion: An Historical Geography of Epidemics in an Island Community*. Cambridge: Cambridge University Press. Reprinted with permission.

the whaler itself were also present. Since, as noted previously, the previous measles epidemic to affect the region was in 1882, many adults were susceptible as well as children. As a result of this mixture of contacts, the epidemic was reinvigorated on a grand scale in the days that followed.

The 1904 outbreak is of special interest as it underlines three factors of prime importance in understanding the spread process. First, it highlights the role of a single infected individual (the index case) whose spatial mobility plays a crucial part in starting an outbreak in a given community. Fishermen (or the crew of whalers in the 1904 outbreak) performed a crucial role in the Icelandic case. Second, it indicates the importance of communal activities which bring susceptibles together at a critical period; the confirmation ceremony held at Eyri church illustrates this point. Third, it describes the spatial counter-measures taken to control the spread of disease: placing ships in quarantine, isolating an infected farmstead, and putting patients into fever hospitals. In addition, the account gives us one of our few indications in the records of reporting errors. In Ísafjörður,

the doctor estimated that there were 1,500 cases, while the data record gives 310, a reporting rate of as low as 20 per cent if the estimate is well founded.

Wave V: August 1928–December 1929

Wave V occurred in the inter-war years. By then, Iceland's population had grown to over 100,000 and its capital city (Reykjavík) had tripled in size to 30,000. The fifth wave (shown in **Figure 2.15A** and B) came hard on the heels of the fourth, separated from it by a gap of only 2 years. It is not surprising to find, therefore, that this wave was both less intense and less prolonged than its predecessor. The total number of reported cases was 5,317 with 16 deaths. The wave had a single peak in January 1929.

The pattern of diffusion through the Icelandic community was distinctive. The starting point in this wave was the medical district of Siglufjarðar on the north coast, with an introduction from Norway into the fishing port. Within the next month, cases were being reported both from other districts in the same part of the north coast,

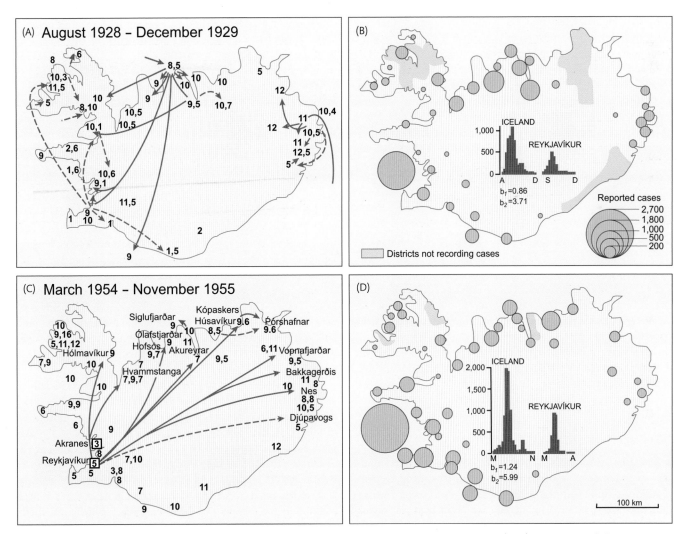

Figure 2.15 Contrasting measles epidemics (waves V and XI). (A, B) Wave V, August 1928 to December 1929. (C, D) Wave XI, March 1954 to November 1955. Maps (A) and (C) show the known vectors of spread based upon physicians' reports from each district. Solid red lines are used for the first year of each epidemic and pecked lines for the second. Maps (B) and (D) give the distribution of reported cases using proportional circles; medical districts not recording cases have been shaded grey. Separate histograms show the time profile of cases both for Iceland as a whole and for Reykjavík.

and from Reykjavík and Vestmannaeyjar (Westman Islands) in the southwest. Three separate subsystems can be identified thereafter: (i) continued spread from the original northern centre in the autumn of 1928 through the remaining northern districts; (ii) secondary spread from Reykjavík in the winter months of 1928–29 to other western and southwestern districts; and (iii) spread between the eastern coastal districts, also in the winter months of 1928–29. The provenance of the third subsystem is not clear, but two small fishing ports were reporting cases in October 1928, presumably stemming from the original Siglufjarðar introduction.

The doctors' reports lay stress on the role of boat crews in passing the disease between the coastal settlements. Even after the wave had expired, quarantine arrangements for ships remained in force. Thus, the Siglufjarðar report for 1932 relates how boats were loaded under the supervision of the police to prevent infected crew members bringing measles ashore. Other reports describe the work of the local 'committee for the prevention of disease' in placing quarantine orders on ships with crews suspected of having the disease.

Wave XI: March 1954–November 1955

This wave (**Figure 2.15C and D**) typifies the period after the American and British occupation in World War II. Not only was the death rate by this date negligible but the capital city Reykjavík now dominated the spread pattern. This reflects the building of a new airport at Keflavík and the growth of air transport and the relative decease in local shipping as a means of passenger transport. Together the three waves show the increasing scale of the epidemics. Wave I was *local*, wave V had a *regional* structure, while wave XI was essentially *island wide*, with only three of the (then) 51 medical districts not reporting cases. The patterns of vectors also show the changing pattern of spread. The first two waves were dominated by ship movements, the third by direct aircraft routes from the capital city.

Overall chain patterns

The search for pathways means probing behind the numbers in the monthly charts to examine the spatial dynamics of each wave. To do this we have to examine the physicians' annual commentaries on the pattern of illness in their districts. This rich source (both as summarized in *Heilbrigðisskýrslur* and in the original records lodged in Iceland's national archives) records the movements of infected people (the so-called *index cases*) which were observed to bring a virus or bacillus into a district. Each known movement has been plotted but such links are strongly concentrated in the first half of the records. We know relatively little about the later decades. Here we separate our findings into (i) international and (ii) internal movements.

International infection chains

Figure 2.16A uses vectors to plot the known international movements of index cases who started measles epidemics in Iceland. The origins of only half of the 16 epidemics are known, covering all the early waves up to 1946 but only two of the post-war waves. In terms of *sources*, five infections can be traced to Norway, two each to Denmark and the Faeroe Islands, and one each to England and the United States. The *landing places* were the island's capital, Reykjavík (five instances) and then, working clockwise round the coast from Reykjavík, two in the northwest, one in the north, one in the east, and Vestmannaeyjar in the south. The last two were

imports by fishing vessels and occurred after the main wave had started.

Internal infection chains

The 16 epidemics each infected, on average, 75 per cent of Iceland's medical districts, ranging from a low of 19 per cent in the 1904–05 outbreak to a high of 90 per cent in that of 1946–48 (**Table 2.1**); over the period, there were 622 individual medical districts infected, some several times over in different epidemics. *In toto*, nearly 90,000 cases of measles were recorded. But we know that in some areas an initial infection died out, only to be rekindled later. While the summary annual reports throw light on some of these links, the full report from each medical practice is retained in Iceland's National Archives. Altogether we were able to identify 170 instances where the donor medical district source of infection for recipient medical districts was clearly recorded. These have been used as the basis for **Figure 2.16B**.

Plotting the index case links between origin and destination medical districts by a straight line is necessary but misleading. Given the difficulty of overland movement, contacts between the coastal settlements have been traditionally reliant on coastal shipping. By 1900, Iceland had a comprehensive network of small harbours, with the only major gap occurring along the southeast coast. The more remote rural areas in the northwest and northeast used to be wholly dependent on coastal shipping for contact with the rest of Iceland, and even this link could be cut by pack ice in severe winters. Around the island, coastal passenger and postal services were established after World War I and, from 1929, were organized by a State Shipping Department (Skipaútgerð ríkisins) but this declined as air and overland traffic increased after 1960.

The most striking aspect of the spatial links when seen as a whole is the extreme seasonal contrast. There were only a handful of recorded movements of index cases during the two winter months with sub-Arctic cold and very short daylight hours. The converse was equally striking. Early summer and midsummer with long daylight hours saw the highest vector movements. May and June alone made up nearly half of the total. If we plot the actual number of measles cases, we see two peaks during the year—one in June and one in December. The December peak reflects the fact that measles in Iceland is a children's disease and contagion is high in both schools and in homes celebrating Christmas. Over time, the summer peak weakened and the winter one strengthened, reflecting Iceland's move from a dominantly rural to urban population.

Through all accounts runs an indication of the economic importance of measles and its relation to the farming and fishing calendars. For example, measles was carried to Mýrdals from Reykjavík in June 1916 and, 'although precautions were not officially taken, many homesteads did their best to protect themselves and tried not to contract the disease at haymaking' (Skipaútgerð ríkisins, cited in Hannesson, 1922, p. 71). At Stokkseyri (southern Iceland), stress is again laid on avoiding loss of manpower at haymaking. Where a community felt the onset of the disease was inevitable, an attempt might be made to bring the infection forward to a more convenient time. Thus, the Borgarfjarðar report for 1916 records that, in May, 'measles attacked 33 to 34 farms; some of them wanted to get it over, and what is more even sought it' (Hannesson, 1922, p. 69).

As with the international records, most records relate to the period before the World War II Anglo-American occupation. Up to

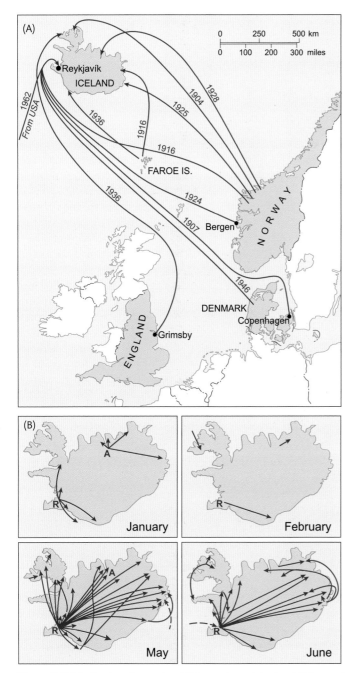

Figure 2.16 Iceland: pathways for all 16 measles epidemics. (A) External links into Iceland where the country of origin is known. (B) Internal pathways for the spread of Icelandic epidemics (1902–88), showing known movements between medical districts for 4 months of the year as recorded in *Heilbrigðisskýrslur*. Links are drawn directly between donor and recipient districts; the actual movements of index cases were likely to be via coastal shipping before 1950, after which air travel became dominant.

Reproduced from Cliff, A.D., Haggett, P., Ord, J.K., Versey, G.R. (1981). *Spatial Diffusion: An Historical Geography of Epidemics in an Island Community*. Cambridge: Cambridge University Press. Reprinted with permission.

passengers. So, three-quarters of the known links relate to the first eight measles waves.

2.5.4 Measles Epidemics as Waves

We look in this section at two aspects of wave structure: (i) *spacing* between the waves and its implications for magnitude, severity, and velocity; and (ii) internal *phases* within waves. While we could draw on the twentieth-century experience of all 16 measles epidemics for analysing chains in section 2.5.3, records for the first two waves do not include a full matrix of months × districts. As a result, some statistics given in this section relate only to the last 14 waves (April 1916–January 1974).

Spacing between waves

Although the study of individual waves gives some idea of the changing character of epidemics, we need to use all the waves if we are to be able to build general models. A clear indication of this is given in **Figure 2.17**. This shows that, over the twentieth century, spacing of the waves became shorter as Iceland's population rose and contacts with the outside world became closer. The average gap between waves in the period from 1896 to 1945 was more than 5 years; between 1946 and 1982, it fell to a year and a half.

Table 2.2 summarizes the differences between the two groups of waves in **Figure 2.17**. The table also gives the results of two sample *t*-tests of means on the differences between the pre- and post-World War II groups. The unequal variances model was used. The primary data appear in **Table 2.1**. For each characteristic, the null hypothesis was that the parameter tested is the same (i.e. difference = 0) for both the pre- and post-war waves.

Although all the differences in the characteristics between the two groups of waves are in the direction which one would intuitively expect, three are statistically significant at the 95 per cent level. Morbidity and mortality from measles fell in the post-World War II period as compared with the first half of the twentieth century. We can speculate that this reflects the impact of general improvements in public health over the century and the effect of mass vaccination campaigns against several vaccine-preventable diseases including measles (see section 6.4 in Chapter 6). The time gap between waves diminished sharply over time reflecting, as we have noted, Iceland's increased international connectedness by air after 1945.

Internal (*SIR*) phases within waves and wave velocity

The spacing or time gaps between successive epidemic waves shown in **Figure 2.17** may be thought of as an *external* measure of speed. It answers the question of how quickly waves arrive in Iceland. The clear answer from **Table 2.2** is that, over time, the time gap between measles epidemic waves fell as waves arrived ever more frequently. Here we look at the related *internal* question: how fast does an epidemic wave travel spatially once it has arrived?

The concept of epidemic velocity has attracted theoretical attention because of its importance for possible preventive measures. Where we are dealing with a simple spatial process with a well-defined wave front, then the physical concept of distance travelled over time may be appropriate. However, where the wave front is not a well-defined line, and where the susceptible population through which the epidemic moves is both discontinuous in space and has sharp variations in intensity, an alternative definition must be sought.

that period very few of the districts were linked by road and, for most land transport, this meant slow journeys by horseback over high cols between scattered settlements in the valleys and fjords. Individual rural doctors were isolated and the presence of a new face (and virus source) was a matter of a boat and its crew or

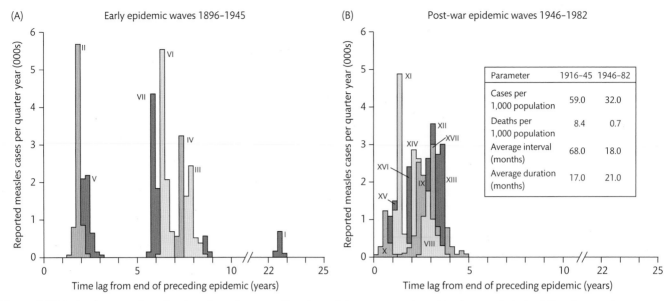

Figure 2.17 Iceland: temporal acceleration of measles waves. Time intervals between measles epidemic waves in Iceland. The diagram shows contrasts between the earlier (widely spaced) and later (closely spaced) measles epidemics over the period 1896–1982.
Reproduced from Cliff, A.D., Haggett, P. (1988). *Atlas of Disease Distributions: Analytical Approaches to Epidemiological Data*. Oxford: Blackwell Reference.

In our early studies, we chose to adhere to classical statistical measures using the frequency distribution of cases measured in the time domain. The simplest measure, the arithmetic mean, $\bar{t}$, indicates the lag in months between the start of the epidemic (the month in which the first case was recorded) and the average time at which cases occur. Thus, in the case of wave I, the first cases occurred in April 1904 while the average occurred 4 months later in August. Applying that simple measure to all districts showed a lower average for the capital city, Reykjavík. In general, this and other velocity measures discussed here might suggest that measles velocity is loosely related to the degree of urbanization—where the density of the susceptible population is higher and, if there is no vaccination, the disease spreads more quickly than it does in more sparsely and less densely populated rural areas.

The other classical measures of standard deviation (s), skewness ($\sqrt{b_1}$), and kurtosis (b_2) are described by Cliff and Haggett (1983, pp. 335–48) and may be interpreted as follows:

1. *Standard deviation*: this measures the spread of cases around the mean, $\bar{t}$. Epidemics in which cases are concentrated around $\bar{t}$ have small values for s and are characteristic of rapidly moving waves. An epidemic in which cases are drawn out over a long period of time are typical of a slow-moving wave and will have a larger value for s.

2. *Skewness*: a positive value for skewness characterizes a wave which has an early peak and a long, slow decline. Conversely, a negative value for skewness typifies a slow case build-up, a late peak, and a rapid decline.

3. *Kurtosis*: epidemics in which cases are highly concentrated in time have large values for b_2, whereas an epidemic which is dissipated over time will have a low value for b_2.

Table 2.3 applies these statistical measures to the two groups of waves defined in Table 2.2. The larger value for $\bar{t}$ for the post-1945 waves suggests they may have spread more slowly through Iceland than those in the first half of the century. We can speculate that this retarding effect was caused by the mass vaccination campaigns against measles after 1957 reducing the spatial density of the susceptible population.

Table 2.2 Sixteen Iceland measles waves, 1904–74. Results of two sample *t*-tests of means, on characteristics of pre- and post-World War II waves. Probabilities *p(t)* are for a one-sided test

Characteristic	Wave group				t-statistic	p(t)
	1905–45		1946–74			
	Mean	Variance	Mean	Variance		
Cases	5,739	6,170,129	5,481	4,091,586	0.22	0.41
Cases/1,000 population	56.5	581.4	32.4	181.4	2.37	0.02
Deaths	89.0	14,943	3.9	12.4	1.84	0.06
Deaths/1,000 cases	15.0	322.5	0.7	0.31	1.96	0.05
Time gap (months)	57.0	839	16.8	123.1	3.46	0.00
Per cent of districts affected	77.2	677.6	74	187.3	0.30	0.38

Statistically significant differences at the 95 per cent level are identified by the dark shading.

Table 2.3 Sixteen Iceland measles waves, 1904–74. Results of two sample *t*-tests of means, on velocity measures of pre- and post-World War II waves. Probabilities *p(t)* are for a one-sided test

Characteristic	Wave group				*t*-statistic	*p(t)*
	1905–45		1946–74			
	Mean	Variance	Mean	Variance		
$\bar{t}$	5.9	1.2	9.5	12.1	−2.93	0.01
s	2.5	1.70	2.9	0.65	−0.69	0.25
Skewness	1.27	0.25	0.89	0.70	1.11	0.14
Kurtosis	4.93	0.65	5.72	7.02	−0.85	0.21

Statistically significant differences at the 95 per cent level are shaded.

But we also have other ways of gauging the spatial velocity of an epidemic wave using the swash–backwash model described in section 1.6.2 in Chapter 1 and applied in section 2.3.3 to examine the spread of influenza epidemics in Cirencester. We look first at an early measles wave and then at the whole sequence of Icelandic waves.

Single wave (wave III, April 1916–May 1917)

This wave was triggered by the arrival in Reykjavík harbour in April 1916 of a ship from Norway, one of whose crew was infected with measles. The wave came nearly 8 years after its predecessor. A scatter of measles notifications had been reported over the intervening years (56 cases in all) but preventive measures were swiftly enforced by local doctors, secondary cases were rare, and no major epidemics had occurred. Wave III, when fully developed, was a major epidemiological event with 4,944 reported cases (an attack rate of 55 per 1,000 population) and 118 deaths (a rate of 23.9 deaths per 1,000 measles cases). It lasted for 14 months, peaked in July 1916, only 4 months after onset, and spread widely over the island infecting all but seven of Iceland's medical districts.

The detailed pattern of its geographical spread has been shown in Chapter 1 in Figure 1.12. For simplicity, the original monthly figures have been aggregated there into 3-month groups based on conventional northern hemisphere seasons (e.g. spring = March, April, May). Cases are shown by concentric circles but the Reykjavík medical district has so many more than other districts that it is shown by an open circle. Districts with 40 or more reported cases are named. Starting in Reykjavík, the disease spread rapidly into northwestern districts and, by the late summer of 1916, was widely dispersed around the island. From this high point the disease contracted in both its intensity and spatial extent over the autumn and winter, finally petering out in the spring of 1917 with its last major strongholds in Akureyrar and Húsavíkur.

The form of the epidemic in the time domain has also been shown earlier in Figure 1.16 in Chapter 1, to which the reader is referred for the following description. We begin with the monthly time series for the number of cases reported and for the number of districts infected: both are illustrated in Figure 1.16A. In each case, the curves are strongly skewed to the left indicating a rapid build-up of both cases and of infected districts. The monthly time series of density of reported cases per infected district is shown as an inset in Figure 1.16B and confirms both early peaking based on Reykjavík and a late, but smaller, surge based on Akureyrar.

Monthly time series of the number of districts newly infected (i.e. when measles cases were *first* recorded) and of the number of districts where infection terminated (i.e. when measles cases were *last* recorded) are shown in Figure 1.16C. Differences between these two series plotted as Figure 1.16D. Note how the differences between the leading and following edges follow the characteristic curves sketched in Figure 1.16C. The mean values for the two series are used to define the swash and backwash stages of wave III in Figure 1.16D. Finally, cumulative curves for the number of newly infected and newly terminated districts used to define susceptible, infective, and recovered districts are shown in Figure 1.16E.

Multiple wave train (waves III–XVI)

Applying the same analysis to the 60-year train of 14 Icelandic measles waves for which data are available in an appropriate form, produces the envelopes of leading and following edges shown in **Figure 2.18**. Since the individual epidemics varied in duration 8 to 27 months and in spatial spread from eight to 47 districts affected (**Table 2.1**), each was standardized to a unitary (0–1) form. The results are plotted in **Figure 2.18A**. They show that the cumulative curves for the newly infected districts (dark orange) are steeper than those for newly terminated districts (light orange), confirming that the swash stages of these waves have collectively moved faster than the backwash stages. The average for the leading edges tends to fall in the sixth month of an outbreak, with the following edge towards the end of the year. In terms of the three integrals, the susceptibles (*S*) make up around one-quarter, the infectives (*I*) around a third, and the recovereds (*R*) the residual space (around 40 per cent) of the phase diagram. That these averages are drawn from a highly volatile series of epidemic behaviours can be seen by looking at the individual traces in **Figure 2.18A**, while **Figure 2.18B** plots the average monthly values for the leading and following edges.

Analysis at the individual wave level appears in **Figure 2.19** which shows the cumulative *SIR* curves for each epidemic. The numbers are the values of the integrals which measure the area under each of the three curves, expressed as a proportion of the total $A \times T$ space of each wave. Comparative wave data are also plotted in **Figure 2.20** which illustrates the three dimensions of the susceptible, infective, and recovered phases for each of the 14 epidemic waves as a ternary diagram. It is notable that the early waves (brown squares) lie broadly to the left of the later (post-World War II) waves on the susceptible phase axis of the diagram. This implies

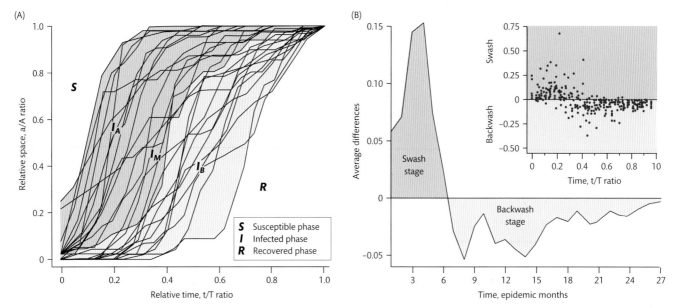

Figure 2.18 Iceland: swash–backwash parameters for 14 measles waves, III–XVI, 1916–74. (A) Leading edge (newly infected) and following edge (newly terminated) cumulative curves for medical districts in each wave. The spatial and dimensional axes have been standardized to unitary length to allow waves of different time duration (*t/T*) and different spatial extent (*a/A*) to be shown comparatively. Each cluster of curves forms an 'envelope' shaded dark orange (*I_A*) for the leading edges and pale orange (*I_B*) for the following edges. The pale purple area (*I_M*) is a zone of overlap between the two envelopes, and represents the switch over from the swash to the backwash stages of the epidemics. (B) Average net values for the swash and backwash stages of the 14 Icelandic measles epidemics by month. The inset graph shows the values for the individual epidemics from which the average curve has been calculated.

Reprinted by permission from Springer Nature, *Journal of Geographical Systems*, 'A swash-backwash model of the single epidemic wave', 8: 227–252. A.D. Cliff, P. Haggett, © 2006.

that the early waves showed a more rapid transition from susceptible to infected phases than later waves.

2.5.5 Widening the Epidemic Range

Study of Iceland's measles waves in the preceding two sections has opened one window on the island's epidemic behaviour. But it is a limited window, bounded in time on both sides: going back in time, by the absence of measles waves (only two known over the course of the nineteenth century) and the poverty of morbidity data. Going forwards into the twenty-first century gives less spatially detailed epidemiological recording, abbreviated doctors' commentaries, and a measles incidence itself greatly reduced by successful vaccination

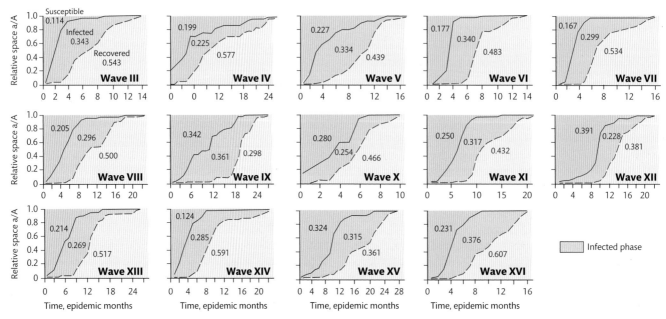

Figure 2.19 Icelandic measles epidemic waves. Superimposed cumulative curves from Figure 2.18 used to define susceptible, infective, and recovered phases of the individual epidemics. The numbers given are integrals which measure the area under each of the three curves as a proportion of the total. As in Figure 2.18, space axes are measured in relative terms.

Reprinted by permission from Springer Nature, *Journal of Geographical Systems*, 'A swash-backwash model of the single epidemic wave', 8: 227–252. A.D. Cliff, P. Haggett, © 2006.

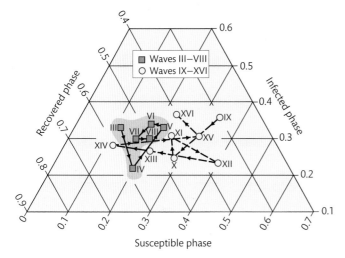

Figure 2.20 Iceland: *SIR* integrals for 14 measles epidemic waves. Values for the susceptible, infective, and recovered phases plotted as a ternary diagram.

Reprinted by permission from Springer Nature, *Journal of Geographical Systems*, 'A swash-backwash model of the single epidemic wave', 8: 227–252. A.D. Cliff, P. Haggett, © 2006.

campaigns. However, we can widen the same temporal window by looking more closely at some of the other infectious diseases which have paralleled the measles epidemics (Cliff, Haggett, and Smallman-Raynor, 2009). We look here at (i) six further diseases, (ii) chain analysis based on contacts, (iii) wave analysis based on morbidity records, and (iv) a geographical stage model based on the seven-disease record. We complete the section with (v) an examination of the epidemiological interactions between the seven diseases ('syndemics').

Six additional infectious diseases

Table 2.4 shows the length of records for measles and six other comparator diseases—influenza, poliomyelitis, rubella, diphtheria, pertussis, and scarlet fever. Each disease is measured from the first month of the first recorded wave to the last month of the final wave. The seven diseases chosen for analysis have common characteristics. All are infectious diseases that spread dominantly by human-to-human contact. All are diseases which had a worldwide distribution in the early years of the twentieth century (scarlet fever largely in the mid and higher latitudes) but which, over the course of the twentieth century, were greatly reduced in geographical range by the introduction of vaccination (see section 6.4 in Chapter 6). All are diseases for which mortality rates have tumbled through improved treatments—most notably by penicillin and other antibiotics produced from the 1940s onwards—which tackle both the primary infection in the case of bacterial diseases and secondary infections in the case of viral diseases.

But, beyond the communality, there are significant differences between the diseases. Four of the seven (influenza, measles, poliomyelitis, and rubella) are caused by viruses that belong to four different virus families. The remaining three diseases are caused by bacteria: pertussis (whooping cough) by *Bordetella pertussis*; diphtheria by a toxin-producing bacillus, *Corynebacterium diphtheriae*; and scarlet fever by an infectious bacterial strain of *Streptococcus*.

Chain analysis based on contacts: epidemic pathways

So far as is feasible, data for the 131 epidemic waves generated by the six comparator diseases were mapped and analysed in the same way as for measles. So, in this section, we report on the results of that analysis with emphasis both on historical trends and space–time patterns; we look at the overall disease patterns as well as those for individual diseases. To avoid repetition, interpretation of both sets of findings is postponed until section 2.5.6.

Again, we began by examining the physicians' annual commentaries on the pattern of illness in their own districts as summarized in *Heilbrigðisskýrslur* and in the original records lodged in Iceland's national archives. In **Figure 2.21** each known movement has been plotted for four of the seven diseases (influenza, measles, pertussis, and rubella). The older records, when populations and travellers were both smaller, are more abundant so that links are strongly concentrated in the pre-World War II period. On the maps, links have been accumulated to quantify epidemic pathways, with the strength of each link indicated by its weight. In interpreting the maps, it is important to note that not all diseases are easy to diagnose nor are index cases readily identified. Diseases with many subclinical cases, for example, poliomyelitis, may be impossible to trace.

These constraints apart, the message from the available cases produces a clear geographical pattern. The upper two maps in **Figure 2.21**, (A) and (B), show links from Reykjavík and reinforce the known role of the capital city in disease transmission. The two lower maps, (C) and (D), plot all other links not involving Reykjavík. The strong local fields around the two regional centres of Akureyrar and Vestmannaeyjar are shown. The four corresponding maps for measles vectors alone show an almost identical pattern and are not included here (but see Cliff et al., 1981, Figure 4.19, pp. 88–9).

Wave analysis: temporal characteristics and velocity

Using the monthly morbidity series for measles and each of the six comparator diseases, we constructed plots of their changing behaviour over time. We review here three groups of findings related to (i) magnitude and intensity, (ii) wavelength, and (iii) velocity.

Magnitude and intensity of epidemic waves

The average size of an Icelandic epidemic over the study period was 4,000 reported cases. But this conceals substantial variations in size from the largest recorded (22,092 cases for the 23rd influenza season of 1937) to the smallest (11 cases for the ninth polio wave of 1954). As with geographical spread (see later), studies of time trends only make sense when results are first standardized on a disease basis. This has been done in **Figure 2.22** where wave magnitude has been plotted over time. That above-average magnitudes tend to occur in the latter part of the century reflects Iceland's larger population, a greater frequency of waves in the latter period, and greater international connectivity via airline traffic.

An alternative approach to epidemic magnitude is to measure each wave's intensity rather than its absolute size. Here, we estimate wave intensity by dividing the number of reported cases by the number of space–time cells; a cell is one medical district reporting in 1 month of an epidemic. This measure allows comparison between waves of different character as the cell permits standardization over waves which are both short and long in time, and which may be either constrained or extensive in space. Four of the diseases show clear falls in

Table 2.4 Iceland: measles and six comparator diseases. Geographical penetration and spatial velocity parameters

Disease	Record length, months[a]	Epidemic waves, number	Average wave duration, months	Average wave spread, districts	Reported cases, number	Seasonality[b]			Velocity[c]					
						Seasonal variability (CV)	Highest trimester (month, % cases)	Lowest trimester (month, % cases)	V-1 Districts per month	V-2 District pop per month	V-3 Skewness	V-4 Leading edge, months	V-5 Leading edge duration, %	V-6 R_{UA}
Influenza (1)	732	61	12.0	30.4	354,071	89.1	2+3+4 = 57%	6+8+9 = 7%	2.53 (1)	7.61 (1)	−0.476 (7)	5.67 (2)	47.3 (7)	0.85 (7)
Poliomyelitis (2)	317	10	13.5	16.0	4,007	81.3	9+10+11 = 51%	3+4+5 = 6%	1.24 (5)	3.63 (5)	0.094 (2)	4.58 (1)	38.3 (6)	1.40 (1)
Rubella (3)	952	15	21.7	28.4	27,300	68.2	11+12+1 = 49%	5+6+7 = 12%	1.40 (4)	4.28 (3)	0.082 (3)	7.78 (4)	37.2 (5)	1.10 (6)
Diphtheria (4)	420	5	70.0	20.6	2,343	57.4	12+1+2 = 45%	8+9+10 = 11%	0.27 (7)	0.57 (7)	0.042 (5)	16.54 (6)	26.8 (1)	1.23 (4)
Pertussis (5)	1,062	17	25.8	31.6	49,331	34.8	3+4+5 = 37%	9+10+11 = 15%	1.44 (3)	4.04 (4)	0.056 (4)	8.21 (5)	33.6 (4)	1.23 (3)
Scarlet fever (6)	804	9	79.1	26.8	10,546	27.0	11+12+1 = 33%	7+8+9 = 18%	0.39 (6)	1.20 (6)	0.034 (6)	27.96 (7)	33.4 (3)	1.23 (3)
Measles (7)	694	14	20.0	43.5	81,236	26.7	12+1+6 = 31%	8+9+10 = 15%	2.30 (2)	6.93 (2)	0.587 (1)	6.02 (3)	29.9 (2)	1.32 (2)
All waves	**1,062**	**131**	**22.7**	**30.1**	**528,884**	**27.3**	**12+1+2 = 35%**	**6+7+8 = 16%**	**1.90**	**5.67**	**−0.131**	**8.14**	**40.1**	**1.05**

[a] Measured from the first month of the first wave to the last month of the last wave. [b] Months coded sequentially (January = 1, February = 2, etc.). [c] Rank of wave velocity given in brackets where 1 = fastest, 7 = slowest. Velocity measures V-1 to V-6 defined in text. CV, coefficient of variation.

Source: Data from Cliff, A.D. Haggett, P., Smallman-Raynor, M.R. (2009). 'The changing shape of island epidemics: Historical trends in Icelandic infectious disease waves, 1902–1988.' *Journal of Historical Geography*, 35, 545–67.

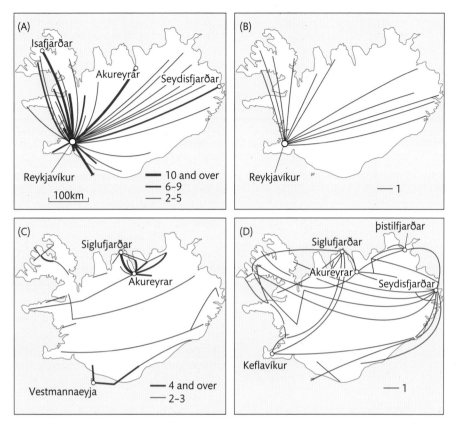

Figure 2.21 Iceland: pathways for seven epidemic diseases. Known pathways for the spread of Icelandic epidemics (1902–88) showing movements between medical districts. The upper two maps (A, B) show pathways linking to the capital city, Reykjavík, while the lower two (C, D) show linkages to other regional centres. As before, links are drawn directly between donor and recipient districts; the actual movements of index cases were likely to be via coastal shipping before 1950 and by air travel thereafter.

Reproduced with permission from Cliff, A.D., Haggett, P., Smallman-Raynor, M.R. (2009). 'The changing shape of island epidemics: Historical trends in Icelandic infectious disease waves, 1902–1988.' *Journal of Historical Geography*, 35, 545–67.

intensity over historical time. That for influenza shows basically no change while polio shows an anomalous rise over its relatively short reporting period. The seventh disease (diphtheria) has only five epidemics so is too short to be usefully included. The dominantly declining intensities for four of the diseases are consistent with the public health improvements associated with vaccination campaigns in Iceland. Influenza vaccination (usually confined to the elderly) has only been partially successful in reducing morbidity and, since it is based on virus strains circulating in the previous years, is unable to protect against the major virus shifts that mark pandemic years.

Wavelength

Various measures of wavelength have been proposed, from the simple to the complex such as spectral decomposition of time series. Here we used the time lag in months between the centre of one epidemic wave and its predecessor wave, taking the mid-point month of each wave as the marker for measurement. A very consistent pattern emerged: with all diseases, waves got closer and closer together over the decades (cf. **Figure 2.17** for measles). This trend is consistent with both the increase in Iceland's population and its increasing susceptibility to viral and bacterial invasions from external sources as transport links improved and its spatial isolation reduced. Influenza was omitted from this analysis; for this disease, we have assumed an unvarying yearly pattern and thus a constant 12-month spacing.

Velocity

As we noted previously, the speed with which an epidemic wave passes through a population is of practical importance in designing control measures; highly contagious diseases which spread rapidly are more difficult to control than their 'slow-burning' counterparts. **Table 2.3** showed that speed can be measured in a number of ways, each of which catches only a part of wave complexity. We now extend our analysis in **Table 2.4** and combine the standard statistical velocity measures of **Table 2.3** with the velocity measures of the swash model to gain a more general picture of the geographical behaviour of infectious disease epidemics in Iceland. In **Table 2.4**, the first eight columns characterize the disease time series studied, including their seasonal patterns. To these are added six further columns with measures of velocity, V-1 to V-6. The first measure (V-1) is the simplest: the number of districts invaded during the course of a wave, divided by wave duration in months. The higher the ratio of districts/month, the faster the wave. Relative wave speed is given in brackets for each disease with 1 = fastest through to 7 = slowest. The second measure (V-2) is closely related but weights the districts invaded by their estimated population to give weighted districts/month. V-3 looks at the history of infected districts by month as a histogram and measures the skewness of the distribution, using the time-weighted version of the standard statistical measure. Skewness is a dimensionless number with high positive values indicating a

(A) Wave magnitude

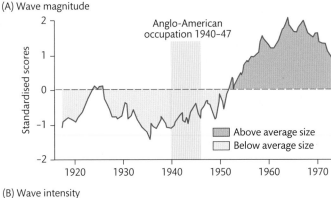

(B) Wave intensity

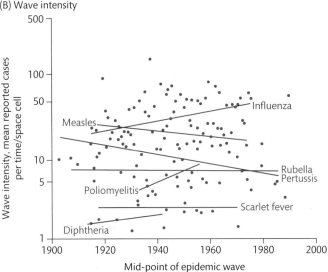

Figure 2.22 Historical trends in wave magnitude and intensity for Icelandic epidemics, 1902–88. (A) Temporal changes in wave magnitude for seven infectious diseases; magnitude is shown as a standardized score on the vertical axis. (B) Trends in wave intensity by disease. Intensity is measured as the average number of reported cases across the seven diseases per occupied space–time cell, weighted by population; a cell is one medical district reporting in one month of an epidemic. Trend lines for each disease based on ordinary least squares regression.

Reproduced with permission from Cliff, A.D., Haggett, P., Smallman-Raynor, M.R. (2009). 'The changing shape of island epidemics: Historical trends in Icelandic infectious disease waves, 1902–1988.' *Journal of Historical Geography*, 35, 545–67.

three. The paradox is due to the fact that it is alone among the seven diseases in being measured on a fixed annual basis while the others are measured on a variable time frame (depending on the duration of the wave in question). Other evidence suggests influenza infectivity is moderate to high (see Table 5.1 in Chapter 5).

Geographical four-stage model

While each of the 131 epidemic waves studied has a unique geographical pattern of spread within Iceland, if we average those patterns, then striking regularities appear. This has been done in **Figure 2.23** by measuring for each district the time lag in months between the onset month for a particular district and the onset month for the first Icelandic district to be infected. The measurements shown here are based on lags for four of the diseases (measles, influenza, pertussis, and rubella) and the results averaged to give the combined delay maps in **Figure 2.23**. Each medical district has been mapped with circles proportional to population size. The numbers indicate the average delay in months from the start of the wave before it reached each medical district. In the first quarter (**Figure 2.23A**), only one settlement appears, the capital Reykjavík with an average delay of 1.8 months. The capital city was either the originating point or near the start of almost all epidemic waves for all four diseases. The second quarter (**Figure 2.23B**) shows intensive local spread around Reykjavík as well as spread to Iceland's second city, Akureyri (with a delay of 5.2 months) on the north coast. The third quarter (**Figure 2.23C**) illustrates spread into almost all the rest of the island. Finally, **Figure 2.23D** identifies the laggard districts with a delay of 9 months or more. These are generally in small and rather isolated settlements with a marked concentration in the northwest (around Ísafjarðar) and eastern fjords (fanning out from the inland centre of Egilsstaða). Here average delays can be up to a year.

These averaged results suggest a strong regional pattern within Iceland that underlies the more random map sequences shown by the individual waves of the four diseases. The diffusion pattern identified shows clear evidence of both hierarchic ('cascade') spread down the Icelandic urban hierarchy but also contagious ('neighbourhood') spread, especially in the southwest corner of Iceland and around the four regional centres.

Links between the seven diseases

One elusive issue that has only occasionally been caught in the epidemiological literature is the question of interactions between infectious diseases. Does an outbreak of disease *A* increase or decrease the likelihood of an outbreak of disease *B* at the same time or slightly after, or are the relationships between them random? The term *syndemics* is used to refer to the concentration of two or more diseases in a population that magnifies (positive comorbidity) or reduces (negative comorbidity) any harmful effects. There is evidence in the literature of both effects—positive in the links between diabetes and the viral agent of COVID-19 (Singer, 2020) and negative in the apparent ability of human rhinoviruses (common cold) to block the replication of the COVID-19 agent (Dee et al., 2021). For a review see Floret (1997), while an historical case study is provided in Herring and Sattenspiel (2007).

The presence of data for seven diseases in Iceland measured on the same recording basis provides an opportunity for some statistical exploration. Ideally, data would be available for the whole 87-year

strong skew of cases towards the start of a wave. The leading edge (V-4) is the average number of months taken for the epidemic to reach each Icelandic district (see equation 1.7 in Chapter 1); the lower the value, the faster the wave. V-5 uses the previous measure (V-4) but converts it to a relative form by standardizing it in terms of the duration of the wave in months; again, the lower this value, the faster the wave. Finally, V-6 is the spatial reproduction number, R_{0_A}, defined in equation 1.14 in Chapter 1 to give a measure of the inherent infectivity of the wave; higher values indicate higher speeds.

In **Table 2.4**, the 'fastest' wave on each of the different measures is shown in brackets. No disease comes first on all six measures. There is considerable variability with four of the seven diseases coming highest on one or other of the measures. If we average across all measures then the 'fastest' disease appears to be the viral disease of measles (cf. Table 5.1 of R_0 values in Chapter 5) and the slowest are two bacterial diseases (diphtheria and scarlet fever). Influenza comes first or second fastest on three measures, but last on the other

(A) First quarter

(B) Second quarter

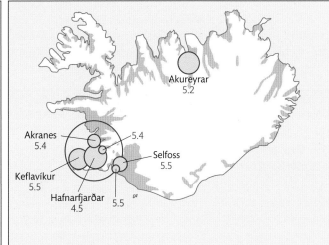

(C) Third quarter

(D) Fourth quarter

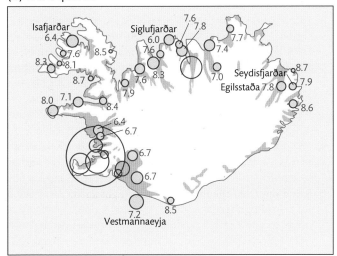
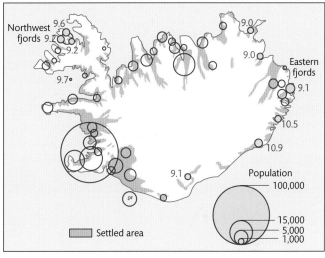

Figure 2.23 Quarterly lag maps of the geographical spread of epidemic waves in Iceland. The maps are based on lags for each medical district for four diseases (influenza, measles, pertussis, and rubella) with circles proportional to population size. Numbers indicate the average delay from the start of the wave in months before it reached each medical district.

Reproduced with permission from Cliff, A.D., Haggett, P., Smallman-Raynor, M.R. (2009). 'The changing shape of island epidemics: Historical trends in Icelandic infectious disease waves, 1902–1988.' *Journal of Historical Geography*, 35, 545–67.

period (1,044 consecutive months) but the variations in the length of records shown in Table 2.4 mean that only parts of the series are available for study. Two windows for comparison can be identified: (i) a *long series* window over 713 consecutive months (September 1914 to January 1974) for five diseases (excluding diphtheria and poliomyelitis); (ii) nested within (i) is a *short series* window over 235 consecutive months (January 1929 to July 1948) for all seven diseases. The long series covers 67 per cent of the full historical record but the short series only 22 per cent.

Correlations between the five and then seven series were conducted using cross-correlation analysis which permits the maximum Pearson correlation coefficient at a given lag to be identified. To allow comparability between seven very diverse series, reported cases for each disease were converted to a standardized monthly series. Table 2.5 gives a summary view of the seven most significant of the 21 potential links at $p \leq 0.01$, the 99 per cent confidence level, with both the average correlation and the lag in months shown. Measles has the highest overall linkage with the other six diseases, influenza the least.

Table 2.5 Iceland: intercorrelations between seven epidemic diseases, 1914–74. Columns 3 and 4 show the maximum correlation (+ or –) at the lag indicated in months (also + or –). Note that the table shows comorbidity as a statistical measure; the possible aetiological connections between the disease patterns remain unknown

Disease	Average correlation with other diseases	Strongest correlation	Lead (+)/lag (–), months with column 1
Measles	0.321	Pertussis +0.68	–13
Pertussis	0.303	Measles +0.68	–13
Scarlet fever	0.273	Rubella –0.43	+17
Rubella	0.242	Scarlet fever –0.43	+17
Poliomyelitis	0.231	Scarlet fever –0.29	+10
Diphtheria	0.209	Pertussis +0.30	+8
Influenza	0.148	Measles –0.18	–16

Source: Data from Cliff, A.D., Haggett, P., Smallman-Raynor, M.R. (2009). 'The changing shape of island epidemics: Historical trends in Icelandic infectious disease waves, 1902–1988.' *Journal of Historical Geography*, 35, 545–67.

In interpreting the findings, we should stress that this shows a statistical and not a causal or aetiological relationship. With diseases that vary greatly in wave characteristics, much will depend on the accident of wave coincidence. The omnipresent influenza has no highly significant relations with any of the others. Where relatively high associations occur (as between measles and pertussis), it may well be that seasonal factors play some part in shackling the series together. Equally, the relatively low values for poliomyelitis may be related to its unique late summer–early autumn peaks.

2.5.6 Discussion: Epidemic Waves in the Icelandic Context

In interpreting the behaviour of epidemic chains and waves in Iceland over this period, we have tried to build bridges between the trends observed and general epidemiological theory as reviewed in Chapter 1. The link to Bartlett's endemicity thresholds (see Figure 1.9, Chapter 1) is striking. But we need also to tease out the way in which Iceland itself has changed over time. We note six points (Cliff, Haggett, and Smallman-Raynor, 2009, pp. 561–66).

1. *Validity of the morbidity evidence.* Analysis has been conducted on the official figures published by the Icelandic health authorities for disease morbidity which in turn are based on individual physicians' reports for each medical district. Reporting of illness depends on a complex of factors in which patient, family, physician, and central health authorities play a part. Not all infections show clear clinical symptoms, not all cases are reported to a physician, not all cases may be correctly diagnosed and reported, and not all diseases are notifiable. Figures are likely to be underestimates, across a wide disease range from measles (which has a high reporting rate based on clear clinical symptoms) to poliomyelitis (a low rate with many subclinical, non-reported cases). There may also be under-reporting in the case of rubella, often regarded as too mild to warrant medical attention and recording before the crucial link to fetal damage was recognized in the 1940s.

   On the positive side, three factors operate. First, Iceland's ratio of physicians to population is very high, its population is highly educated and awareness of the fatal history of epidemic diseases in the island is high. Reporting rates are high by international standards. Second, the very high number of cases for some of the diseases suggests that the general shape of the epidemic (if not its fine detail) is likely to be correct. Third, the statistical measures used in the analysis are largely non-parametric and depend on the presence or absence of a reported case rather than the specific number.

2. *The context of public health changes.* The epidemic waves observed occurred during a period of remarkable change in Icelandic public health. Over the 80 years, all seven diseases showed marked falls in their severity as judged by mortality. Thus, of the 14 measles waves, the first seven waves accounted for 263 deaths (6.06 deaths per 1,000 cases), but the last seven only 18 deaths (0.47 deaths per 1,000 cases). Vaccination saw the elimination of poliomyelitis from the island (from 1963), as well as the virtual elimination of diphtheria, measles, pertussis, and scarlet fever as causes of childhood death. In that context, the persistence of waves and the trends towards increased

magnitude seem puzzling. The answer to the paradox may lie in the dominance of the two diseases which together make up over half of the waves and four in five of reported cases. Influenza was and remains a largely untamed epidemic disease which, in pandemic years, generated a huge burden of cases in the post-war period. Measles, despite the major reductions brought about by MMR (measles, mumps, and rubella) vaccination, continued to generate many cases and has never quite reached the elimination goals set in the 1960s.

3. *The role of long-run demographic changes.* At the start of our study period (1902), we estimate the population of Iceland at 79,000; by 1988 it had grown to 252,000. But the threefold growth was not evenly distributed across age groups. Instead, the proportion of younger people, below the age of 20 years and most likely to be victims of the seven diseases, had grown from 38 to 45 per cent. Still more striking were the geographical changes. Here, growth had been preponderantly in urban areas while rural districts had either stagnated or, in the most remote districts, lost population (see Figure 2.12B and C). Extraordinarily, Iceland's largest city, the capital, Reykjavík, located in the southwest corner of the island, had seen its share of the total population quadruple, from 10 per cent to 40 per cent. Both changes increased the density of the susceptible childhood populations and marginally augmented the likelihood of person-to-person transmission of infection. Over the period, spatial remoteness provided an ever-weakening shield against infection as larger settlements grew and smaller ones contracted.

4. *The reinforcing effect of educational changes.* Schools have always played a critical role in the transmission of childhood diseases by bringing together susceptible subgroups of the population stratified by age. In Iceland, the state did not take over responsibility for providing education until 1907 when school attendance was made compulsory for children aged 10–14 years. At the start of our study period, two-thirds of rural districts were served by ambulatory teachers who moved from one isolated settlement and farmstead to another, normally on horseback. In the inter-war period, more small boarding schools, often with only two or three teachers, were built to serve more populous areas.

   The transport improvements which accompanied Anglo-American occupation in World War II were followed by a phasing out of the ambulatory system and replacement by larger residential schools with older children being flown weekly into Reykjavík from around the island to attend specialist schools. Over the 80-year study period, the age range of compulsory education was widened, reinforcing the trend for children to become less geographically isolated and for the potential for child-to-child contact to increase. *Ceteris paribus* educational changes would by themselves have encouraged a more rapid spread of infectious diseases through the school age population. The hierarchical pattern of disease spread evident in Figures 2.21 and 2.23 is consistent with these educational changes.

5. *Shifts in dominant transport modes.* One of the direct impacts of the Anglo-American occupation in World War II was to accelerate the shift away from reliance on coastal transport. Epidemics in the study period were occurring in a context of revolutionary changes in dominant transport modes. Before World War I, passenger movements were heavily dependent on shipping which,

apart from the mail boats with their weekly, fortnightly, or even less frequent calls, were highly informal. Services improved with the establishment of a State Shipping Department (Skipaútgerð ríkisins) in 1929 but all coastal shipping could be interrupted in severe winters by sea ice floes blocking fjord entrances. Overland transport was originally largely local and by horseback. With the first imported motor vehicle (1913), road gravelling and bridge-building were improved but the road system remained fragmented. The first round-the-island gravel road had to await the work of American forces in the 1940s. Even by the end of the study period, weatherproofed roads were confined to the environs of regional centres.

Revolutionary change in contact patterns had to wait for air transport. This had an uncertain start in 1937 with a single float-plane based at Akureyri, was reorganized in 1940 as Flugfélag Íslands and moved to Reykjavík with a fleet of four aircraft. By 1942, these were providing a valuable service to outlying communities. Business journeys which previously depended on the weekly or less frequent mail boats were sharply cut; a day's business in Reykjavík now involved a day or two rather than the previous week or more away. A second company, Loftleiðir, began operation in 1944 and within 2 years international flights were established to Scotland and Denmark using Catalina flying boats. International links were strengthened by 1950 when the new airfield at Keflavík became a critical refuelling point for European and American airlines on their (then) multistage transatlantic flights around, rather than across, the North Atlantic. Volumes of air travel increased exponentially; Iceland now has the highest domestic per capita movements for any European country. Conversely, sea passenger movements have fallen steadily since 1960. Unlike shipping and road transport which retains its ring structure, the airline system is hierarchic in character with services to the main regional hubs predominating.

6. *The impact of World War II*. The main discontinuity in Iceland's history during this period was in the 1940s when the country moved from Danish dependency to independence. But as **Figures 2.17** and **2.20** demonstrate, such breaks were epidemiological as well as constitutional. After the German invasion of Denmark in World War II, a British force arrived at Reykjavík in May 1940 to forestall German occupation and to establish a convoy protection base to help vital Allied shipping movements in the North Atlantic. The force consisted of approximately 25,000 men, mainly based in and around Reykjavík. The main result was the building of a major airfield on the (then) outskirts of the city, which is still used for domestic flights, and further airfields at Flói and Hornafjörður. It also established a naval base at Hvalfjörður in July 1941. Tripartite agreement between Iceland, the United Kingdom, and the United States followed. The first American troops arrived in July 1941 and grew to 60,000 strong. They built a new airfield and large military base at Keflavík on the Reykjanes peninsula west of Reykjavík and progressively took over the British bases at Reykjavík and Hvalfjörður. A round-the-island road was completed for the first time in the island's history. British troops left Iceland in spring 1946 and the Americans in May 1947. But the United States retained interest in Keflavík (until 2006) as a Cold War base, maintaining a small force of troops (600–1,000) plus a large

civilian contingent. Although contacts between the military and the civil population were strictly limited by stringent sets of regulations, some links of epidemiological importance are likely to have occurred. Despite the absence of direct evidence from classified military medical records, we speculate that the large foreign presence which, at its peak made up a quarter of the total island population, provided microbial sources that replaced the previous epidemiological links with Denmark and Norway. It is perhaps no accident that some of the changes observed mentioned previously have a hinge-line (**Figure 2.22A**) which appears to fall around the 7-year band of the Anglo-American occupation from May 1940 to May 1947.

2.6 Conclusion

In this chapter, we have shown how the careful observational epidemiology of local doctors in two very different environments—country general practice in the United Kingdom and medical districts in Iceland—can shed valuable light on the processes whereby individual cases of disease can develop into full-blown epidemics. The contact tracing that frequently accompanies such observational work also allows a much greater understanding of the geographical parameters of spread within and between families, and between spatial units.

In 1998, Dr John Horder summarized the contribution of research in general practice to British medicine in the following terms:

> I have been collecting documents for 50 years, so here is a copy of the Steering Committee's [subsequently the Research Committee of the RCGP] report. It must be quite a rare document now. There's one paragraph I'd like to read. It's the first one about research:
>
> 'From many letters which have been received by the Steering Committee and from publications and correspondence which have appeared in the medical journals, it is clear that there is a reawakening of interest in research work by doctors in general practice and in the possibilities of applying modern principles of scientific investigation into the problems of general practitioners. That important advances in medical knowledge can be made by general practitioners has been demonstrated beyond doubt by men such as Jenner, Withering, Thracker, Budd, Mackenzie, Pickles. [And, being a Londoner, I would add Parkinson.]
>
> But much of the field in which these men carried out their exploratory work still remains uncultivated since a great proportion of the conditions met by family doctors never reaches the hospitals in which present day medical research tends to be concentrated.' (Horder, in Tansley et al., 1998, p.79)

Just as the records of local doctors are being re-evaluated for their epidemiological significance, so the records, prepared by local physicians, of countries like Iceland which have uniquely long time runs of geocoded disease data have attracted research from many disciplines for their ability to inform synoptic views of changes over time and space in infectious disease incidence. Our analysis of the detailed spatial monthly records of the remarkable island of Iceland in the time window between 1902 and 1988 shows that it has documentary resources that reward such study. During this 87-year period, spatially detailed records for seven leading infectious diseases allow the historical geography of 131 discrete epidemic waves (with a recorded total of >0.5 million cases) to be reconstructed. Changes in epidemiological behaviour over this period and between the seven diseases have been documented and major trends in wave spacing, wave velocity, and wave geography identified. These changes can be related both to epidemiological theory and to aspects of the changing historical geography of the island—its long-run demographic changes, the accompanying educational changes, the switch in dominant transport modes, and the short-term disruptions related to World War II. This confirms that understanding changes in the infectious disease patterns within a region need to be set against the broad canvas of the historical geography of its susceptible population.

In the next chapter, we turn from local area studies and shift up the geographical and temporal scale to begin our consideration of epidemic disease patterns at the global level and over centuries.

Global Origins and Dispersals

CONTENTS

3.1 Introduction

Recent decades have borne witness to a curious paradox in the history of epidemic diseases. On the one hand, there has been a steady fall in mortality from the classic infectious diseases, culminating in the 1970s in the global eradication of one of the world's most dreaded killers (smallpox). On the other hand, within the same decade a new pandemic disease, HIV/AIDS, emerged that seemed likely to kill in the next two decades as many victims as had smallpox in all the previous decades of the twentieth century. Nor was HIV/AIDS alone. To it we can add such apparently new infectious diseases as Legionnaires' disease and Lyme disease, plus the outbreaks of African tropical diseases caused by the Lassa, Marburg, and Ebola viruses (**Table 3.1**). The re-emergence of old scourges, such as malaria and tuberculosis, confirms the two contrasting faces of human infectious diseases in the early decades of the twenty-first century.

The paradox raises two questions. First, how do epidemic diseases emerge? And can we trace their geographical origins to any particular part of the world? Second, why do more diseases appear to be emerging now? And how far does this crudescence relate to the unprecedented changes in the global environment? To approach such questions implies a shift in gear compared with Chapter 2. There, we concentrated on painting on a small, even a miniature, canvas: individual doctors' practices, small islands, and relatively narrow time spans. The brush we used in painting an epidemic was fine-tipped with even individual index cases identified. In the present chapter, we set those constraints aside. The palette will now be expanded; doctors' practices and small islands will be replaced by world regional and global questions, narrow time bands will be extended backwards to the origins of human populations, and forwards to the end of the present century. The fine-tipped brush will be put aside and replaced by a broad and coarse paint brush.

3.1.1 Historic Transitions in Disease Emergence

McMichael (2004) provides us with a useful framework for conceptualizing the evolving relationship of humans and microbes over the millennia. In brief, McMichael identifies four historic transitions that, since the initial advent of agriculture and livestock herding, have promoted the emergence and re-emergence diseases. These four transitions, each associated with a progressive increase in the

Table 3.1 Sample emerging diseases in the human population by year of first recognition

Year	Disease
1967	Marburg virus disease
1968	Influenza A (H3N2)
1969	Lassa fever
1975	Legionnaires' disease
1976	Ebola virus disease
1981	HIV/AIDS
1991	Venezuelan haemorrhagic fever
1993	Hantavirus pulmonary syndrome
1994	Brazilian haemorrhagic fever
1996	New-variant Creutzfeldt–Jakob disease (vCJD)
1997	Avian influenza A (H5N1)
1998	Nipah virus infection
2003	Severe acute respiratory syndrome (SARS)
2009	Influenza A (H1N1/09)
2012	Middle East respiratory syndrome (MERS)
2019	Coronavirus disease 2019 (COVID-19)

geographical scale of operation (local → continental → intercontinental → global), are:

1. *First historic transition (5,000–10,000 years ago)*: a local transition when early agrarian-based settlements brought humans into contact with sylvatic enzootic pathogens. Close and prolonged exposure to domesticated animals and urban pests (e.g. rodents and flies) resulted in the cross-species transmission of the ancestral agents of many modern-day human infectious diseases, including influenza, measles, smallpox, tuberculosis, and typhoid.

2. *Second historic transition (1,500–3,000 years ago)*: a continental-level transition, fuelled by the military and trade contacts of early Eurasian civilizations which resulted in the cross-civilization transmission of infectious agents. In the wake of this historical transition, a trans-European 'equilibration' of infectious agents occurred and the diseases became endemic to the population.

3. *Third historic transition (200–500 years ago)*: an intercontinental transition associated with European expansion, resulting in the trans-oceanic spread of infectious agents. This transition began with the discovery of the Americas and continued for some three centuries or more with the trans-Atlantic slave trade and European explorations of the Asia-Pacific region.

4. *Fourth historic transition (present day)*: a global transition in which demographic, environmental, behavioural, and technological factors have led to the appearance of apparently new diseases in the human population.

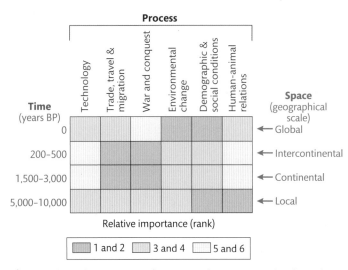

Figure 3.1 Rank importance of six principal environmental and social factors on the emergence of infectious diseases by historical period. Principal environmental and social factors are grouped by rank of importance (rank 1 = most important). Time periods relate to each of four historic transitions in disease emergence as defined by McMichael (2004): (i) first historic transition (5000–10,000 years before present (BP)); (ii) second historic transition (1500–3000 years BP); (iii) third historic transition (200–500 years BP); and (iv) fourth historic transition (present day). Note the sequential increase in the geographical scale of developments from the first (local) to the fourth (global) transition.

Reproduced with permission from Cliff, A.D., Smallman-Raynor, M.R., Haggett, P., Stroup, D.F., Thacker, S.B. (2009). *Infectious Diseases. Emergence and Re-emergence: A Geographical Analysis*. Oxford: Oxford University Press. Source: Data from McMichael, A.J. (2004). 'Environmental and social influences on emerging infectious diseases: Past, present and future.' *Philosophical Transactions of the Royal Society* B, 359, 1049–58.

For each of the four transition periods, (1)–(4), **Figure 3.1** provides an indication of the relative importance of six principal social and environmental factors in the disease emergence complex. Reading from the bottom of the diagram, the most important influencing factors (ranks 1 and 2) shifted over the millennia from (i) a local focus on human–animal relations and demographic and social conditions at 5,000–10,000 years before present; through (ii) continental and intercontinental trade, travel, migration, war, and conquest at 1,500–3,000 and 200–500 years before present; to (iii) the global environmental change and demographic and social conditions of the present day.

In this chapter, we focus on the first and fourth of these great transitions. Our examination begins, in section 3.2, at the dawn of civilization and the emergence of the great herd diseases that have plagued humankind for millennia. We then turn, in section 3.3, to the present day and the global changes associated with the phenomenon of newly emerging diseases in the human population. Examples of international epidemics spawned by the fourth transition are examined in section 3.4, while the great pandemics of apparently new diseases (including novel strains of influenza A virus, HIV/AIDS, and coronavirus disease 2019 (COVID-19)) are treated in Chapters 4 and 5.

3.2 The First Historic Transition: The Question of Disease Origins

Weiss (2001) observes that there are two possible origins of human microbial pathogens: (i) co-evolution with human emergence from primate ancestors and (ii) the crossover of pathogens from animals to humans. Co-evolving microbes typically exert a low mortality upon their hosts. Examples include members of the herpesvirus family, in which individual viruses in humans are genetically similar to those of host species that are closest to us in evolution. Most human infections have, however, originated with an animal source and crossed the species to humans. Early examples of human infectious diseases of animal origins, with estimated dates of cross-over events, are provided in Table 3.2.

There has been a continuous exchange of infective organisms between humans and other animals, with the outcome of the exchange being determined by climatic, social, and other conditions. Contact with animals increased under agriculture, both with domestic animals (e.g. cattle, sheep, goats, pigs, and horses) and with intruders attracted to human settlements (e.g. rats, mice, ticks, fleas, and mosquitoes). Owing to the species-specific nature of these infections, many of the pathogens to which humans were exposed did not result in infection. Occasionally, however, one would gain a foothold. Then, successful transmission between people would set the stage for the establishment of a human pathogen. For example, measles virus may have emerged from an infection of dogs (distemper) or ruminants (rinderpest), while the rhinoviruses which cause the common cold may have been derived from horses. It is possible that the human form of the tubercle bacillus derived from the bovine form, while the water buffalo may have been the original source of leprosy, the cow of diphtheria, and the monkey of syphilis. Plague may have arisen as an inapparent infection of gerbils in eastern Asia.

Table 3.2 Examples of human infectious diseases of animal origin

Disease	Microbe	Animal source	Date of cross-over
Malaria	Protozoan	Non-human primate	~8000 BC
Measles	Virus	Sheep, goat, or dog	~6000 BC
Smallpox	Virus	Ruminant?	>2000 BC
Tuberculosis	Mycobacterium	Ruminant?	>1000 BC
Plague	Bacterium	Rodent	AD 541, AD 1347, AD 1665
Dengue	Virus	Non-human primate	~AD 1000
Yellow fever	Virus	Non-human primate	AD 1641
'Spanish' influenza	Virus	Bird, pig	AD 1918
AIDS/HIV	Virus	Non-human primate	~AD 1950

Reproduced with permission from Cliff, A.D., Smallman-Raynor, M.R., Haggett, P., Stroup, D.F., Thacker, S.B. (2009). *Infectious Diseases. Emergence and Re-emergence: A Geographical Analysis.* Oxford: Oxford University Press. Source: Data from Weiss, R.A. (2001). 'The Leeuwenhoek Lecture 2001. Animal origins of human infectious disease.' *Philosophical Transactions of the Royal Society B,* 356, 957–77.

3.2.1 The Limits of the Historical Evidence

As we move backwards through time, we continue to find diseases that have plagued the human population for all of recorded history (Table 3.2). For these diseases, two lines of reconstruction are possible. The first is historical. Because of problems of accurate identification and recording conventions it is difficult to press back the statistical record of disease activity much before the mid-nineteenth century. There are a few exceptions, notably in the historical statistics gathered for some large cities such as London (Landers, 1993) and some unique Japanese records (Jannetta, 1987). If quantitative evidence is scarce, however, there are other historical and pre-historical sources to draw upon.

Palaeopathological evidence

Studies of many thousands of mummies in various locations around the world have revealed a long series of diseases that cover virtually every modern medical and surgical speciality (Živanović, 1982). Traces of infectious diseases have been found, including scars resulting from smallpox, skin infections, and specific diseases such as tuberculosis and leprosy. Oxenham et al. (2004) have studied skeletal remains from Northern Vietnam to determine the role of the transition from sedentary, foraging, coastally orientated economies to centralized chiefdoms (with attendant development and intensification of agriculture, trade, metal technologies, warfare, and population) in the emergence and increase in infectious diseases. While skeletal evidence for infectious diseases was absent from the period prior to 5,000 years before present, more than 10 per cent of samples from the metal period (3,300–1,700 years before present) yielded evidence of lesions consistent with either infectious diseases or immune system disorders. More generally, palaeopathological studies have presented evidence for an increase in the frequency of infectious diseases with changes in settlement patterns and the subsistence economy in parts of the Americas, Asia, Europe, and Oceania (Oxenham et al., 2004).

Since the 1990s, molecular palaeopathology (the detection of ancient microbial DNA from skeletal and mummified tissue) has provided an additional approach to the study of infectious disease agents in historic times (Zink et al., 2002). This approach has resulted in the detection of a variety of bacterial, protozoal, and viral agents in ancient tissues, including *Mycobacterium tuberculosis, Mycobacterium leprae, Yersinia pestis,* and *Plasmodium falciparum* (Table 3.3).

The written record

Once we enter the period of the written record, still more diseases come to the fore. In addition to Biblical references and the writings of ancient Egypt, medical treatises from the ancient Greek, Roman, Indian, Chinese, and Arab civilizations describe diseases which we try to pair with their modern counterparts (Table 3.4). One of the great epidemics of classical times was the Plague of Athens, described by Thucydides (460?–395? BC) in Book II of his celebrated *History of the Peloponnesian War* (431–404 BC). Thucydides' account describes an epidemic which (i) occurred in two distinct waves, (ii) had a devastating impact with a mortality of around one-third, (iii) appeared to cause immunity in those affected in the first wave, and (iv) affected animals as well as humans. Identifying the cause of the Plague of Athens has given rise to a lively academic debate, with a list of 30 or so contending diseases ranging from typhus fever, smallpox, typhoid fever, and bubonic plague through to measles and influenza. Others have argued that the disease may have been 'antique plague' or some other malady which no longer occurs; see Cliff, Smallman-Raynor, Haggett, et al. (2009, pp. 50–3). Indeed, the history of disease is studded with epidemics that we can no longer trace. In late medieval and early modern England, for example, the so-called English Sweating Sickness spread in epidemic form on just five occasions (1485, 1508, 1517, 1528–29, 1551) before disappearing from the epidemiological scene (Creighton, 1891–94, Vol. I, pp. 237–81). Just what it was, where it came from, and why it disappeared are not known.

3.2.2 The McKeown Model and Geographical Speculation

An alternative approach to probing into disease origins in which the evidence is obscured is to transpose our present understanding of disease processes into past environments.

Table 3.3 Sample infectious disease agents detected by molecular analysis of ancient human specimens

Disease agent	Human specimen			References
	Type	Location	Approximate date	
Trypanosoma cruzi	Mummified remains	Northern Chile & southern Peru	7050–3000 BC	Aufderheide et al. (2004)
Trypanosoma cruzi	Mummified remains	Northern Chile	2000 BC	Guhl et al. (1999)
Mycobacterium tuberculosis	Mummified body	Egypt	1550–1080 BC	Nerlich et al. (1997)
Corynebacterium spp.	Mummified head	Egypt	1550–1080 BC	Zink et al. (2001)
Escherichia coli	Bog body	Northwest England	300 BC (2 BC–AD 119?)	Fricker et al. (1997)
HTLV-I	Mummified remains	Northern Chile	AD 500	Li et al. (1999)
Mycobacterium leprae	Bone sample	Bethany, Jordan	AD 600	Rafi et al. (1994)
Mycobacterium leprae	Skeletal remains	Hungary	Tenth century AD	Haas et al. (2000)
Mycobacterium tuberculosis	Mummified body	Southern Peru	AD 1000–1300	Salo et al. (1994)
Mycobacterium leprae	Skeletal remains	Seville, Spain	Twelfth century AD	Montiel et al. (2003)
Human papillomavirus 18	Mummified body	Naples, Italy	AD 1503–68	Fornaciari et al. (2003)
Yersinia pestis	Skeletal remains of plague victims	France	AD 1590 & 1722	Drancourt et al. (1998)
Treponema pallidum	Skeletal specimen	Easter Island	AD 1760	Kolman et al. (1999)
'Spanish' influenza A	Tissues from influenza victims	USA	AD 1918	Reid et al. (1999), Tumpey et al. (2005)

Reproduced with permission from Cliff, A.D., Smallman-Raynor, M.R., Haggett, P., Stroup, D.F., Thacker, S.B. (2009). *Infectious Diseases. Emergence and Re-emergence: A Geographical Analysis*. Oxford: Oxford University Press.

Table 3.4 Sample epidemics in Antiquity, 2000 BC–AD 500

Year	Epidemic/disease	Afflicted population/area
Biblical and Ancient Egyptian references		
c.1715 BC	t3nt '3mw (Plague? Typhus? Tularaemia?)	Eastern Nile Delta
c.1492–1425 BC (?)	Ten Plagues of Egypt: Plague 6 (Anthrax? Ecthyma? Glanders?)	Egyptian Empire
c.1335–1295 BC	The 'Hittite plague' (Tularaemia?)	Eastern Mediterranean
c.1190 BC	Plague of Ashdod (Bubonic plague? Dysentery? Tularaemia?)	Philistines at Ashdod, Gath, and Ekron
c.701 BC	Plague of the Assyrian army (Bubonic plague? Dysentery?)	Assyrian army at Jerusalem or Pelusium
c.588–587 BC	Starvation (accompanied by disease?)	Jerusalem
Ancient Greece		
c.1200 BC	Literary reference to undetermined disease	Greek army outside Troy
480 BC	Plague of Xerxes (Bubonic plague? Dysentery?)	Persian army
430–425 BC	Plague of Athens (multiple hypotheses on aetiology)	Athens and Southern Greece
c.410 BC	Thasian epidemic (Mumps)	Thasos
c.400 BC	'Cough of Perinthus' (Diphtheria? Influenza? Whooping cough?)	Perinthus
396 BC	Smallpox?	Carthaginian army at Syracuse
Rome and the Roman Empire		
451 BC	Roman Pestilence of 451 BC (Anthrax? Tuberculosis?)	Romans and Aequians
390 BC	?	Gaul army besieging Rome
212 BC	Influenza?	Carthaginian, Roman, and Sicilian Armies at Syracuse
88 BC	?	Army of Octavius at Rome
AD c.125	Plague of Orosius	Roman army at Utica
AD 165–180	Plague of the Antonines/Galen (Smallpox? Measles?)	Roman Empire (and beyond)
AD 251–266	Plague of Cyprian (Smallpox? Measles?)	Roman Empire (and beyond)
AD 425	?	Hun army advancing on Constantinople

Reproduced with permission from Smallman-Raynor, M.R., Cliff, A.D. (2004). *War Epidemics: An Historical Geography of Infectious Diseases in Military Conflict and Civil Strife, 1850–2000*. Oxford: Oxford University Press. Source: Data from Smallman-Raynor and Cliff (2004, Table 2.2, p. 69), with additional information from Marr and Malloy (1996), Kohn (1998) and Trevisanato (2004, 2007a, b).

Biological arguments

McKeown (1988) has argued that it was the growth of cities made possible by settled agriculture which was the primary early engine of the exchange of infections between animals and man. Early man was exposed to infectious diseases (especially zoonoses), but living in small groups, the disease agents could not be sustained by the susceptible population. Thus, in the early phase of human existence, from the Pleistocene up to about 8000 BC, infectious diseases due to microorganisms that were specifically adapted to the human species—including the great herd diseases of the historical period—were non-existent. There were a few exceptions among the viral diseases (herpes simplex and chickenpox) and bacterial and protozoal diseases (tuberculosis, leprosy, and treponematosis), all of which are characterized by latency and recurrence. The situation changed when humans began to live in large groups. The phase shift in community size began about 6,000 years ago, when large cities began to appear with the first great civilizations. This development was itself dependent upon improved farming techniques especially irrigation. As McKeown (1988, p. 51) notes, 'Remarkably, we owe the origin of most serious infectious diseases to the conditions which led to our cultural heritage, the city states made possible by the planting of crops in the flood plains of Mesopotamia, Egypt and the Indus Valley'.

The massing of large populations served to facilitate the spread of airborne and other infections, while the hygienic conditions that followed the introduction of agriculture made it possible for new diseases to appear and existing diseases to become more serious. Hygienic conditions began to be important—especially those associated with the handling of food and water and the disposing of excreta and waste. Cholera, McKeown notes, emerged when villages and village water supplies were established, while malaria became serious when the size of human populations and the opportunities for breeding of vectors increased with advances in agriculture. Tuberculosis emerged as an important disease with the development of large cities, while intestinal infections (typhoid, dysentery, salmonella) resulted from the contamination of food and water.

Archaeological implications

For each of the communicable crowd diseases, of which measles, poliomyelitis, and smallpox are prime examples, we noted in Chapter 1 that there exists a critical community size which is required to ensure endemic persistence of the disease—only above the population threshold for the disease will there be sufficient susceptibles and infectives in circulation to maintain the person-to-person transmission chains of infection. Drawing on the evidence in section 1.4.3 in Chapter 1, if we use an estimate of approximately 250,000 as a working figure for the size of our human virus-sustaining population for diseases such as measles and poliomyelitis (Cliff and Haggett, 1990; Smallman-Raynor et al., 2006), then we must ask where and when such clusters developed. Table 3.5 gives a simplified summary of the major centres so far revealed by archaeological research (Haggett, 1979). Given the dates in Table 3.5 then, in terms of timing, person-to-person 'civilized' types of transmissible infectious diseases could not have established themselves much before 3000–2700 BC and the emergence of the urban cultures of Egypt (Nile Valley) and Sumer (Mesopotamia). On this basis, Figure 3.2 provides a hypothetical reconstruction of the dispersal of one such disease (poliomyelitis) from this early possible hearth in the Near/Middle East. Similar reconstructions have been proposed for measles (Cliff et al., 1993, pp. 46–52) and smallpox (Cliff et al., 2004, p. 38).

In subsequent centuries, as other parts of the world also became seats of urban civilizations, continuous infectious chains became possible elsewhere. First here, then there, one or another disease organism invaded the ecological niche that increasing human density provided for it.

3.3 The Fourth Historic Transition: Disease Implications of Global Change

Although the investigation of disease origins and dispersals has an innate fascination, their study is not merely one of antiquarian interest. Disease patterns are changing at an unprecedented rate today and raise our second question: why do more diseases appear to be emerging now than in the past, and how far is this phenomenon related to the unprecedented changes in the global environment? In addressing these questions, we fast-forward several thousand years to the modern day and McMichael's *fourth historic transition* (section 3.1.1) in the relationship of humans and disease microbes.

3.3.1 Disease Emergence Factors

Morse (1995) identifies six factors that have facilitated the emergence (and re-emergence) of infectious diseases in recent times. These factors are as follows:

1. *Ecological changes*, including those due to economic development and land use. These can precipitate the emergence of infectious diseases by placing people in contact with a natural reservoir or host of an unfamiliar (to humans) but already present infection.

Table 3.5 Main urban nuclear centres as revealed by archaeological research

Type	Zone	Locations	Dates
Primary Nuclear Areas	Fertile Crescent (Middle East)	Nile Valley, Mesopotamia (Tigris-Euphrates Valley), Indus Valley, Hwang Valley	3000–1300 BC
	America	Yucatan Peninsula, Central Mexico, Peru, Niger Valley	AD 500–1300
Secondary Nuclear Areas	Southern Europe	Aegean Peninsula and islands, Italian Pensinsula	2000–400 BC
	South and East Asia	Mekong Valley, Japan, Central Burma, Ceylon	AD 600–1100

Source: Data from Wheatley, P. (1971). *The Pivot of the Four Quarters: A Preliminary Enquiry into the Origins and Character of the Ancient Chinese City.* Edinburgh: University of Edinburgh Press.

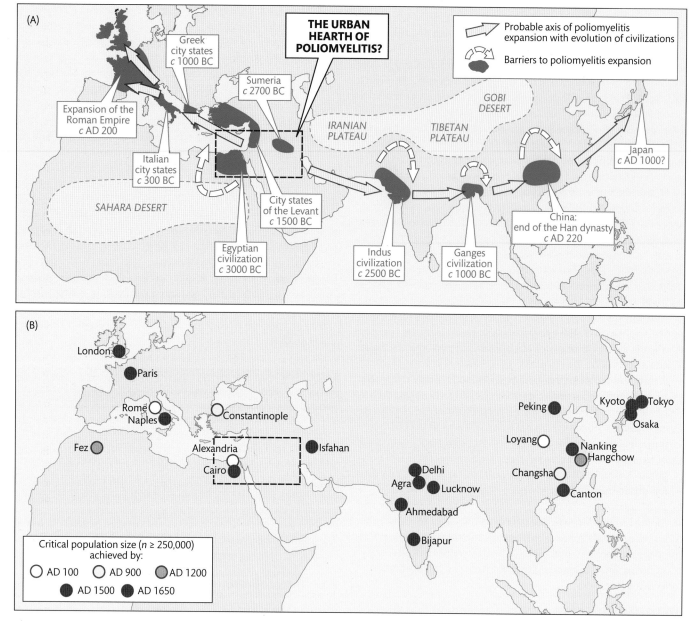

Figure 3.2 Hypothetical reconstruction of original hearth of poliomyelitis and its probable spread. (*Upper*) Probable axis of poliomyelitis diffusion and barriers to expansion. (*Lower*) Evolution of settlements at or above the critical community size for poliomyelitis (taken here at 250,000, the mid-point size estimate in Eichner et al., 1994).

Reproduced from Smallman-Raynor, M.R., Cliff, A.D., Trevelyan, B., Nettleton, C., Sneddon, S. (2006). *Poliomyelitis. A World Geography: Emergence to Eradication*. Oxford: Oxford University Press.

This contact may arise by increasing proximity or by changing conditions so that an increased microbe population results. Examples include schistosomiasis (dams), Rift Valley fever (dams, irrigation), Argentine haemorrhagic fever (AHF; agriculture), Korean haemorrhagic fever (agriculture), Lyme disease (deforestation/reforestation), and hantavirus pulmonary syndrome (HPS; weather anomalies in the United States).

2. *Human demographics and behaviour*, including societal events, population growth, migration, war and civil conflict, urban decay, sexual behaviour, and drug use. Example consequences include the introduction and spread of HIV and other sexually transmitted infections, and the spread of dengue. The United

Nations estimates that, by 2025, 65 per cent of the world's population will live in cities. The process of urbanization, especially in developing countries, heightens the opportunity for the introduction of once-isolated infections in rural areas to large urban agglomerations. Thus, dengue haemorrhagic fever is common in some cities of Asia, where the high prevalence is attributed to the proliferation of open containers for water storage which provide breeding grounds for the mosquito vector.

3. *International travel and commerce*, including the worldwide movement of goods and people. Examples include airport malaria, the dissemination of mosquito vectors, the introduction of cholera into South America, and the dissemination of *Vibrio*

cholerae O139. Classic historical examples include the introduction of bubonic plague to Europe from Asia along the Silk Road in the fourteenth century, the carriage of yellow fever and its mosquito vector, *Aedes aegypti*, to the Americas in the sixteenth and seventeenth centuries associated with the importation of slaves from West Africa, and, in the nineteenth century, the dispersion of cholera around the world from its focus in the Ganges plain. Similar histories are being repeated. Rats have carried hantaviruses virtually worldwide while, from 1982, the Asian tiger mosquito, *Aedes albopictus*, has been introduced to the United States, Brazil, and parts of Africa with shipments of used tyres from Asia and has been associated with the spread of several viral diseases.

4. *Technology and industry*, including the globalization of food supplies, changes in food processing, organ and tissue transplantation, immunosuppressive drugs, and widespread use of antibiotics. Examples include *Escherichia coli* contamination of foodstuffs, bovine spongiform encephalopathy, and variant Creutzfeldt–Jakob disease. The concentrating effects associated with blood and tissue products have served to disseminate infections such as HIV and hepatitis B.

5. *Microbial adaptation and change*, including microbial evolution and selection in the environment. Examples include antigenic drift in influenza A virus, the emergence of antibiotic-resistant bacteria, and drug-resistant parasites. On rare occasions, the evolution of a fresh variant of a disease agent may result in the new expression of a disease. One example is the epidemic of Brazilian purpuric fever in 1990, associated with a newly emerged variant of *Hemophilus influenzae*, biogroup *aegyptius*. Manifestations of group A streptococci, including necrotizing fasciitis, may also fall within this category.

6. *Breakdown in public health measures*, including the curtailment or reduction in prevention programmes, inadequate sanitation, and vector control measures. Examples include the re-emergence of tuberculosis in the United States, cholera in refugee camps in Africa, and the resurgence of diphtheria in the former Soviet Union in the 1990s.

These various factors operate at different stages of the emergence process, with several factors often working in combination to precipitate the appearance of a disease agent in the human population. We illustrate here the impact of four such changes: demographic growth and relocation of the human population (section 3.3.2), globalization and the collapse of geographical space (section 3.3.3), global land-use changes (section 3.3.4), and climate change and variability (section 3.3.5).

3.3.2 Growth and Relocation of the Human Population

The Neolithic revolution in agriculture that occurred 10,000–12,000 years ago is thought by archaeologists to be the key change that permitted the human population to live in permanent settled clusters. Over the succeeding millennia the human population has increased by roughly three orders of magnitude, from 10^7 to now approaching 10^{10}. The earlier totals are inevitably rough but a figure of 250 million humans at the start of the Current Era, doubling to 500 million by AD 1600 would be widely supported. With the advent of national population censuses from the late eighteenth century,

global figures also become more reliable. The world total of approximately 1 billion in 1805 had doubled to approximately 2 billion by 1925, approximately 4 billion by 1975 and approximately 8 billion by 2020; see Table 1.3 in Chapter 1.

From the viewpoint of disease evolution, the changes in overall host totals, striking though they are, have less significance than the concentration of that population into a hierarchy of high-density clusters (villages, towns, metropolitan areas). As discussed in section 1.4.3 in Chapter 1, the links between the growing size of human settlements and epidemic behaviour was investigated in a series of classic papers by the statistician, Maurice Bartlett (Bartlett, 1957, 1960). He found that the endemic threshold population (i.e. the size of a population cluster required to maintain measles in endemic form) was of the order 250,000–300,000. Subsequent research has shown that the threshold for measles, or indeed for any other infectious disease, is likely to be rather variable with the threshold influenced by population densities and vaccination levels. But nevertheless, the threshold principle demonstrated by Bartlett remains intact (Cliff et al., 2000, pp. 85–118).

The impact of population growth in providing clusters in the host population where an infectious disease can be maintained endemically is illustrated in **Figure 3.3** for a single country. This shows the growing number of cities within the conterminous United States that meet the 250,000–300,000 Bartlett threshold for measles endemicity over a 120-year period. In **Figure 3.3A**, the number of cities in 1870 was only six, four along the Atlantic seaboard plus Chicago and St. Louis in the Midwest. Subsequent maps show the steady growth in number and geographical spread at intervals of roughly a human generation (30 years). By 1990 (**Figure 3.3E**), the number had increased tenfold to 63 and the geographical spread was coast to coast with heavy concentrations in the southern states. The American story of increasing numbers of 'endemic cities' is repeated worldwide, and they have also shifted in location; it is that spatial shift to which we now turn.

Geographical shifts in clusters

The spatial distribution of the world's largest cities over recent decades is shown in **Figure 3.4**. Each dot on the world map represents a massive human settlement, a city or metropolitan area with a population estimated to be not less than 5 million people (i.e. 20 times greater than the measles threshold used on the United States maps in **Figure 3.3**). The maps show the growth of the urbanized world at four cross-sections over a 60-year period, 1955–2015. Just after World War II, the world had only 11 of these megacities. As **Figure 3.4A** indicates, they were predominantly northern hemisphere and mid-latitude in location, with Tokyo, Japan (13.7 million), as the largest. Together, the megacities totalled 80 million and made up less than 3 per cent of an estimated world population of 2.7 billion.

Over the next 20 years, the pattern shifted only a little (**Figure 3.4B**, with 18 megacities and a combined population of 170 million). There had been especially high growth in Latin America and south Asia. By 1995, the number of megacities had doubled in number (**Figure 3.4C**) and the total population in them had also doubled to 343 million. Again, growth was especially rapid in Latin America, but now Africa, India, and China were also expanding very quickly.

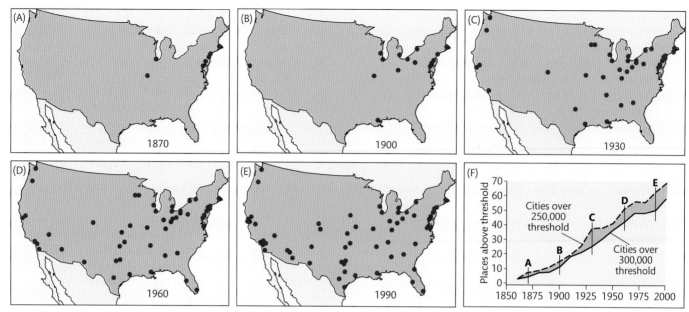

Figure 3.3 Changes in the number of settlements meeting the Bartlett threshold for measles endemicity in the conterminous United States. (A)–(E) Maps at 30-year intervals over the period 1870–1990. (F) Graph of changing number of cities meeting the threshold, 1850–2000.

Reproduced with permission from Cliff, A.D., Smallman-Raynor, M.R., Haggett, P., Stroup, D.F., Thacker, S.B. (2009). *Infectious Diseases. Emergence and Re-emergence: A Geographical Analysis*. Oxford: Oxford University Press. Source: Data from United States Bureau of the Census: Tables for Population of the 100 Largest Urban Places, 1850–1990.

Growth in megacities has continued apace since 1995. The world had passed the 50 cities mark by 2005 and the 60 cities mark by 2015 (**Figure 3.4D**). By 2020, megacities had a combined population of 854 million, comprising 11.2 per cent of an estimated global population of 7.6 billion. In other words, by 2020, one in nine of the world's people were resident in one of its megacities.

The changes in the resident population of megacities are shown in a time framework in **Figure 3.4E**, while their changing geography

as measured by latitude and average year-round temperature are examined in **Figure 3.4F**. On latitude, megacities range from St. Petersburg, Russia (60°N) as the most poleward to Jakarta, Indonesia (6°S) as the most equatorward. Over the 60 years, the average location of megacities has shifted equatorwards by 11° of latitude, from 39° (equivalent to that of Madrid) to 28° (that of Delhi).

If we now take the average temperature of cities over a year, this ranges from Moscow, Russia (4°C) to Khartoum, Sudan (29°C).

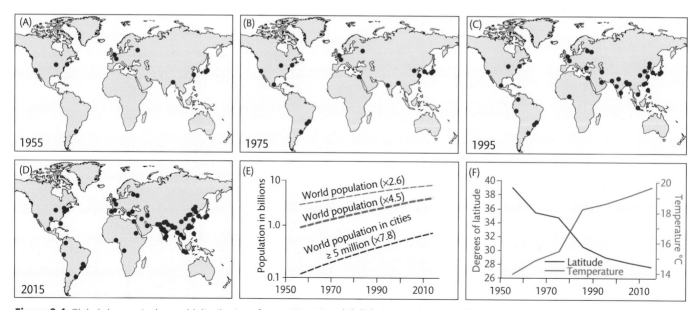

Figure 3.4 Global changes in the world distribution of megacities. Maps (A)–(D) show the location of cities with 5 million or more inhabitants in 1955, 1975, 1995, and 2015. (E) Graph of population changes over the period 1955–2015. (F) Graph of changes in the average location of megacities in terms of latitude and temperature over the period.

Reproduced with permission from Cliff, A.D., Smallman-Raynor, M.R., Haggett, P., Stroup, D.F., Thacker, S.B. (2009). *Infectious Diseases. Emergence and Re-emergence: A Geographical Analysis*. Oxford: Oxford University Press. Source: Data on city sizes from United Nations Population Division.

Over the 60 years, the average for all megacities has shown an increase of 5.7°C—from 13.9°C (typical of Istanbul, Turkey) in 1955 to 19.6°C (typical of Lima, Peru) by 2015. This shift of nearly 6°C needs to be seen against the global warming trend over the same period of about 0.5°C. In other words, the relative geographical shift in population has outpaced global warming some 12-fold as a source of 'population warming'.

Implications for disease emergence

One implication of the above findings is that the battle against epidemic diseases will be increasingly fought in urban (and tropical urban) rather than rural arenas. But the disease implications of urbanization are complex. Positive effects from improved sanitation or better access to healthcare facilities have to be set against the negative effects from increased risk of disease contacts through crowding and pollution.

In the last four decades, the world's population has more than doubled. **Figure 3.5A** plots as a histogram the present latitudinal distribution of population along a pole-to-pole latitude continuum. It shows a marked concentration in the northern mid-latitudes. But that situation is changing. It is expected that some 94 per cent of population growth over the next 20 years will occur in economically developing countries (**Figure 3.5C**). Present and future growth will shift the balance of world population towards the tropics and low latitudes with their wider range of diseases. This redistribution will also increase the average temperature of the global population by around +1°C, from 17°C to 18°C (even assuming no increase from

global warming). This concentration will place more people than at any time in the world's previous history in areas of high microbiological diversity, potentially exposing a greater share of the world's population to the disease hazards of the tropics (**Figure 3.5B**).

3.3.3 Globalization and the Collapse of Geographical Space

In section 1.2.2, in Chapter 1, we highlighted the epidemiological implications of developments in travel and transportation in recent centuries. The broad statistical trend for movement over the last 200 years for an individual country is given in **Figure 3.6**. This plots, for France since 1800, the average kilometres travelled daily by people (i) by particular transport mode and (ii) by all modes. For the former we see how one mode reaches a peak and declines to be overtaken by a successor but the combined movement total keeps on growing. Since the vertical scale is logarithmic, the graph demonstrates that, despite changes in the mode used, average travel increased exponentially over the period, broken only by the two World Wars—a rise of over 1,000-fold in mobility.

Historical changes in travel patterns have been shown in a different but equally interesting way by Bradley (1989). He compared the travel patterns of four successive generations of the Bradley family: his great-grandfather, his grandfather, his father, and himself (**Figure 3.7**). The life-time travel track of his great-grandfather around a village in Northamptonshire, England, could be contained within a square with sides of only 40 km. His grandfather's map was still limited to southern England, but it now ranged as far as London

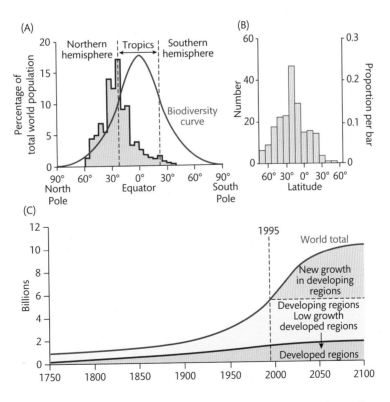

Figure 3.5 Global population growth in relation to latitude. (A) Geographical distribution of population (shaded histogram) by 5° latitudinal bands north and south of the equator. The biodiversity curve is approximate and does not make allowance for the global distribution of humidity. (B) Latitudinal variation in the number of infectious diseases. (C) Course of global population growth for the period from 1750 projected forward to 2100.

Reproduced with permission from Cliff, A.D., Smallman-Raynor, M.R., Haggett, P., Stroup, D.F., Thacker, S.B. (2009). *Infectious Diseases. Emergence and Re-emergence: A Geographical Analysis*. Oxford: Oxford University Press. Source: Data from Haggett (2000, fig. 3.7, p. 85); Cliff, Haggett, and Smallman-Raynor (2000, fig. 7.1, p. 296).

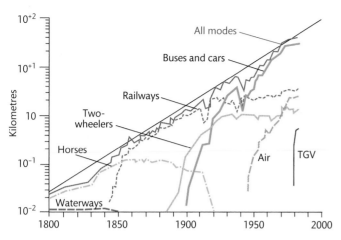

Figure 3.6 Increased spatial mobility of the population of France over a 200-year period, 1800–2000. The vertical scale is logarithmic so that increases in average travel distance by all transport modes is shown to be increasing exponentially over time. TGV, high-speed train (Train à Grande Vitesse).

Source: Data from Grubler, A. (1990). *The Rise and Fall of Infrastructures: Dynamics of Evolution and Technological Change in Transport*. Heidelberg: Physica-Verlag.

has increased tenfold in each generation so that Bradley's own range is 1,000 times wider than that of his great-grandfather.

The precise rates of population flux or travel both within and between countries are difficult to catch in official statistics. But most available evidence suggests that the flux over the last few decades has risen at an accelerating rate. An immediate and important effect is the possible exposure of the travelling public to a greater range of diseases than they might meet in their home country. The relative risks encountered in tropical areas by travellers coming from western countries (data mainly from North America and Western Europe) have been estimated by Steffen (World Health Organization, 1995). These suggest a spectrum of risks from unspecified traveller's diarrhoea (a high risk of 20 per cent) to paralytic poliomyelitis (a very low risk of <0.001 per cent).

Epidemiological impacts of sea travel

For most of human history, long-distance travel was dominantly water dependent. From the nineteenth century, the succession of technological changes in ships that generally made them faster, larger, and safer is largely one of the development of steam navigation and its succession over sail (Fletcher, 1910; Rowland, 1970). Although the practical use of steamships can be traced to the early years of the century, a number of fundamental advances from 1860 increased dramatically the speed and efficiency of ocean-going steamers. The impact of these improvements on voyaging times is shown in **Figure 3.8**. This plots the changes in travel times by sea over two major oceans. Graph (A) shows crossing times from

and could be contained within a square with sides of 400 km. If we compare these maps with those of Bradley's father (who travelled widely in Europe) and Bradley's own sphere of travel (worldwide), then the enclosing square has to be widened to sides of 4,000 km and 40,000 km, respectively. In broad terms, the spatial range of travel

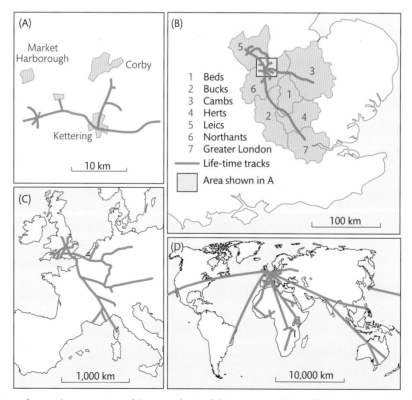

Figure 3.7 Increasing travel over four male generations of the same family. (A) Great-grandfather. (B) Grandfather. (C) Father. (D) Son. Each map shows in a simplified manner the individual's 'life-time tracks' in a widening spatial context, with the linear scale increasing by a factor of 10 between each generation.

Reproduced from Bradley, D.J. (1989). 'The scope of travel medicine.' In: R. Steffen, H.O. Lobel, J. Haworth, and D.J. Bradley (eds.), *Travel Medicine: Proceedings of the First Conference on International Travel Medicine, Zürich, Switzerland, 5–8 April 1988.* Berlin: Springer Verlag, 1–9.

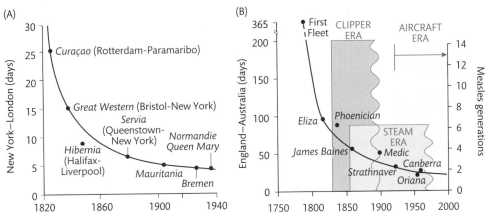

Figure 3.8 Time changes in intercontinental travel by sea transport. (A) Transatlantic travel between Europe and North America, 1820–1940. (B) Travel between England and Australia, 1788–2000. The solid lines show the exponential decline in travel times. A measles generation is defined as 14 days.
Reproduced with permission from Cliff, A.D., Smallman-Raynor, M.R., Haggett, P., Stroup, D.F., Thacker, S.B. (2009). *Infectious Diseases. Emergence and Re-emergence: A Geographical Analysis*. Oxford: Oxford University Press. Source: Data from Davies (1964, fig. 91, pp. 508–9); Cliff and Haggett (2004, fig. 1A, p. 89).

Europe across the North Atlantic over a 120-year period. A 3-week journey by sailing ship in 1820 had been reduced to a 4-day crossing by passenger liner by 1940. Graph (B) shows the time in days for sea travel from Britain to Australia from the sailing of the First Fleet in 1788. The vertical axis of the graph has two scales, measuring travel times in days (left-hand vertical axis) and—as an epidemiological exemplar—measles virus generations (right-hand vertical axis). We define a measles generation (or serial interval) as 14 days, the typical time between the observation of symptoms of measles in one case and the observation of symptoms in a second case directly infected from the first (see Figure 1.1 in Chapter 1).

The solid lines on both graphs in **Figure 3.8** depict an exponentially declining trend in voyage times. As the early decades of the nineteenth century passed, so the size and speed of ships on both routes increased. On the England–Australia run, the periods encompassing the clipper era (1830s–1890s) and the steam era (from the 1850s) are indicated for reference. By 1840, clippers had reduced the voyage time to 100 days and, by the first decade of the twentieth century, steamers had halved the voyage time again. In terms of measles virus generations, the reduction was from six to three, greatly increasing the chance of infections surviving on board and of infectives causing outbreaks in Australia.

The Pacific island of Fiji provides a practical example of the way in which the technological change from sailing ship to steamship eroded the epidemiological isolation of once remote populations. In the late nineteenth century, Fiji was one of a series of tropical islands whose climate and soils were ideal for growing sugar cane, a crop in soaring demand in Europe. In the post-slavery period, a new source of labour (India) and a new form of bondage (indentured labour) provided a solution to the demand for labour generated by Fiji's burgeoning sugar plantations.

Between 1879 and 1920, Indian immigrant ships made 87 voyages to Fiji carrying nearly 61,000 indentured emigrants. The main routes followed are mapped in **Figure 3.9A**. This illustrates an important distinction between voyages by sailing ships (used between 1879 and 1904) and steamships (used between 1884 and 1916). To take advantage of prevailing winds, sailing ships followed the route south of Australia and took 70–90 days for the voyage. Steamships used the more direct Torres Strait north of Australia and halved the

sailing ship times; they were also able to carry a larger number of immigrants.

Since measles was an endemic disease in India, it is not surprising that cases among the Indian labourers were recorded on departure, although there were checks in the camps both at Calcutta and Madras (the two exit ports) before embarkation. Indeed, measles was detected on one-third of all vessels on departure from India, and this proportion of 'infected' voyages remained constant over the period. These are shown in **Figure 3.9B** in which each voyage is plotted in terms of the time taken and the passenger size of each vessel.

For the smaller and slower sailing ships, around one-third of the vessels carrying labourers left India with infectives on board but in no instance did the measles virus survive the journey. By the end of the voyage, those infected had either recovered or died and the long chain of measles generations needed to maintain infection (up to six on slower voyages) was broken. But, for the faster and larger steamships, **Figure 3.9B** reveals a very different situation. Ships on one-third of the voyages still carried infectives on departure and, in 11 instances, the virus continued to thrive on arrival in Fiji. The larger susceptible population and shorter travel times (as few as two generations on the fastest voyages) ensured the virus persisted to pose a potential threat at the receiving end. Only intensive quarantine guaranteed that the experience of the disastrous 1875 measles epidemic in Fiji was not repeated (Cliff and Haggett, 1985).

Air transportation and global transmission networks

Like travel times by sea in the nineteenth century, the story of air transportation in the twentieth century is one of exponentially diminishing journey times, with exponentially increasing speeds and growing carrying capacities. However, the collapse of geographical space has not been uniform. It is the distance between major centres, notably the world's great cities, that has been cut most dramatically. The ability of long-distance aircraft to 'overfly' intermediate locations (which previously served as necessary refuelling places along the route) has now made these places relatively less accessible. Thus, the shrinking world is marked by (i) reducing travel times between major centres, balanced by (ii) unchanging or reducing accessibility for minor centres off the well-beaten transport tracks.

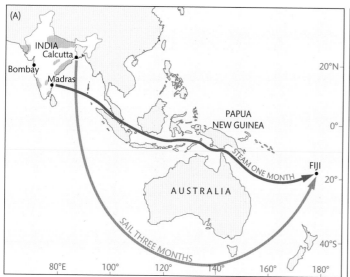

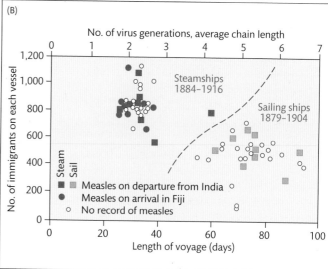

Figure 3.9 Measles transfer from India to Fiji. (A) Routes from India to Fiji via sailing ships and steamships. (B) Vessels carrying immigrants between India and Fiji, 1879–1916, categorized by length of voyage in days and in measles virus generations (14-day periods), type of vessel, and measles status. Reproduced with permission from Cliff, A.D., Smallman-Raynor, M.R., Haggett, P., Stroup, D.F., Thacker, S.B. (2009). *Infectious Diseases. Emergence and Re-emergence: A Geographical Analysis.* Oxford: Oxford University Press. Source: Data from archival research by Cliff and Haggett (1985; see also 2004, fig. 4, p. 94).

In addition to increased speed, the increasing size in terms of passenger numbers also needs to be taken into account. Bradley (1989) postulates a hypothetical situation in which the chance of one person in the travelling population having a given communicable disease in the infectious stage is 1 in 10,000. Assume that, with a 200-seat aircraft, the probability of having one infected passenger on board (x) is small, say 0.02, and the number of potential contacts (y) is 199. If we assume homogeneous mixing, this gives a combined risk factor (xy) of 3.98. If we double the aircraft size to 400 passengers, then the corresponding figures are $x = 0.04$, $y = 398$, and $xy = 15.92$. In other words, *ceteris paribus*, doubling the aircraft size increases the risk from the flight fourfold, although in practice such probabilities would be modulated by the air circulation technology used. Thus, new generations of wide-bodied jets present fresh possibilities for disease spread, not only through their flying range and their speed, but also from their size.

One impact of recent disease emergence episodes such as severe acute respiratory syndrome (SARS) (section 3.4.2) has been to focus on global modelling of spread on very large and very complex networks. This worldwide air transport network is growing but, in the early twenty-first century, consisted of 3,880 airports (Figure 3.10). In terms of graph theory, the network may be thought of as a weighted graph with $V = 3,880$ vertices which are connected by $E = 18,810$ edges, each with a weight w_{ij} related to passenger flow between airports i and j. Flows along some links are very small so that the network can be pruned to 3,100 airports and 17,182 links while retaining 99 per cent of total flow. Colizza et al. (2006a) show that a relatively small number of airports and pairs make up a very large share of the total traffic; conversely, a large number of small airports and lightly used links make up only a small fraction of worldwide air transport network activity.

A number of epidemiologists have studied the worldwide air transport network as a spatial framework for predicting the potential spread of infectious diseases. Simulations of intervention strategies by imposing travel restrictions within the network have given mixed results;

Colizza et al. (2006a, 2006b, 2007) suggest the procedure is worthwhile but Cooper et al. (2006) concluded that international travel restrictions do little to reduce the rate of spread globally. Rather, they suggest that local interventions at source aimed at reducing transmission are more likely to reduce the rate of spread. These views are supported by Hollingsworth et al. (2006) using a simplified global model.

Epstein et al. (2007) concluded from their modelling of pandemic influenza that air travel restrictions could be useful less in

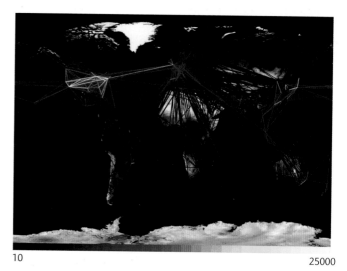

10   25000

Figure 3.10 The world airline network at the millennium. A simplified representation of the global aviation network at the start of the present century showing direct civil aviation routes between the world's largest 500 international airports, as measured by passenger traffic. Each line on the map represents a direct connection between airports. Although the map shown represents only one in eight of international airports it captures over 95 per cent of international civil aviation traffic. Reproduced with permission from Hufnagel, L., Brockmann, D., Geisel, T. (2004). 'Forecast and control of epidemics in a globalized world.' Copyright (2004) *Proceedings of the National Academy of Sciences, USA*, 101, 15124–9.

ameliorating the pandemic than in buying time to develop and deliver vaccines and in developing other protective measures (e.g. public education, social distancing among susceptibles, and emergency hospital arrangements; see Chapter 5). They also found that travel restrictions could be harmful in circumstances where the delay achieved through travel restriction simply pushed the peak into a high epidemic season where local transmission is likely to be greater. The increasing range and capacity of computer simulation models to 'mimic' the behaviour of epidemic waves on a spatially intricate world and national stage now means that quite sophisticated strategies for dealing with potential pandemic events can be tested and revised. That some results are clearly counterintuitive (e.g. some plausible intervention strategies actually exacerbate morbidity rates) underlines the need for continuing work in this area. Grais et al. (2003), in their simulation studies of the spread of a Hong Kong type of influenza through a network of 52 global cities, emphasize how short the time can be for effective public health interventions.

While simulation on airline networks is a powerful investigative tool, it needs to be backed up by specific epidemiological studies of the actual movement of infected passengers. We know, for example, that the country-wide dispersal of HIV-1 in the United States in the early 1980s can in part be attributed to the activities of an early case, so-called Patient 0, an HIV-infected airline steward (**Figure 3.11**) (Smallman-Raynor et al., 1992). At a population-wide, rather than individual level, Brownstein et al. (2006) have presented evidence that the grounding of airplanes in the United States after 11 September 2001 delayed the dynamics of influenza during the 2001–02 season by approximately 2 weeks. This conclusion has been challenged by Viboud et al. (2006).

3.3.4 Environmental Changes, I: Global Land Use

Diseases originate, spread, and persist or wither, within a specific environmental context. For the entire time during which humans have lived on the Earth, this environmental context has changed and, viewed from the beginning of a new millennium, all the available evidence suggests that the environment is set to change further

and faster than at any other time in human history. Anthropogenic environmental changes and ecological modifications that promote the emergence and resurgence of infectious diseases are numerous and include deforestation and reforestation, road construction, agricultural development, dam building, irrigation and water control schemes, coastal zone degradation and wetland modification, mining and urbanization, and macro- and micro-climate change and variability (Morse, 1995; Patz et al., 2000, 2004; McMichael, 2004). As Patz et al. (2004, p. 1092) observe, these changes and modifications can, in turn, provoke a 'cascade effect' of habitat fragmentation, ecosystem degradation and biodiversity loss, pollution, poverty, and human migration that serve to amplify the risks of disease emergence and spread (Table 3.6).

Of the several factors identified in Table 3.6, we illustrate here the effects of agricultural development and deforestation and reforestation. The effects of climate change and variability are examined in section 3.3.5.

Agricultural development: Argentine haemorrhagic fever

Agricultural development is one of the key ways by which people alter their environment, and it is a prominent driver of disease emergence and resurgence—not least by increasing the risk of human exposure to the pool of disease agents harboured by both wild and domestic animals (Morse, 1995; McMichael, 2004; Patz et al., 2004). In parts of Asia, for example, post-war developments in rice production have favoured an increase in Hantaan virus-carrying rodents (*Apodemus agrarius*), with a corresponding increase in the incidence of Korean haemorrhagic fever in farm workers. Likewise, integrated systems of pig, duck, and rice agriculture in south-East Asia have been posited as sources of human exposure to avian influenza A viruses, raising the spectre of the emergence of new human pandemic strains of the virus (section 3.4.1). The implementation of crop irrigation systems, the replacement of forests with farmland, and climate-induced shifts in agricultural production can all result in new habitats that are supportive of disease microbes, their vectors, and reservoirs. Thus there have been documented increases in the

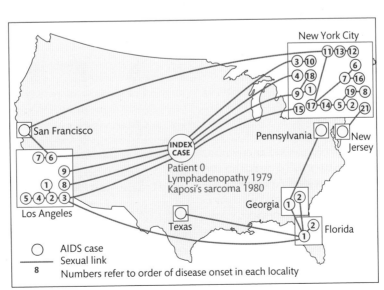

Figure 3.11 Contact network of 'Patient 0' in the early stages of the HIV/AIDS epidemic in the United States. Each circle represents an AIDS case, with the known links between cases indicated. Numbers refer to the order of disease onset in each location.

Reproduced from Smallman-Raynor, M.R., Cliff, A.D., Haggett, P. (1992). *London International Atlas of AIDS*. Oxford: Wiley.

Table 3.6 Environmental changes and disease emergence

Facilitating factor	Sample diseases	Sample geographical regions
Agricultural development	Argentine haemorrhagic fever (AHF)	Americas (South)
	Korean haemorrhagic fever (KHF)	Western Pacific
Water control and irrigation	Dracunculiasis	Africa
	Filariasis	Africa/Eastern Mediterranean
	Japanese encephalitis	Western Pacific
	Malaria	Africa
	Onchocerciasis	Africa
	Rift Valley fever	Africa/Eastern Mediterranean
	Schistosomiasis	Africa/Eastern Mediterranean/Western Pacific
Deforestation and reforestation	Lyme disease	Americas (North)/Europe
	Malaria	Americas (South)
	Nipah viral disease	Western Pacific
Climate change and variability	Cholera	Africa/South-East Asia
	Dengue	Americas (South)/South-East Asia/Western Pacific
	Hantavirus pulmonary syndrome (HPS)	Americas
	Malaria	Americas (South)/South-East Asia
	Nipah viral disease	Western Pacific
Natural disasters	Diarrhoeal diseases	Americas (North)/South-East Asia
	Malaria	South-East Asia

Reproduced with permission from Cliff, A.D., Smallman-Raynor, M.R., Haggett, P., Stroup, D.F., Thacker, S.B. (2009). *Infectious Diseases. Emergence and Re-emergence: A Geographical Analysis*. Oxford: Oxford University Press. Source: Data from Morse, S.S. (1995). 'Factors in the emergence of infectious diseases.' *Emerging Infectious Diseases*, 1, 7–15; and McMichael, A.J. (2004). 'Environmental and social influences on emerging infectious diseases: Past, present and future.' *Philosophical Transactions of the Royal Society B*, 359, 1049–58.

incidence of lymphatic filariasis (Harb et al., 1993), malaria (Sogoba et al., 2007), Rift Valley fever (Wilson, 1994), and schistosomiasis (Malek, 1975) in association with the development of crop irrigation schemes in Africa. The spread of Lyme and other tick-borne diseases has been associated with the implementation of agricultural land set-aside policies in the European Union (Süss et al., 2008) and, as described in more detail here, the emergence of AHF with the establishment of crop cultivation in South America (Morse, 1995).

Argentine haemorrhagic fever is an acute febrile disease that occurs in a geographically circumscribed area of the Argentine pampas in South America. Clinical and epidemiological details are provided by Heymann (2015, pp. 47–8). Here we note that the disease in humans presents as a clinical syndrome that includes manifestations of renal, cardiovascular, haematological, and neurological involvement, with a case-fatality rate of 15–30 per cent in untreated cases. The specific agent of the disease is Junín virus. It belongs to the New World (Tacaribe) arenavirus complex, of which Guanarito virus (Venezuelan haemorrhagic fever), Machupo virus (Bolivian haemorrhagic fever), and Sabiá virus (Brazilian haemorrhagic fever) are also known to be pathogenic for humans. The reservoirs of these viruses are rodents of the family *Cricetidae*, each with an ecologically determined range that limits the geographical distribution of the associated diseases (Downs, 1993). Junín virus is shed in the secretions and excretions of infected rodents, and the principal route of transmission to humans is by inhalation of contaminated aerosol particles (Jahrling, 1997).

The currently recognized endemo-epidemic area of AHF lies between latitudes 33–37°S and longitudes 59–65°W, extending across a large and heavily cultivated area of the Humid Pampas in northern Buenos Aires and La Pampa Provinces and southern Córdoba and Santa Fe Provinces. The first detailed account of AHF was provided by R.A. Arribalzaga (1955) who described the clinical features of an apparently new epidemic disease in the Pampas of northern Buenos Aires Province in 1953 and 1954. As the map sequence in **Figure 3.12** shows, the endemo-epidemic area has expanded markedly since that time. New endemic areas were identified in central Buenos Aires, southern Córdoba, and northern La Pampa in the mid-to-late 1960s (**Figure 3.12B**), with the total endemo-epidemic area expanding to over 120,000 km² by the mid-1980s (**Figure 3.12C–E**). Further expansion, concentrated along the north-central perimeter of the zone in **Figure 3.12E**, has subsequently been documented by Enria et al. (2008).

The emergence and spread of AHF is intimately associated with the adoption of agricultural activities that favour the rodent reservoirs of Junín virus, and which bring the rodents and their excreta into contact with humans. High rodent densities in the endemo-epidemic area are correlated with the cultivation of grains (especially maize), with the concentration of AHF among grain harvesters so well recognized that the condition is colloquially referred to as 'stubble disease' (Mettler, 1969). Against this background, Viglizzo et al. (2004) note that the pampas has a relatively short farming history, having remained as native grassland until the latter part of the nineteenth century. In the twentieth century, the extensive conversion of grassland to maize cultivation provided an environment in which *Calomys* rodents could flourish, increasing the opportunities for the zoonotic transmission of Junín virus and the emergence of an apparently new viral disease in the human population (Morse, 1995; McMichael, 2001; Hui, 2006).

Deforestation and reforestation: Lyme disease

Changes in global forest cover are linked to disease changes in complex ways. Among the many interconnected factors, ecological changes that have followed on from the massive deforestation of tropical and temperate areas over the last century—and which have heightened the risk of human exposure to the zoonotic pool—have been identified as key drivers of disease emergence and resurgence (Patz et al., 2004). Deforestation, and the reverse process of reforestation, have been directly associated with the emergence and resurgence of several vectored and non-vectored infectious diseases (**Table 3.6**). Among the vector-borne conditions, high levels of malarial infection have been encountered by settlers who have followed the logging roads into Amazonia. As the ecology of an area changes, so the vector species may also change. Some vectors may convert from a primarily zoophilic to a primarily anthropophilic orientation as contact with humans increases, while those settlers new to an area may lack protective immunity to the local diseases and/or familiarity with the practices that would serve to limit the risks of pathogen transmission. In turn, as human population density increases, so the opportunity for exchange and transmission of disease microorganisms rises (Patz et al., 2000, 2004).

Lyme disease provides an archetypal example of the role of temperate reforestation as a facilitating factor in the emergence of a newly identified disease. The disease is caused by certain bacteria of the genus *Borrelia*. The bacteria are transmitted to humans via

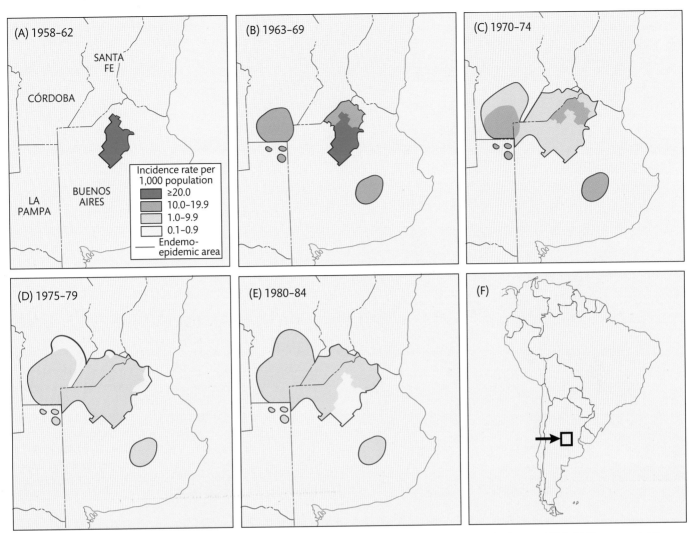

Figure 3.12 Argentine haemorrhagic fever (AHF): geographical expansion of the recognized endemo-epidemic area, 1958–84. The maps plot the geographical extent of the recognized endemo-epidemic area in (A) 1958–62, (B) 1963–69, (C) 1970–74, (D) 1975–79, and (E) 1980–84. Infected areas are shaded according to the AHF incidence rate (per 1,000 population) in a given time period.

Reproduced with permission from Cliff, A.D., Smallman-Raynor, M.R., Haggett, P., Stroup, D.F., Thacker, S.B. (2009). *Infectious Diseases. Emergence and Re-emergence: A Geographical Analysis*. Oxford: Oxford University Press. Source: Data from Maiztegui et al. (1986, Figure 1 and Table 1, pp. 150–1).

the bite of species of tick belonging to the genus *Ixodes*. Deer, in turn, serve as important maintenance hosts for adults of the vector species. Clinically, the disease manifests as a multisystem disorder that, in its early stages, manifests as cutaneous lesions at the point of inoculation. Within weeks or months, some untreated patients develop neurological and cardiac abnormalities and recurrent arthritic attacks of the knees and other large joints. Finally, months or years after primary infection, patients may develop late-stage symptoms of infection, including degenerative skin disorders and neurological and articular changes. Prompt antibiotic treatment of early disease is usually effective (Heymann, 2015, pp. 363–6).

Although Lyme disease is now known to be widespread on several continents, its first recognition as a distinct clinical entity was in the course of a localized outbreak in the United States in the mid-1970s. In 1975, the Connecticut State Health Department was informed of an unusual number of cases of childhood arthritis in the town of Old Lyme. Investigations revealed that the cases formed distinct clusters in rural, wooded areas and that a characteristic rash was displayed in

a number of patients (Steere et al., 1977). The syndrome was found to be more prevalent in areas to the west of the Connecticut River where much of the farmland had been allowed to revert to woodland and where deer were plentiful. Children commonly used the woods for recreation, particularly in the summer months. It was several years later that a bacterium, isolated from the gut of *I. scapularis* ticks in the endemic area and named *B. burgdorferi*, was confirmed as the agent of Lyme disease in humans (Benach et al., 1983; Steere et al., 1983).

Since Lyme disease became notifiable in the United States in 1991, it has become the most commonly recorded arthropod-borne disease in the country. The major foci of reported disease activity are mapped for a sample year (2005) in **Figure 3.13** and include: (i) the Atlantic coast, from Massachusetts to Maryland; (ii) the upper Midwest, including Wisconsin and Minnesota; and (iii) the Pacific coast, intermittently from southern California to northern Washington.

Factors associated with the emergence of Lyme disease as a significant public health problem in the United States, and which would

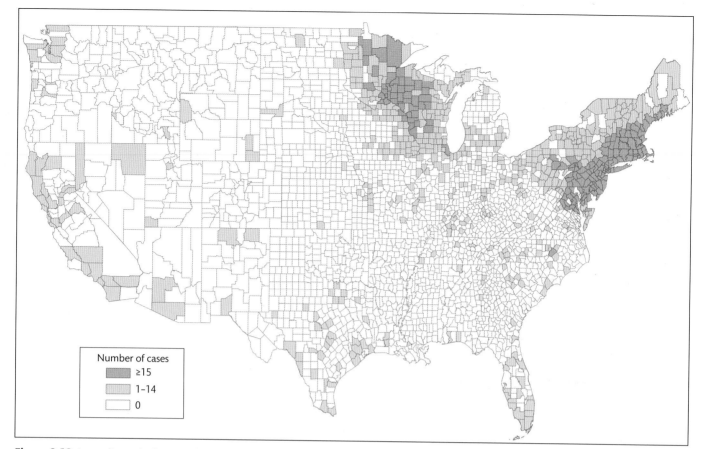

Figure 3.13 Lyme disease in the United States, 2005. The map shades counties from which cases of Lyme disease were reported in the sample year. Reproduced with permission from Cliff, A.D., Smallman-Raynor, M.R., Haggett, P., Stroup, D.F., Thacker, S.B. (2009). *Infectious Diseases. Emergence and Re-emergence: A Geographical Analysis.* Oxford: Oxford University Press. Adapted from Centers for Disease Control and Prevention (2007, p. 59).

account for the primary foci of disease activity in Figure 3.13, are reviewed by Barbour and Fish (1993), Spielman (1994), and Steere (1998). In earlier centuries, demand for trees as fuel for domestic and industrial purposes, coupled with the extension of agricultural activities, rendered much of the eastern United States virtually treeless. From the early twentieth century, however, the transfer of agriculture to the Great Plains resulted in the reforestation of vast regions of the eastern United States. The abundance of deer increased in parallel with that of woodland. In turn, the invasion of reforested areas by *Ixodes* ticks initiated the appearance of Lyme disease. As Steere (1998, pp. 222–3) explains:

> The emergence of Lyme disease in the United States in the late twentieth century is thought to have occurred primarily because of ecological conditions favorable for deer ... As farmland in the northeast reverted to woodland, the habitat for deer improved: the natural predators were gone, the number of deer increased dramatically, they migrated to new areas, and federal programs protected them. With the advent of the automobile and super-highways, rural and suburban areas, where deer now lived, became populated with large numbers of susceptible urbanites who had never been exposed to the spirochete.

Similar processes of reforestation and increased deer abundance have been witnessed across the North Temperate Zone, resulting in the development of deer-infested stands, interspersed with houses, in North America and Europe (Spielman, 1994, p. 154).

3.3.5 Environmental Changes, II: Climate Change and Variability

Climate is inextricably linked to human health. Extremes of climate—of cold or heat—can have direct impacts on the health of humans, typically manifesting in temperate latitudes as excess morbidity and mortality from hypothermia (winter months) and heat stroke (summer months). But climate can also have indirect impacts by influencing such factors as levels of atmospheric pollution, the operation of agricultural and marine systems, the distribution of disease vectors and pathogens, and patterns of human activity and behaviour. Viewed in historical perspective, short-, medium-, and long-term swings in climate have had pronounced impacts on the geographical occurrence of many old human diseases. And, very occasionally, the same climatic swings have been implicated as precipitating factors in the appearance of previously unknown pathogens in the human population (Table 3.6).

Dimensions of climate change

The Intergovernmental Panel on Climate Change (IPCC) was established by the World Meteorological Organization and the United Nations Environment Programme in 1988. Since inception, the remit of the IPCC has been to review the published scientific literature relating to the processes of human-induced climate change, the impact of these changes on human societies, and the responses that could be implemented to ameliorate the effects (Githeko and

Woodward, 2003). Among the principal conclusions of the fifth IPCC *Assessment Report*, published in 2014, the combined land and ocean surface temperature of the Earth warmed by 0.85°C (range: 0.65–1.06°C) between 1880 and 2012 (Intergovernmental Panel on Climate Change, 2014). This warming has been accompanied by changes in the magnitude and/or frequency of a range of hydro-meteorological and oceanographic phenomena, including wind intensity, drought, heavy precipitation and flood events, hurricane intensity, and sea level rises (Intergovernmental Panel on Climate Change, 2007, 2014). Future scenarios for climate change are speculative, although the IPCC project that the surface temperature of the Earth will continue to rise during the twenty-first century under all assessed emission scenarios (Intergovernmental Panel on Climate Change, 2014).

Potential health impacts of long-term climate change

Climate change can have diverse impacts on human health via multiple pathways (McMichael et al., 2003). According to Volume II of the IPCC's *Fifth Assessment Report*, the principal health effects of climate change to mid-century include the increased likelihood of injury and death due to heat waves and fires, the increased incidence of foodborne and waterborne diseases, the increased risk of undernutrition in low-income regions and a general increase in the risk of vector-borne diseases. While climate change can be expected to have some positive health impacts (e.g. a reduction in cold-related mortality in temperate latitudes), the IPCC predicts that 'Globally, the magnitude and severity of negative impacts will increasingly outweigh positive impacts' (Intergovernmental Panel on Climate Change, 2014, p. 69).

Of the likely effects of climate change on infectious diseases, particular attention has focused on the possible impact of global warming scenarios on vector-borne diseases; see, for example, Giesen et al. (2020) and Rocklöv and Dubrow (2020). Although the effects of climate on the physical and biotic controls on vectors, pathogens, and vertebrate hosts are complex, the IPCC anticipates that increased mean temperatures and changes in precipitation will serve to alter (primarily, to extend) the geographical range of a number of vector-borne diseases, including dengue, Lyme disease, malaria, and tick-borne encephalitis. An early illustration of the projected effects on one of these diseases (dengue) is provided by Patz et al. (1998) who use three climate general circulation models to generate the estimated changes in dengue transmission potential shown in **Figure 3.14**. Each circulation model provides evidence of a projected increase in biting-mosquito numbers but, as the maps show, there is considerable variation in the specific spatial pattern of increase.

Short-term climate variability: hantavirus pulmonary syndrome

Climate variability on temporal scales of days, seasons, and years is an inherent characteristic of climate, regardless of whether or not the system is subject to long-term climate change. The El Niño–Southern Oscillation (ENSO) is the name given to quasi-periodic inter-annual climate variability that arises from changes in sea temperature (El Niño) and atmospheric pressure (Southern Oscillation) in the Pacific Basin. ENSO events are linked to worldwide weather changes. During an ENSO event, a typical increase in the average global temperature of 0.5°C is accompanied by heterogeneous

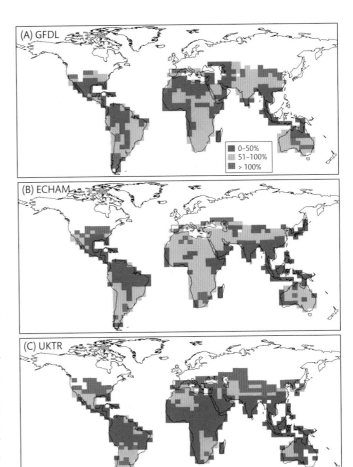

Figure 3.14 Global climate change models and potential dengue expansion. Results of the application of three general circulation models of climate to estimate the increase in dengue average annual epidemic potential due to global warming. The general circulation models were developed by research groups working in (A) the United States (GFDL), (B) Germany (ECHAM), and (C) the United Kingdom (UKTR). Maps of projected changes in dengue transmission potential, presented as percentage increases on baseline values, are illustrated for each model. All three models predict substantial increases based on a temperature rise of 1.16°C, but the specific geographical distribution of these increases differs from model to model.

Reproduced from Patz, J.A., Martens, W.J.M., Focks, D.A., Jetten, T.H. (1998). 'Dengue fever epidemic potential as projected by general circulation models of global climate change.' *Environmental Health Perspectives*, 106, 147–53. Reproduced from *Environmental Health Perspectives* with permission from the authors.

effects on regional patterns of precipitation. Past ENSO events have been associated with droughts in parts of Central and South America, Southern Africa, South and South-East Asia, and the Western Pacific. Conversely, areas at risk of excess rainfall have been observed in parts of North and South America, Central and East Africa, and South Asia. Although the potential impact of long-term global climatic change on ENSO events remains uncertain, it is anticipated that such developments will result in greater extremes of dry weather and heavy rainfall, thereby increasing the risk of ENSO-related droughts and floods (Kovats, 2000; Kovats et al., 2003).

ENSO-related changes in temperature and precipitation can affect the abundance and distribution of pathogens, arthropod vectors and intermediate hosts, and the pattern of human and arthropod behaviour and land use. Rarely, however, is there a simple association between changes in these variables and disease incidence. In a review of the scientific literature, 1980–2002, Kovats et al. (2003) identified 21 reports of a temporal relationship between ENSO and human infectious diseases (including Barmah forest virus disease, cholera, dengue, malaria, plague, Rift Valley fever, Ross River virus disease, and visceral leishmaniasis) in countries of the WHO Africa, Americas, Eastern Mediterranean, South-East Asia, and Western Pacific Regions.

The complex relationship between climate variability and disease emergence is well illustrated by HPS in the south-western United States in the 1990s. Rodents are the natural reservoir of the agent of HPS (Sin Nombre virus), with the primary route of human exposure via contact with rodents and their excreta—a transmission process analogous to that described for AHF in section 3.3.4. HPS presents as a prodromal febrile phase (chills, myalgia, headache, abdominal pain) followed by a pulmonary phase (coughing and rapid development of respiratory deficiency). The crude fatality rate is 40–50 per cent. Geographically, the risk of HPS extends across the New World, with sporadic cases and outbreaks due to one or more HPS-causing viruses having been reported in countries of both North and South America (Heymann, 2015, pp. 245–9).

HPS was first described in the spring of 1993 when it manifested as an outbreak of fatal respiratory illness in the Four Corners region of the southwestern United States; the states that constitute the index region (Arizona, Colorado, New Mexico, and Utah) are identified by the heavy border in **Figure 3.15A**. The earliest recognized cases were recorded among Native Americans in New Mexico, with investigations in neighbouring states and elsewhere yielding evidence of a total of 42 cases (including 26 deaths) by October 1993. The case distribution, with a primary focus on the Four Corners region, is represented by the proportional circles in **Figure 3.15A**. Early suspicions that a virus was involved in the aetiology of the disease were confirmed when a novel hantavirus, later named Sin Nombre virus, was isolated from case patients. Environmental investigations yielded evidence of the same virus in deer mice (*Peromyscus maniculatus*) in the outbreak area, and the deer mouse is now recognized as the natural reservoir of Sin Nombre virus (Hughes et al., 1993; Centers for Disease Control and Prevention, 2008).

Why did HPS emerge, apparently for the first time, in the Four Corners region in the spring of 1993? And what factors could account for the periodic outbreaks of HPS that have occurred in the index region in subsequent years? Possible answers to these questions can be found in the hypothesized link between HPS activity and ENSO-related patterns of climate variability (Epstein, 1995; Engelthaler et al., 1999). The link is summarized in the trophic cascade model in **Figure 3.16**. The model hinges on the observed tendency for ENSO events to yield excess levels of rainfall in the southwestern United States. From this starting point, **Figure 3.16** depicts a chain-like sequence of events in which the environmental trigger (the ENSO event of 1991–93) resulted in a short-term climate response (above-average precipitation, December 1992–March 1993) and an associated rodent habitat response (increased vegetation and food) that favoured an explosive increase in local populations of deer mice. As Engelthaler et al. (1999, p. 88) explain, these developments may have:

> increased the likelihood of more rodent-to-rodent contact, rodent-to-human contact, and viral transmission … In addition, as rodent

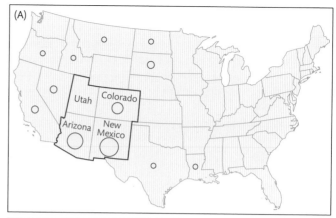

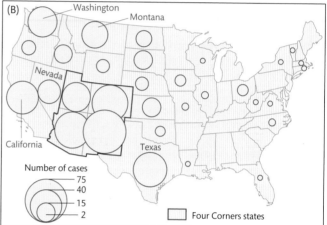

Figure 3.15 Cases of hantavirus pulmonary syndrome by reporting state, United States. Cumulative cases to (A) 21 October 1993 and (B) 26 March 2007. The Four Corners states (Arizona, Colorado, New Mexico, and Utah) are indicated.

Reproduced with permission from Cliff, A.D., Smallman-Raynor, M.R., Haggett, P., Stroup, D.F., Thacker, S.B. (2009). *Infectious Diseases. Emergence and Re-emergence: A Geographical Analysis*. Oxford: Oxford University Press. Source: Data from Centers for Disease Control and Prevention (1993, Figure 1, p. 816; 2008).

populations surpassed the carrying capacity of their local environments and precipitation plummeted, available food may have been depleted, resulting in rodent population stress. Increased stress likely increased rodent-to-rodent contact, as rodents competed for food and water, and increased rodent-to-human contact, as rodents moved into new, potentially less stressful environments, such as homes and peridomestic structures.

Studies of subsequent outbreaks of HPS in the Four Corners region have highlighted the possible role of ENSO-related climate variability as a serial environmental trigger of disease activity. Based on evidence for an extended period of 16 years, 1991–2006, Cliff, Smallman-Raynor, Haggett, et al. (2009, pp. 407–14) demonstrated that ENSO events (and associated increases in precipitation) presaged HPS outbreaks in Four Corners by an average of one year. The same analysis also demonstrated an in-phase relationship between extreme drought and HPS cases. This latter finding is consistent with the hypothesized role of below-average precipitation in the post-ENSO period as an immediate trigger mechanism for (i) heightened rodent population stress and (ii) the consequent spread of Sin Nombre virus to the human population (**Figure 3.16**).

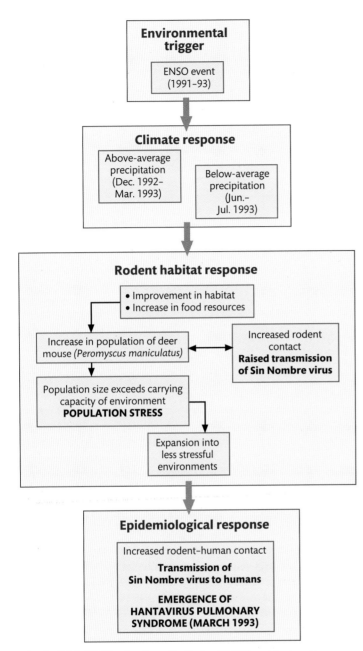

Figure 3.16 El Niño–Southern Oscillation (ENSO) and the trophic cascade model of the emergence of hantavirus pulmonary syndrome in the Four Corners states of the United States, 1993.

Reproduced with permission from Cliff, A.D., Smallman-Raynor, M.R., Haggett, P., Stroup, D.F., Thacker, S.B. (2009). *Infectious Diseases. Emergence and Re-emergence: A Geographical Analysis*. Oxford: Oxford University Press.

3.4 Newly Emerging Diseases: International Epidemics

One prominent feature of some recently emerging diseases has been their propensity to spread across international borders. In this section, we examine a sample of international epidemic events that have stopped short of global pandemics. These events are 'bird flu' associated with the influenza A (H5N1) virus (section 3.4.1), SARS associated with SARS coronavirus (CoV; section 3.4.2), and the

2013–16 epidemic of Ebola virus disease in West Africa (section 3.4.3). Global pandemic events of newly emerging diseases are examined in Chapters 4 and 5.

3.4.1 Bird Flu: Avian Influenza A (H5N1)

On Thursday, 15 May 1997, a 3-year-old boy was admitted to a Hong Kong hospital with a fever, sore throat, and cough of 6 days' duration. The child's condition deteriorated rapidly, with acute respiratory distress, multi-organ failure, and death on the 12th day of illness. An atypical influenza virus, recovered from the child's upper respiratory tract, was typed as avian influenza A (H5N1)—a novel and highly pathogenic virus of poultry that had been identified first in China the previous year (Centers for Disease Control and Prevention, 1997, 1998). Further 'dead-end' jumps of H5N1 from birds to humans were recorded in Hong Kong in late 1997 and again in early 2003 (Claas et al., 1998; Peiris et al., 2004). But it was the unprecedented events of the winter of 2003–04 that raised international concerns over H5N1 to a new level. Beginning in the latter part of 2003, poultry-based outbreaks of avian influenza, caused by genetic variants of the H5N1 virus, erupted in geographically disseminated form in East Asia. From this early epicentre, the isochrones in **Figure 3.17** trace the rapid westwards spread of the virus in avian species to Siberia, Europe, the Middle East, and Africa by June 2006.

The epizootic wave

The rapid spatial expansion of the epizootic wave in **Figure 3.17** was linked to a rarely observed phenomenon in the epizootiology of avian influenza: the apparent ability of migratory wildfowl to carry H5N1 in a highly pathogenic form over extended distances, and to seed the virus along principal flyways. The first substantial evidence of the phenomenon came in late April 2005, when a mass die-off of some 6,000 migratory birds was recorded at the Qinghai Lake nature reserve (a major rendezvous and breeding site for birds on Asia–Siberia migratory routes) in central China. The source of H5N1 which sparked the die-off is unknown, although an importation with bar-headed geese (*Anser indicus*) arriving from areas of enzootic infection via one of the Asian flyways is suspected (Liu et al., 2005; Chen et al., 2006). From here, Qinghai-like viruses began to appear in northern and northwestern China, Mongolia, and, to the west, Siberia and the Black Sea region. The latter location, in turn, served as a bridgehead for the carriage of H5N1 by migratory waterfowl to countries of southern, central, and northern Europe, Eastern Mediterranean, and West Africa in the early months of 2006. At about the same time, outbreaks of H5N1 also began to be reported from parts of South Asia and the Middle East, including Afghanistan, India, Iran, Iraq, and Pakistan.

Human infections

Beginning in late October 2003—coincident with the inferred time of onset of the epizootic spread of H5N1 in domestic poultry in East Asia—sporadic human cases of severe respiratory illness began to present at hospitals in Hanoi and neighbouring provinces of northern Vietnam. Among the series of 14 suspicious cases, a 12-year-old girl from Ha Nam Province, admitted to hospital in Hanoi on 27 December, was subsequently identified as the first WHO-confirmed human case of avian influenza A (H5N1) associated with the nascent

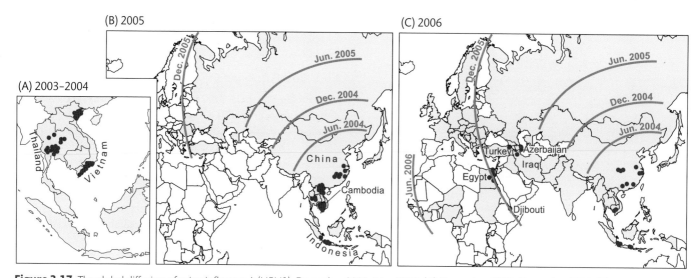

Figure 3.17 The global diffusion of avian influenza A (H5N1), December 2003–May 2006. (A) December 2003–December 2004. (B) January–December 2005. (C) January–May 2006. Countries in which avian influenza A (H5N1) had been confirmed in wild birds and/or poultry by the end of each time period are shaded blue. Isochrones show the approximate position of the epizootic wavefront at 6-monthly intervals. Circles plot, by time period, the geographical distribution of the 216 WHO-confirmed human cases of avian influenza A (H5N1) reported to 18 May 2006.
Redrawn from Smallman-Raynor and Cliff (2008, Figure 7, p. 568). Smallman-Raynor, M.R., Cliff, A.D. (2008). 'The geographical spread of avian influenza A (H5N1): Panzootic transmission (December 2003–May 2006), pandemic potential and implications.' *Annals of the Association of American Geographers*, 98, 553–82.

epizootic (World Health Organization, 2004).[1] From this putative beginning, a global total of 861 WHO-confirmed cases of human infection (including 455 deaths; case-fatality rate 53 per cent) had been documented from 17 countries of Asia and Africa by mid-October 2020 (World Health Organization, 2020a). The clinical and epidemiological dimensions of these human infections are outlined by Heymann (2015, pp. 313–22), where evidence consistent with bird-to-human, environment-to-human, and limited, non-sustained, human-to-human transmission (**Figure 3.18**) is summarized.

The circles in **Figure 3.17** plot the geographical incidence of the early WHO-confirmed human cases of H5N1 infection. Cases were confined to East Asia in the period to December 2004 (**Figure 3.17A**), with major clusters of disease activity in northern and southern Vietnam and central Thailand associated with strongly defined peaks of epizootic activity. Notwithstanding the rapid westwards movement of the epizootic wavefront, cases remained concentrated in East Asia in 2005 (**Figure 3.17B**), with Cambodia, Indonesia, and, by the end of year, China reporting their first confirmed human infections. Finally, trailing the epizootic wavefront, human cases of the disease were reported for the first time in countries of Europe (Azerbaijan and Turkey) and the Eastern Mediterranean (Djibouti, Egypt, and Iraq) in the period January–May 2006 (**Figure 3.17C**).

In deciphering the evolution of the disease pattern in **Figure 3.17**, Smallman-Raynor and Cliff (2008) note that the spatial pattern of human cases has tracked—albeit imperfectly—the spatial pattern of

poultry-based H5N1 outbreaks. Evidence of human infection due to contact with migratory waterfowl and other wild birds has been reported on only rare occasions (see, e.g. Gilsdorf et al., 2006), and no human cases of avian influenza A (H5N1) have been documented in countries for which outbreaks have been limited to wild bird species. Thus, the pattern highlights the pivotal role of poultry in the pan-continental extension of human infection with H5N1.

Epidemiological facets: age distribution

One especially noteworthy epidemiological feature of WHO-confirmed human cases of the disease is the skewed distribution towards children and young adults, with relatively few cases in older age categories (World Health Organization, 2006b). To illustrate the phenomenon, the box-and-whisker plots in **Figure 3.19** are based on a sample of 169 (77 males and 92 females) of the first 216 documented human cases and show the age distribution of patients by sex (A), year of report (B), patient outcome (C), and country (D). The mean age of the 169 sample cases was 19.8 years (median 18.0; range 0.3–75.0), with estimated age-specific case rates per million population of 0.15 (0–9 years), 0.15 (10–19 years), 0.13 (20–29 years), 0.08 (30–39 years), and 0.02 (≥40 years). The skewed age distribution is reflected in each field of **Figure 3.19**, with the third quartiles of the plots (Q_3, defined by the box tops) demarcating an age band (30–35 years) above which proportionally very few cases (<10 per cent overall) occurred.

Behavioural factors that increase the risk of H5N1 exposure in younger persons, including the engagement of children and young adults in the slaughter, de-feathering, and cooking of poultry, have been proposed by the WHO as one determinant of the skewed age distribution in **Figure 3.19** (World Health Organization, 2006b). Biological mechanisms, too, might account for the apparent selective demographic targeting of H5N1. A hyperactive immune response has been reported from studies of the pathogenesis of H5N1 in Vietnamese patients (de Jong et al., 2006) and might account for

[1] An earlier WHO-confirmed human case of avian influenza A (H5N1), with symptom onset on 25 November 2003, has been retrospectively identified by Chinese scientists. The patient (a 24-year-old male in military service) was hospitalized with a severe respiratory illness in Beijing, China, and died on 3 December 2003. It was initially suspected that the patient was infected with the SARS virus. Stored specimens from the man tested positive for H5N1 (Zhu et al., 2006).

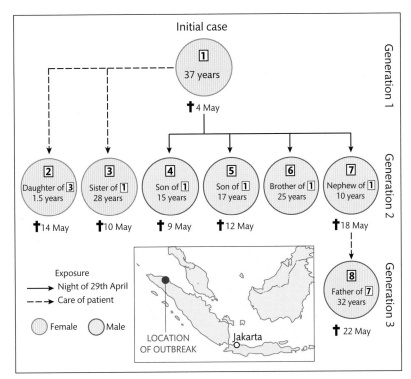

Figure 3.18 Extended family cluster of avian influenza A (H5N1) in the villages of Kubu Simbelang and Kabanjahe, North Sumatra, Indonesia, April–May 2006. Confirmed (n = 7) and probable (n = 1) cases are represented by circles (coded 1–8). The vectors indicate inferred routes of virus exposure. The age, date of death, and relationship of cases are indicated. The inset map gives the location of the cluster.

Reproduced from Smallman-Raynor, M.R., Cliff, A.D. (2008). 'The geographical spread of avian influenza A (H5N1): Panzootic transmission (December 2003–May 2006), pandemic potential and implications.' *Annals of the Association of American Geographers*, 98, 553–82, copyright © The Association of American Geographers, reprinted by permission of Informa UK Limited, trading as Taylor & Francis Group, www.tandfonline.com on behalf of The Association of American Geographers, www.aag.org. Source: Data from Butler, D. (2006). 'Family tragedy spotlights flu mutations.' *Nature*, 442, 114–15.

the apparently higher levels of severe disease in younger subjects. Finally, we note that a biological model of geographically widespread immunity in persons born prior to 1969 (i.e. ~35 years prior to the onset of the currently recognized epizootic in domestic poultry) might also account for some of the demographic pattern in **Figure 3.19** (Smallman-Raynor and Cliff, 2007).

Pandemic potential

This capacity of the H5N1 virus to cross the species barrier, and to cause severe disease and death in humans, has raised concerns over the pandemic potential of the virus. In the words of the late Dr Lee Jong-wook, former Director-General of WHO, the advent of the H5N1 virus moved the world 'closer to a further [influenza] pandemic than … at any time since 1968' (World Health Organization, 2005b, p. 3). In recognition of the heightened concern, WHO currently classifies the world at Phase 3 of the operative six-phase system of global pandemic alert for influenza as it relates to the H5N1 virus:

> In Phase 3, an animal or human-animal influenza reassortant virus has caused sporadic cases or small clusters of disease in people, but has not resulted in human-to-human transmission sufficient to sustain community-level outbreaks. Limited human-to-human transmission may occur under some circumstances, for example, when there is close contact between an infected person and an unprotected caregiver. However, limited transmission under such restricted circumstances does not indicate that the virus has gained the level of transmissibility among humans necessary to cause a pandemic. (World Health Organization, 2020b, unpaginated)

As Alvarado de la Barrera and Reyes-Terán (2005) observe, the occurrence of a pandemic of human influenza is dependent on three conditions: (i) a new influenza virus emerges, (ii) the new virus has the ability to cause disease in humans, and (iii) the new virus can spread from human to human in an efficient and sustained manner. The H5N1 virus currently meets conditions (i) and (ii), but not the transmissibility condition (iii). Reassortment events and adaptive mutation are generally recognized as the principal mechanisms by which increased transmissibility among humans might arise. As the WHO (2005a) observes, the risk that the H5N1 virus might acquire the ability to spread efficiently from human to human via either mechanism will persist as long as the opportunities for human infection occur. As the highly pathogenic H5N1 virus is now considered to be enzootic in avian species in some parts of Asia, this risk is likely to continue for the foreseeable future.

3.4.2 Severe Acute Respiratory Syndrome, 2003–04

Coronaviruses are a large group of viruses that, for the most part, circulate among bats, pigs, camels, cats, and some avian species. Occasionally, CoVs may spill over to humans. Several human CoVs are currently recognized, some of which are a common cause of mild upper respiratory tract infections (Song et al., 2019). Three human CoV diseases, however, have emerged in the last two decades that have been associated with potentially severe respiratory disease and death:

- SARS due to SARS-CoV, first identified in 2003.
- Middle East respiratory syndrome (MERS) due to MERS-CoV, first identified in 2012.

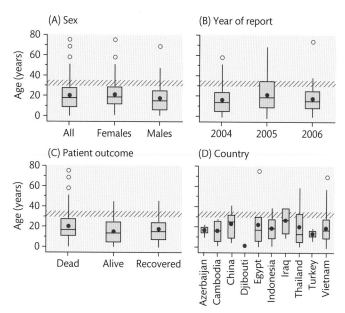

Figure 3.19 Age distribution of confirmed human cases of avian influenza A (H5N1), December 2003–May 2006. Box-and-whisker plots show the age distribution of cases by (A) sex, (B) year of report, (C) patient outcome, and (D) country. The horizontal line and bullet mark in each box give, respectively, the median and mean age of cases. The variability in age is shown by plotting, as the outer limits of the shaded box, the first and third quartiles, Q_1 and, Q_3, of the ages. Whiskers encompass all ages that satisfy the criteria $Q_1 - 1.5(Q_3 - Q_1)$ (lower limit) and $Q_3 + 1.5(Q_3 - Q_1)$ (upper limit). Points beyond the whiskers denote outliers. Information in graph (C) is based on the recorded status of patients according to WHO sources, with the category 'alive' formed to include patients that were last reported as hospitalized (alive) or discharged (recovered). The age category 30–35 years (shaded band) is marked on each graph for reference.

Reproduced from Smallman-Raynor, M.R., Cliff, A.D. (2007). 'Avian influenza A (H5N1) age distribution in humans.' *Emerging Infectious Diseases*, 13, 510–12.

- COVID-19 due to SARS-CoV-2, first identified in the latter months of 2019.

While MERS had been identified in 27 countries and had caused 866 recorded deaths worldwide as of 31 January 2020, human-to-human transmission has largely been restricted to family groups and healthcare settings and the associated virus has not threatened to spread in pandemic form (World Health Organization, 2020c). In contrast, the viruses associated with SARS and COVID-19 have demonstrated an ability for rapid and sustained human-to-human transmission and have sparked international epidemic (SARS) and pandemic (COVID-19) events. In the present section, we consider the international epidemic of SARS that occurred in 2002–03—the first and only recorded occurrence of the disease to date. The on-going global pandemic of COVID-19 is examined in Chapter 5.

The SARS outbreak

Severe acute respiratory syndrome was the first emerging infectious disease of the twenty-first century with the potential to become a global pandemic. It was caused by a previously unknown CoV subtype (SARS-CoV), which crossed the species barrier with subsequent human-to-human transmission. From November 2002 to July 2003, 8,096 SARS cases and 774 deaths were reported from

29 countries and areas. More than 95 per cent of cases occurred in 12 countries of the Western Pacific Region. Mainland China was the worst affected with 5,327 cases. Healthcare workers accounted for some 20 per cent of SARS cases worldwide. Globally, the case-fatality rate was estimated at around 15 per cent, increasing to more than 55 per cent for people above 60 years of age (Ahmad and Andraghetti, 2007).

The principal tools used to limit the spread of the SARS outbreak were contact tracing, quarantine, and isolation. Such traditional intervention methods had not been used on such a scale for several decades and legislative changes were required in many countries to facilitate the approach (Rothstein et al., 2003). The WHO was strongly interventionist in leading the global response. Over the longer run, as the characteristics of the causative CoV were established, it became clear that it had a relatively modest transmissibility between humans (basic reproductive number, R_0, of 2–5) when compared to some other disease agents (see Table 5.1 in Chapter 5) and that peak infectiousness followed the onset of clinical symptoms. These characteristics conspired to make the simple public health measures used initially, such as isolating patients and quarantining their contacts, very effective in the control of the epidemic (Anderson et al., 2004).

Geographical diffusion

Figures 3.20 and 3.21 show the geographical diffusion process. One of the index cases in the international spread process was a 72-year-old man. The patient had been taken ill on China Airways flight CA112 from Hong Kong to Beijing, China, on 15 March 2003. On the flight, he transmitted the SARS virus to a number of fellow travellers seated near him (**Figure 3.20A**) (Olsen et al., 2003; Whaley, 2006). The aircraft was a Boeing 737-300 which can typically carry up to 126 passengers; on this flight there were 112, with eight crew members. The index case had stayed at the Metropole Hotel in Hong Kong. Subsequent tracking confirmed that 22 fellow passengers and two crew members were infected by this index case, four of whom eventually died. Studies of other flights with SARS cases on board showed within-plane virus spread on only four of 35 flights, so CA112 may be viewed to be an extreme event on the virus spreading scale.

Rapid onwards spread of the virus occurred because many of the fellow travellers, now infected, flew on to Taipei, Singapore, Bangkok, and Inner Mongolia (**Figure 3.20C**). Onwards geographical spread continued so that, by May 2003, cases of SARS were occurring worldwide, driven by international air travel (**Figure 3.21**).

Intervention strategies

Perspectives on the SARS response at the global and national levels are provided by the WHO (2006a). In the absence of a vaccine or effective therapies, the options for intervention within a country were limited to public health measures. There are essentially six intervention categories, namely (i) restrictions on entry to the country and screening at the point of arrival for fever; (ii) isolation of suspected cases; (iii) the encouragement of rapid reporting to a healthcare setting following the onset of defined clinical symptoms, with subsequent isolation; (iv) rigorous infection control measures in healthcare settings; (v) restrictions on movements within a country (restricting travel, limiting congregations such as attendance at

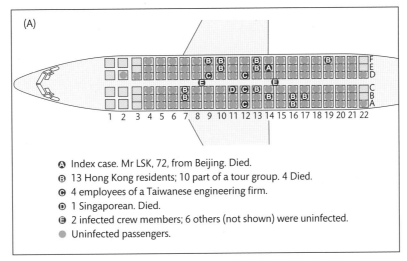

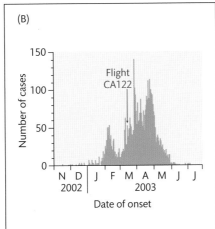

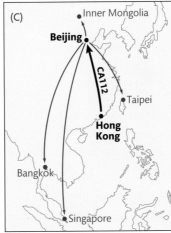

Figure 3.20 Pattern of SARS spread, 2003, by aircraft. (A) Contacts within an aircraft cabin. SARS infections on Flight CA112 from Hong Kong to Beijing, 15 March 2003. (B) SARS epidemic curve, November 2002–July 2003 showing fuelling of the curve by flight CA112 and its sequelae. (C) Subsequent movement of infected passengers.

Reproduced with permission from Cliff, A.D., Smallman-Raynor, M.R. (2013). *Infectious Disease Control: A Geographical Analysis from Medieval Quarantine to Global Eradication.* Oxford: Oxford University Press. Source: Data from Whaley, F. (2006). 'Flight CA112: Facing the spectre of in-flight transmission.' In: S. Omi (ed.), *SARS: How a Global Epidemic was Stopped.* Manila: WHO (Western Pacific Region), 149–54.

school); and (vi) contact tracing and isolation of contacts (Anderson et al., 2004; Ahmad and Andraghetti, 2007). **Figure 3.22** uses symbols and shading to indicate which interventions were used in each of the countries chiefly affected.

Affected countries fell into two distinct categories: *category 1*, countries with local SARS transmission (Canada, mainland China, Hong Kong, Singapore, Taiwan, and Vietnam) and *category 2*, countries with imported SARS cases (the United States, Thailand, Malaysia, and Australia). The category 1 countries recorded 98 per cent of the world's cases (Ahmad and Andraghetti, 2007, p. 7). Once the presence of SARS was realized, a number of mechanisms were implemented to control transmission in the affected countries. In addition to legislative responses that rendered SARS a notifiable disease, all countries set up SARS task forces and committees at the central and regional levels for coordinating intensified surveillance, response, and communication activities. In addition, with the exception of Vietnam and Canada, all the category 1 countries implemented mandatory quarantining of contacts; no category 2 countries did so. Category 1 countries instituted active tracing of close

contacts. Mandatory home quarantining of contacts of cases (actual and suspected) was commenced in category 1 except for Vietnam and Canada. Voluntary home quarantining occurred in Canada and category 2 countries. Vietnam implemented institutional quarantine at affected sites. Eventually, the various public health measures used were sufficient to cause the epidemic to die out in the middle of 2003.

3.4.3 Ebola Outbreaks in Africa

Ebola virus disease is a severe viral illness that was first recognized in the course of virulent outbreaks in the mid-1970s. The mode of transmission of Ebola virus is via person-to-person contact with infected blood, secretions, organs, or semen; healthcare workers are at high risk of infection. The period of communicability is as long as blood and secretions contain virus. Susceptibility appears to be general and observed case-fatality rates generally range between 30 and 90 per cent. Fruits bats are suspected to be a reservoir of Ebola virus although, in the case of epidemics, it has usually been possible to trace the source back to a human or non-human primate index case and no further (Heymann, 2015, pp. 173–8).

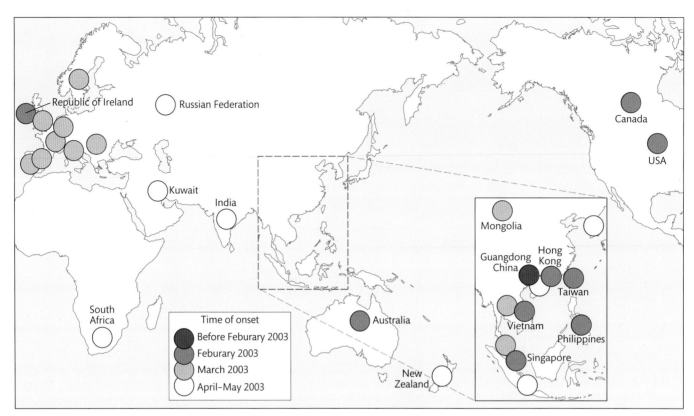

Figure 3.21 Global spread of SARS, November 2002–May 2003. Sequence of appearance of probable SARS cases in 29 countries and major administrative regions. Timings are based on the date of onset of the first recorded case in a given geographical area.

Reproduced with permission from Cliff, A.D., Smallman-Raynor, M.R. (2013). *Infectious Disease Control: A Geographical Analysis from Medieval Quarantine to Global Eradication.* Oxford: Oxford University Press. Source: Data from World Health Organization (2005c). *Summary of Probable SARS Cases with Onset of Illness from 1 November 2002 to 31 July 2003.* Geneva: WHO.

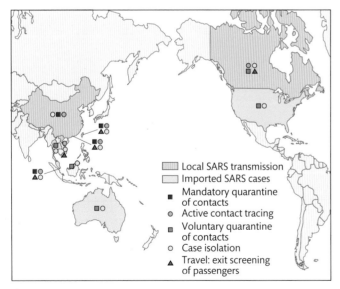

Figure 3.22 SARS control measures, 2002–03. Symbols and shading are used to indicate the main public health control measures adopted in each of the ten countries principally affected. There is a clear difference between countries with local SARS transmission, where mandatory quarantine and vigorous contact tracing were undertaken to try to break the chains of infection, and the more permissive approach in countries with solely imported cases.

Reproduced with permission from Cliff, A.D., Smallman-Raynor, M.R. (2013). *Infectious Disease Control: A Geographical Analysis from Medieval Quarantine to Global Eradication.* Oxford: Oxford University Press. Source: Data from Ahmad and Andraghetti (2007, Tables 1–7, pp. 13, 15, 17, 20–1, 23, 25, 27).

Ebola outbreaks in Africa: West Africa (2013–16)

Documented outbreaks under natural conditions have been limited to certain countries of the WHO Africa Region and Sudan (in the WHO Eastern Mediterranean Region). The disease was first recognized in 1976 when it caused near-simultaneous outbreaks associated with greater than 600 documented cases in two districts 150 km apart: (i) the Maridi region of southern Sudan and (ii) the Bumba Zone of Équateur province in northern Zaire (International Commission, 1978; WHO/International Study Team, 1978). With the exception of further limited occurrences in Zaire and Sudan in the late 1970s, Ebola virus largely retreated as the cause of documented human disease, re-emerging in the form of a series of outbreaks of varying magnitude from the mid-1990s (**Figure 3.23**). Then, in 2014, the first cases were reported to the WHO as the vanguard to the catastrophically large outbreak in West Africa. Although initial case reports occurred in March 2014, researchers in Guinea believe the index case actually occurred in December 2013 in the village of Meliandou, Guéckédou Prefecture, Guinea.

The Meliandou outbreak developed quickly from the index case (**Figure 3.24**) and, on 8 August 2014, 33 weeks into the longest, largest, and most widespread Ebola outbreak on record, the WHO declared the epidemic to be a Public Health Emergency of International Concern. As described by Briand et al. (2014, p. 1181), a Public Health Emergency of International Concern is an instrument of the International Health Regulations, a legally binding agreement made by 196 countries on the containment of major international health

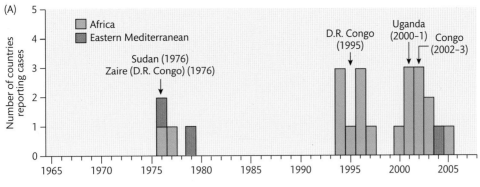

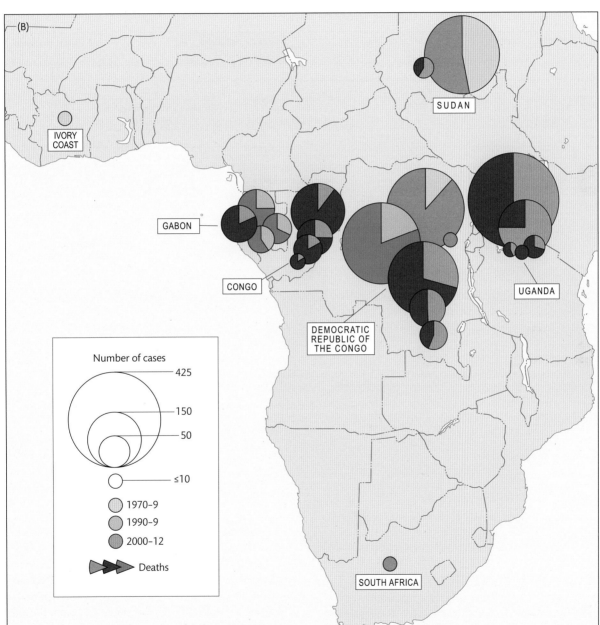

Figure 3.23 Ebola virus disease, 1976–2012: geographical and temporal patterns of reported outbreaks in Africa. (A) Number of countries reporting cases annually. (B) Location of outbreaks. Circle sizes are proportional to the number of reported cases with the proportion of deaths shown by the circle slices.

Reproduced with permission from Smallman-Raynor, M.R., Cliff, A.D. (2018). *Atlas of Refugees, Displaced Populations, and Epidemic Diseases. Decoding Global Geographical Patterns and Processes Since 1901.* Oxford: Oxford University Press.

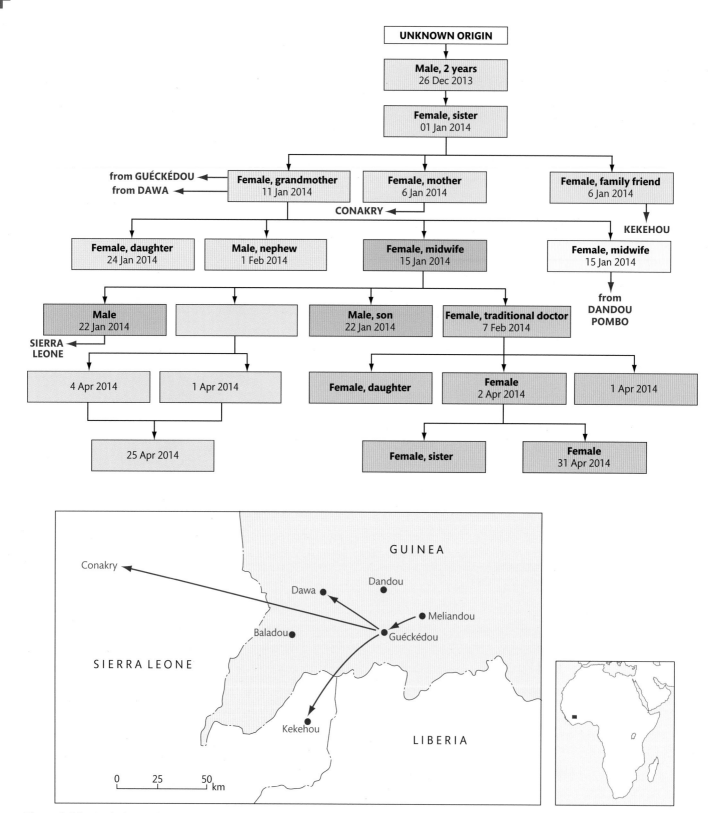

Figure 3.24 Guéckédou Prefecture, Guinea, West Africa: early stages of the West African outbreak of Ebola virus disease. (*Upper*) The diagram shows the person-to-person transmission chains of laboratory-confirmed cases of the disease from an index case in Meliandou Village, Guéckédou Prefecture, Guinea. Four generations of virus transmission are shown, ranging from early localized spread to later, longer-distance transmission outside the immediate source area and to other West African countries. Where known, spread within different family units is identified by different colour shadings. (*Lower*) Geographical realization of the contact tracing network.

Reproduced with permission from Smallman-Raynor, M.R., Cliff, A.D. (2018). *Atlas of Refugees, Displaced Populations, and Epidemic Diseases. Decoding Global Geographical Patterns and Processes Since 1901.* Oxford: Oxford University Press. Source: data from WHO Department of Pandemic and Epidemic Diseases. http://www.who.int/csr/disease/ebola/ebola-6-months/guinea/en/, accessed 6 December 2020.

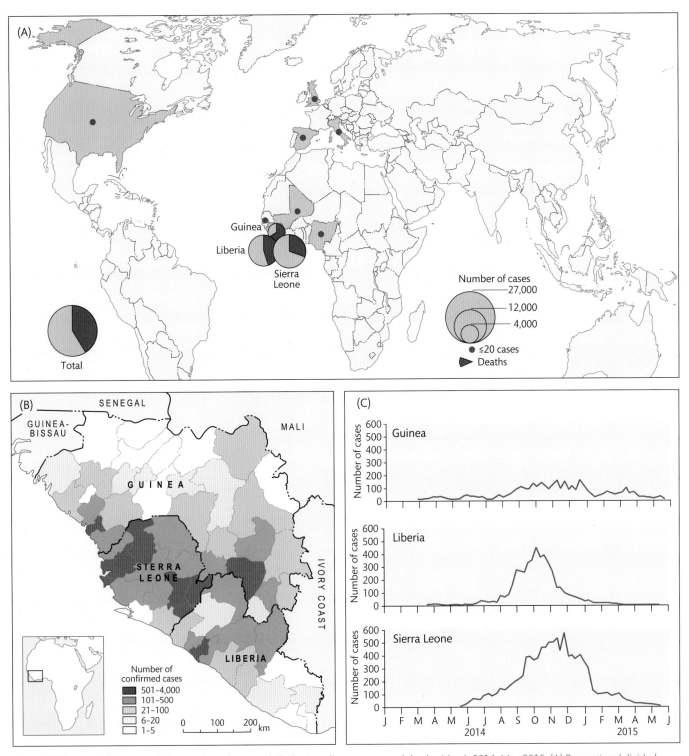

Figure 3.25 West Africa: cumulative number of reported Ebola virus disease cases and deaths, March 2014–May 2015. (A) Proportional divided circles are used to show the number of cases and deaths reported by all countries that have reported cases. (B) Choropleth shading is used to show the cumulative number of cases by district in the three principally affected countries (Guinea, Liberia, and Sierra Leone). (C) Temporal distribution of cases.

Reproduced with permission from Smallman-Raynor, M.R., Cliff, A.D. (2018). *Atlas of Refugees, Displaced Populations, and Epidemic Diseases. Decoding Global Geographical Patterns and Processes Since 1901.* Oxford: Oxford University Press. Source: Data from World Health Organization (2015a). *Ebola Situation Report, 6 May 2015.* Geneva: WHO. http://apps. who.int/ebola/en/current-situation/ebola-situation-report-6-may-2015

threats. By 31 May 2015, the cumulative number of confirmed, probable, and suspected cases had reached 27,181 with 11,162 deaths (Figure 3.25), and the epidemic had seriously affected three countries—Guinea, Liberia, and Sierra Leone. Six countries (Mali,

Nigeria, Senegal, Spain, the United Kingdom, and the United States) had reported a case or cases imported from a country with widespread and intense transmission, carried there by returning health workers and travellers. Among the core countries, the outbreak was officially declared to be over in Liberia on 9 May 2015, although the tail of the epidemic continued until June 2016.

In parallel with the West African outbreak, the seventh reported outbreak of Ebola virus disease in the equatorial African country of the Democratic Republic of Congo began on 26 July 2014. This simultaneity raised the question of whether the two outbreaks were linked, and this has been investigated by Maganga et al. (2014). The Democratic Republic of Congo outbreak began in Inkanamongo village in the vicinity of Boende town in Équateur province and was confined to that province. A total of 69 suspected, probable, or confirmed cases were reported between 26 July and 7 October 2014, including eight cases among healthcare workers, with 49 deaths. The reported weekly case incidence peaked in the weeks of 17 and 24 August and fell sharply thereafter. Genome sequencing indicated the outbreak to be caused by a local virus and was unrelated to the contemporaneous events in West Africa.

Future threats

Since the West African outbreak, several further Ebola outbreaks have been reported in sub-Saharan Africa. The most recent outbreak—and the second largest on record—ended in the Democratic Republic of Congo in late June 2020, having been associated with 3,470 cases and 2,287 deaths (World Health Organization, 2020d). While the cumulative total number of recorded human cases of Ebola virus disease is small in a global context, the potential threat from the disease is high (Feldmann, 2014). As seen in the West African outbreak of 2013–16, international importation of the disease into Europe and North America by healthcare workers and travellers has underlined the potential threat of the disease beyond the assumed endemic areas.

3.5 Conclusion: Looking Forwards to 'Disease X'

Such have been the recent concerns over the emergence of apparently new infectious diseases in the human population that, in 2015, the WHO began preparations for so-called Disease X—a placeholder name for a disease that had yet to appear in the human population and which could spread around the world and claim the lives of millions (see Table 1.6 in Chapter 1). Disease X now sits alongside a number of other emerging diseases (including COVID-19, Ebola and Marburg virus diseases, MERS and SARS, henipaviral diseases, Rift Valley fever, and Zika) as a priority for the WHO's 'R&D Blueprint' for preparedness and response to highly infectious pathogens (World Health Organization, 2020e). As described in this chapter, recent experience indicates that an understanding of the geographical processes that underpin the emergence and spread of new infectious diseases can only assist in anticipating and, ultimately, reducing the global threat posed by any future Disease X.

4

Pandemics, I
Pandemics in History

CONTENTS

4.1 Introduction

Despite being part of everyday vocabulary, the term 'pandemic' (from the Greek *pan* [all] + *-dēmos* [people]) defies a simple and commonly agreed definition (Morens et al., 2009). While the term is usually reserved in the scientific literature for certain infectious disease events, it has gained colloquial use in public health communications and the media to describe health events of a non-infectious aetiology (as in the 'obesity pandemic'). According to The International Epidemiological Association, a pandemic is defined as:

> An epidemic occurring over a very wide area, crossing international boundaries, and usually affecting a large number of people. Only some pandemics cause severe disease in some individuals or at a population level. (Porta, 2008, p. 209)

Thus a pandemic is imprecisely defined by its geographical extent and the size of the affected population, and it is independent of such considerations as severity, virology, and population immunity (Kelly, 2011).

4.1.1 Evolution of the Term Pandemic

One of the earliest references to a pandemic in the English language can be traced to 1666 and the first edition of Gideon Harvey's *Morbus Anglicus*. In this work, Harvey (1666, p. 3) used the term to describe the endemic nature of pulmonary tuberculosis ('which instances do evidently bring a Consumption under the notion of a Pan|demick, or Endemick … (a disease always reigning in a Countrey)'). Morens et al. (2009, p. 1018) note that, throughout the seventeenth and eighteenth centuries, 'the terms epidemic and pandemic were used vaguely and often interchangeably in various social and medical contexts' and it was only in the late nineteenth century that the term pandemic began to gain traction in its modern sense. August Hirsch (1883–86, Vol. I), for example, described a 'true pandemic' as an event that occurred 'over a great part of the globe', adding that 'influenza takes an exceptional place among the acute infective diseases; no other of them has shown so pronounced a pandemic character as influenza' (p. 18). According to the same source, other 'true' pandemic events included malarial diseases (e.g. in 1557–58, 1823–27, 1855–60), yellow fever (e.g. in 1796–98, 1819–20, 1839, 1852–53), and, perhaps more conventionally to a modern observer, cholera and plague (p. 228). A few years later, Creighton (1891–94, Vol. I, p. 402) applied the term to the 'universal epidemic' of influenza in 1557—'one of the great historical waves of influenza'. In the twenty-first century, the WHO has applied the term to the rapid global spread of such novel viral agents as influenza A (H1N1/09)

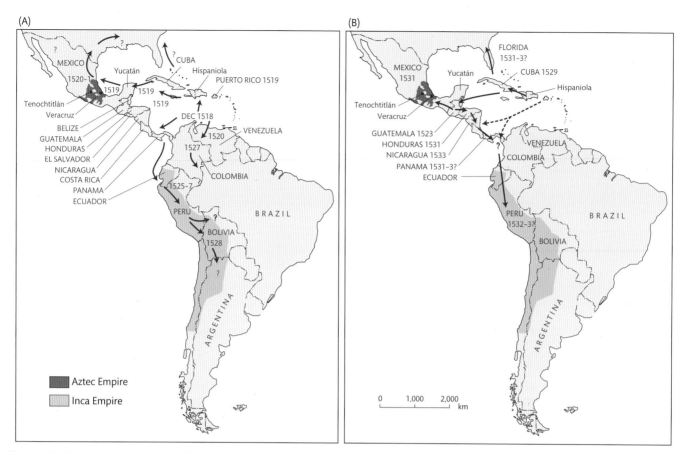

Figure 4.1 Epidemic transmission and the Spanish conquest of the Americas. Vectors trace the diffusion of the smallpox 'pandemic' of 1518–28 (A) and the measles 'pandemic' of 1531–34 (B). The geographical extents of the Aztec and Inca civilizations at about the time of European contact are indicated for reference.

Reproduced with permission from Smallman-Raynor, M.R., Cliff, A.D. (2004). *War Epidemics: An Historical Geography of Infectious Diseases in Military Conflict and Civil Strife, 1850–2000*. Oxford: Oxford University Press.

(2009–10) and SARS-CoV-2 (2020–) (World Health Organization, 2009, 2020f).

4.1.2 Pandemics in History

Accepting the imprecise definition of a pandemic, disease historians and others have described many infectious disease events of greater or lesser geographical extent as pandemic events. Popular listings of pandemics include, for example, the Plague of Athens (430–425 BC), the early-contact epidemics of smallpox and measles in the Americas in 1518–34 (Figure 4.1), and, as described in section 3.4.2 in Chapter 3, the international outbreak of SARS in 2003–04 (History.com, 2021). It remains the case, however, that certain diseases have become synonymous with the term pandemic in the epidemiological literature. These diseases are influenza, plague, cholera, HIV/AIDS, and, most recently, COVID-19. Table 4.1 provides a summary overview of 36 pandemics or probable pandemics of these five diseases over the last 15 centuries.

In forming Table 4.1, we note that the date brackets of some pandemic events vary from one source to another. This is especially noteworthy in the instance of cholera (see Cliff, Smallman-Raynor, Haggett et al., 2009, table 2.6, p. 85), for which the date brackets provided by Wilson and Miles (1975) have been adopted here. Subject to this caveat, the pandemic record begins with the 'Plague of Justinian' (First Plague Pandemic) in the sixth century AD, ends with

the ongoing (at the time of writing) global pandemics of HIV/AIDS and COVID-19, and includes 24 influenza, seven cholera, and three plague pandemics. The combined duration of these events is approximately 400 years, with the onset of a new pandemic occurring, on average, every 40–50 years. It is also apparent that the number of pandemic events increases substantially from around 1500 AD, with the onset of a new pandemic occurring, on average, every 10–20 years in the modern era. While this apparent acceleration in pandemic frequency may in part reflect the uncertainties that attach to the early disease record and the apparent paucity of events in the Middle Ages, it also reflects the increased opportunities for pandemic transmission in relation to factors such as international travel, global integration, and urbanization in the modern era; see sections 1.2.2 and 3.3.3 in Chapters 1 and 3, respectively.

Even the vaguest estimates of global morbidity and/or mortality are lacking for most of the events in Table 4.1. For some countries, however, it is possible to piece together sufficient information to provide a broad indication of relative severity. Thus, for those pandemics that are known to have affected England and Wales and for which relevant information is available, the right-hand columns in Table 4.1 give indicative estimates of deaths and death rates per 100,000 population. In terms of death rates, a full five orders of magnitude separate the least severe (influenza pandemic of 2009–10; 0.3 deaths per 100,000 population) from the most severe ('Black Death',

Table 4.1 Sample pandemic events in history

Year	Disease	Notes	England and Wales Deaths[1]	Death rate per 100,000
540s–590s	Plague	First Plague Pandemic ('Plague of Justinian'). Estimated 30–50 million deaths worldwide[2]	–	–
1330s–1380s	Plague	Second Plague Pandemic ('Black Death'). ~50 million deaths in Africa, Asia, and Europe[3]	1–3 million [est.]	20,000–60,000[4]
1510	Influenza	First recognition of influenza as a pandemic disease. 'Few recognized deaths'[5]	<400 [est.]	<15[6]
1557	Influenza	'One of the great historical waves of influenza'[7]; 'highly fatal'[8]	500–1,000 [est.]	15–30[6]
1580	Influenza	General diffusion over the East, in Africa and in Europe[9]; 'apparently highly fatal'[8]	<600 [est.]	<15[6]
1593	Influenza	General diffusion[9]	<700 [est.]	<15[6]
1729–30	Influenza	'May have become truly worldwide'[10]; 'high attack rates and high mortality'[11]	?	?
1732–33	Influenza	'Seemingly a general diffusion over the globe'[12]; 'high attack rates and high mortality'[11]	?	?
1761–62	Influenza	General diffusion[13]; 'by no means so severe or so fatal as the disease [influenza] of … 1733'[14]	<1,100 [est.]	<15[6]
1767	Influenza	Widely diffused over North America and Europe[13]; 'fatal to a very few old and infirm persons'[15]	<1,100 [est.]	<15[6]
1781–82	Influenza	General diffusion over the Eastern Hemisphere[16]; 'extremely high attack rates but negligible mortality'[11]	<1,200 [est.]	<15[6]
1788–89	Influenza	General diffusion over the Western Hemisphere (1789–1790)[16]	<1,200 [est.]	<15[6]
1802–3	Influenza	England and Wales—very mild disease[6]	<1,300 [est.]	<15[6]
1817–23	Cholera	First Cholera Pandemic. 100,000 deaths in Java, Indonesia[17]	–	–
1826–37	Cholera	Second Cholera Pandemic. ~230,000 deaths in Russia (1830–31).[18] ~150,000 deaths in Egypt (1831)[19]	21,641[20]	~170
1830–33	Influenza	General diffusion[21]; 'extremely high attack rates but low mortality'[11]	3,900–5,800 [est.]	30–45[6]
1836–37	Influenza	Diffusion in the Eastern Hemisphere[22]; 'extremely high attack rates but low mortality'[11]	2,100–4,200 [est.]	15–30[6]
1846–62	Cholera	Third Cholera Pandemic. In the United States (1849), death rate <10 per cent of the population[23]	73,390[24]	~450
1847–48	Influenza	Generally diffused over the Eastern Hemisphere[25]	12,844[26]	30–45[6]
1850–51	Influenza	Generally diffused over the Western and Eastern Hemispheres[25]	3,532[26]	<15[6]
1850s–1950s	Plague	Third Plague Pandemic. 10 million deaths in India to 1918[27]	–	–
1855	Influenza	General prevalence in Europe[28]	3,568[26]	15–30[6]
1857–58	Influenza	Wide diffusion over the Western and Eastern Hemispheres[29]	3,187[26]	<15[6]
1864–75	Cholera	Fourth Cholera Pandemic. >0.7 million deaths worldwide; ~50,000 deaths in the United States (1866)[30]	14,378[31]	~70
1874–75	Influenza	Widely spread over the Western and Eastern Hemispheres[32]	694[26]	<15[6]
1883–96	Cholera	Fifth Cholera Pandemic. ~60,000 deaths in Spain (1884); ~342,000 deaths in Russia (1892–93)[33]	–	–
1889–90	Influenza	'Russian influenza'. ~1.0 million estimated deaths worldwide[34]	4,578[26]	15–30[6]
1899–1923	Cholera	Sixth Cholera Pandemic. >3.3 million deaths in India (1900–09)[35]	–	–
1899–1900	Influenza	England and Wales—severe disease[6]	>14,400 [est.]	>45[6]
1918–19	Influenza	'Spanish' influenza. 25–50 million deaths worldwide[36]	180,000[37] [est.]	~480
1957–58	Influenza	'Asian' influenza. >1 million estimated deaths worldwide[38]	~20,000[38] [est.]	~48
1961–75	Cholera	Seventh (El Tor) Cholera Pandemic	–	–
1968–69	Influenza	'Hong Kong' influenza. 1–4 million estimated deaths worldwide[38]	~30,000[38] [est.]	~70
1981–	HIV/AIDS	~33.0 million deaths worldwide (1981–2019)[39]	21,029[40]	~40
2009–10	Influenza	~0.3 million estimated deaths worldwide[41]	138[42]	~0.3
2020–	COVID-19	~125.8 million cases and ~2.8 million deaths reported worldwide as of 27 March 2021[43]	116,880[44]	~197

[1] Recorded deaths unless indicated as estimates [est.]. [2] Than (2014). [3] World Health Organization (2000). [4] Hatcher (1994). [5] Morens, Taubenberger, et al. (2010, p. 1442). [6] Eichel (1922). [7] Creighton (1891–94, Vol. I, p. 402). [8] Taubenberger and Morens (2009, p. 190). [9] Hirsch (1883–86, Vol. I, p. 8). [10] Patterson (1986, p. 14). [11] Taubenberger and Morens (2009, p. 191). [12] Hirsch (1883–86, Vol. I, p. 9). [13] Hirsch (1883–86, Vol. I, p. 10). [14] Thompson (1852, p. 77). [15] Thompson (1852, p. 85). [16] Hirsch (1883–86, Vol. I, p. 11). [17] Pollitzer (1954, p. 429). [18] Kohn (1998, p. 272). [19] Shousha (1948, p. 353). [20] Creighton (1891–94, Vol. I, p. 13). [21] Hirsch (1883–86, Vol. I, pp. 821–2). [22] Hirsch (1883–86, Vol. I, p. 14). [23] Kohn (1998, p. 337). [24] Creighton (1891–94, Vol. II, pp. 843, 852). [25] Hirsch (1883–86, Vol. I, p. 16). [26] Parsons (1891, p. 3). [27] Kohn (1998, p. 261). [28] Hirsch (1883–86, Vol. I, p. 16). [29] Hirsch (1883–86, Vol. I, p. 17). [30] Kohn (1998, pp. 11–12). [31] Creighton (1891–94, Vol. II, p. 852). [32] Hirsch (1883–86, Vol. I, p. 17). [33] Kohn (1998, pp. 12, 273). [34] Shally-Jensen (2010, p. 1510). [35] Kohn (1998, pp. 13, 274). [36] Johnson and Mueller (2002). [37] Registrar-General for England and Wales (1920, pp. 3–7). [38] Honigsbaum (2020, p. 1824). [39] World Health Organization (2020g). [40] Public Health England (2020a), data for 1981–2018. [41] Liu, Kuo, and Shih (2020, p. 329). [42] Donaldson et al. (2009), pandemic-related deaths (June–November 2009). [43] World Health Organization (2020h). [44] United Kingdom Government (2020), cumulative to 27 March 2021.

Second Plague Pandemic; 20,000–60,000 deaths per 100,000 population) events. It is also apparent from **Table 4.1** that high-mortality events are relatively rare. So, in addition to the extreme instance of the 'Black Death', only four events were associated with death rates greater than 100 per 100,000 population: the cholera pandemics of 1826–37 (~170/100,000) and 1846–62 (~450/100,000), the 'Spanish' influenza pandemic of 1918–19 (~480/100,000), and, most recently, the COVID-19 pandemic (~197/100,000, to 27 March 2021). Most other pandemic events, including the majority of influenza pandemics, yielded death rates of well below 50 per 100,000 population.

Against this background, consecutive sections of the present chapter explore the pandemic geography of four of the five diseases in Table 4.1, namely plague (section 4.2), cholera (section 4.3), influenza (section 4.4), and HIV/AIDS (section 4.5). The novelty, severity, and dynamism of the COVID-19 pandemic lends it a special place in our treatment and is examined in Chapter 5.

4.2 Pandemic Plague

Plague is a zoonosis caused by the bacillus *Yersinia pestis*. The natural vertebrate reservoirs of *Y. pestis* are wild rodents. The disease in humans occurs as a result of (i) intrusion into the zoonotic (sylvatic) cycle, or (ii) by the entry of sylvatic rodents or their infected fleas into human habitats. It is widely assumed that the most frequent source of exposure resulting in human disease worldwide has been the bite of infected rodent fleas (especially *Xenopsylla cheopis*, the oriental rat flea). Recent studies, however, have pointed to the possible role of human ectoparasites (including the human flea and the body louse) as plague vectors in past times (Dean et al., 2018). Plague occurs in two major forms. Bubonic plague is caused by the bite of an infected flea and manifests as a painful swelling of the lymph glands ('buboes'). Bacteraemia and septicaemia often follow, as may secondary pneumonia. Primary pneumonic plague (contracted through exposure to the airborne exhalations of patients with primary pneumonic plague or the secondary pneumonia of bubonic plague) manifests as severe malaise, frequent cough with mucoid sputum, severe chest pains, and rapidly increasing respiratory distress. The incubation periods are usually 1–7 days (bubonic plague) and 1–4 days (primary pneumonic plague). Untreated bubonic plague has a case-fatality rate of 50–60 per cent; untreated primary pneumonic plague is almost invariably fatal (Heymann, 2015, pp. 456–65).

4.2.1 Early History

Human plague is a disease of considerable antiquity. References to plague-like diseases can be traced back to the twelfth century BC, while Jean-Pierre Papon, cited in Simpson (1905), provides a chronological list of 41 possible plague epidemics in the empires and nations of the Mediterranean Basin in the pre-Christian era. In later times, the 44th book of the *Collectanea* of Oribasius, dating from the fourth century AD, includes an excerpt from the writings of Rufus of Ephesus (*fl.* first century AD) that makes mention of a certain disease as '*pestilentes bubones maxime letales et acuti, qui maxime circa Libyam et Ægyptum et Syriam observantur*' (cited in Hirsch, 1883–86, Vol. I, p. 494). The accompanying clinical description leaves no doubt that the malady was bubonic plague, prompting Simpson (1905, p. 5) to conclude that:

> The evidence is sufficient to establish the fact that plague is of great antiquity and that it prevailed in Libya, Egypt, and Syria at an early period of the world's history when these countries on the southern and eastern shores of the Mediterranean played a leading part in the civilisation of the day and their towns were important centres of commerce.

Consistent with these observations, an examination of the archaeoentomological, archaeozoological, and biogeographical evidence led Panagiotakopulu (2004) to hypothesize that Pharaonic Egypt was the most probable place of origin of bubonic plague as an epidemic disease.

While the plague epidemics of antiquity appear to have been relatively geographically confined, the history of the disease from the early Middle Ages is dominated by three great pandemic cycles, each of 50–100 years' duration and each resulting in the spread of *Y. pestis* across much of the civilized world.

4.2.2 The First Plague Pandemic: The Plague of Justinian (540s–590s)

The sixth century AD is generally recognized as marking the first pandemic cycle of human bubonic plague. An eyewitness account of the emergence and initial spread of the pandemic and its particular coincidence with Byzantine military operations during Emperor Justinian's wars with the Goths and the Persians is provided by the Byzantine historian, Procopius (AD *c.*500–?). According to Procopius, plague first came to light among the Egyptians at Pelusium in 541. From there, the disease:

> divided and moved in one direction towards Alexandria and the rest of Aegypt, and in the other direction it came to Palestine on the borders of Aegypt; and from there it spread over the whole world … And this disease always took its start from the coast, and from there went up to the interior. (Procopius, ii.22, transl. Dewing, 1914, p. 455)

Plague reached Byzantium in the spring of 542 where, during the height of the 4-month visitation, 'the tale of the dead reached five thousand each day, and again it even came to ten thousand and still more than that' (Procopius, ii.23, transl. Dewing, 1914, p. 465).

It seems reasonable to infer that the epidemic spread outwards from Byzantium with the movements of soldiers who were deployed in operations against the Italian Goths to the west and the Persians to the east; see Kohn (1998). We learn from Procopius that plague 'fell … upon the land of the Persians and visited all the other barbarians besides' (Procopius, ii.23, transl. Dewing, 1914, p. 473). The same source (ii.24) cites the appearance of the disease among the former peoples both as a precipitating factor in Persian efforts to treat for peace in 543 and as an immediate spur for the Roman Byzantine forces to invade Persarmenia. More generally, Russell (1972) suggests that the epidemic resulted in a contraction of the European Mediterranean population by some 25 per cent. With later recrudescences, the pandemic caused a regional population decline of some 50–60 per cent in the period to 570 and it has been viewed as a major contributor to the political and military decline of the classical Mediterranean civilizations.

4.2.3 The Second Plague Pandemic: The Black Death (1330s–1380s)

In terms of its grip on the public imagination, the Black Death remains one of the most visible symbols of the power and influence of

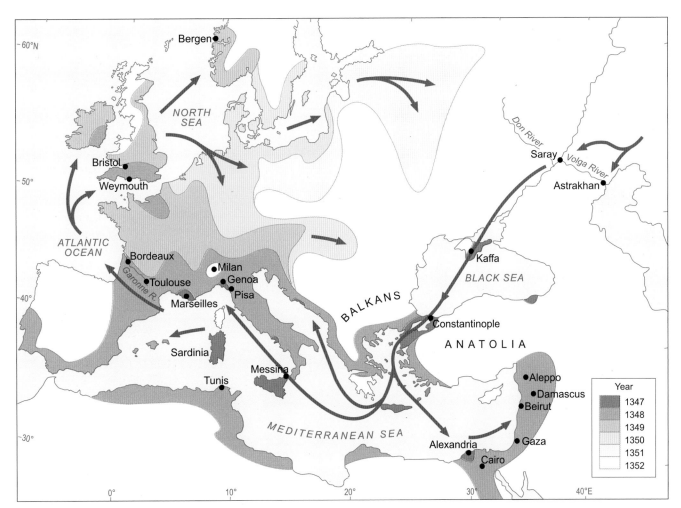

Figure 4.2 Spread of the Black Death, 1347–52. Vectors show the main routeways by which bubonic plague diffused from Central Asia, via the Ukrainian city of Kaffa, to the Mediterranean and Northern Europe. The Mongol–Italian conflict of the mid-1340s, centred on the Genoan occupation of Kaffa, facilitated the spread of the disease from the Black Sea to the Mediterranean ports of Genoa, Venice, and elsewhere.
Reproduced from Cliff, A.D., Haggett, P., Smallman-Raynor, M.R. (2004). *World Atlas of Epidemic Diseases*. London: Arnold.

epidemic disease. In 1346, Europe, Northern Africa, and the Levant (the westward parts of the Middle East) had a population of the order of 100 million (McEvedy, 1988). Within a decade, nearly a quarter of them had died and the population rise that had marked the evolution of medieval society had come to an abrupt end. Although not all historians agree, the cause of what was known as the Great Dying or the Great Pestilence (it was only later that the term 'Black Death' emerged) is generally accepted to have been *Y. pestis* which, a full eight centuries after its first pandemic cycle in the human population, again spread across the Eurasian landmass (Raoult et al., 2000).

The spatial origins and full geographical extent of the Black Death still remain to be determined. There are two main competitors for the dubious honour of being the source: (i) an origin east of the Caspian, possibly in eastern Mongolia, Yunnan, or Tibet; and (ii) an origin south of the Caspian in Kurdistan or Iraq. The first is suggested by Arabic sources and by the fact that plague is still enzootic there in various populations of wild rodents. From either of these sources, plague might have spread along the Mongol trade routes east to China, south to India, and west to the Black Sea ports.

Whatever the dispute about the origins, the westward trajectory of the pandemic into and across Europe is well established

(**Figure 4.2**). It reached the Crimea from Central Asia in the winter of 1346–47 and Constantinople by early spring 1347. From there, it moved in two directions: (i) counter-clockwise into the Eastern Mediterranean and the Levant and (ii) clockwise through the western Mediterranean and Europe. As the time-contours in **Figure 4.2** indicate, most of Europe was affected before the main wave of the pandemic finally subsided in 1352.

4.2.4 The Third Plague Pandemic (1850s–1950s)

The several centuries of heightened outbreak activity that followed the Second Plague Pandemic (1330s–1380s) were superseded, from the mid-eighteenth century, by an apparent geographical retreat of *Y. pestis* to permanent enzootic foci in Central Asia and East Africa. The period of epidemiological quiescence, however, came to an end in the latter half of the nineteenth century as the disease re-emerged in the form of the Third Plague Pandemic.

The global diffusion of the Third Plague Pandemic is reconstructed in **Figure 4.3**. The ultimate origin of the pandemic can be traced to west Yunnan, China—part of the vast enzootic focus of the disease in the Central Asia Highland—in the mid-1850s. From here, plague spread slowly at first, through China, eventually to

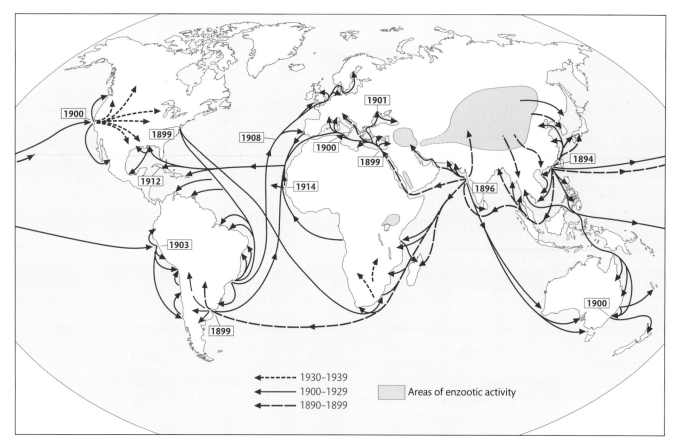

Figure 4.3 Global spread of the Third Plague Pandemic, 1850s–1950s. Vectors show the diffusion of plague from permanent enzootic foci in Central Asia and East Africa.

Reproduced with permission from Smallman-Raynor, M.R., Cliff, A.D. (2012). *Atlas of Epidemic Britain: A Twentieth Century Picture*. Oxford: Oxford University Press. Source: Data from Rodenwaldt and Jusatz (1954–61, Map III/87).

reach the port cities and international shipping hubs of Canton and Hong Kong in 1894. Details of the subsequent rapid global spread of the disease from these centres are provided by Pollitzer (1954) and Rodenwaldt (1952–61) but, fuelled by late nineteenth-century developments in the size, speed, and efficiency of steamships, Figure 4.3 shows that plague had circumnavigated the world by 1910. As Raettig (1954–61, p. III/33) observes of this period: 'New foci of sylvan plague arose everywhere ... lying between 20°C summer isotherms of the northern and southern hemispheres and in which it was possible for the plague causative agents to be transmitted from the rats of the harbour towns to the wild rodents in the vast steppes and semi-desert regions.'

The global time series of reported plague cases associated with the main phase of pandemic transmission, 1899–1953, is plotted in **Figure 4.4**. The curve displays a rapid growth to a sharp peak in 1911, with pronounced fluctuations superimposed on a steady and progressive decline in reported disease incidence over the next several decades. By the 1950s, Raettig (1954–61, p. III/33) could report that the pandemic was finally drawing to a close: 'Statistics of the infection show that the prognosis is a favourable one, as plague is receding in all the foci which are still active. The vast pandemia ... is dying out.' A final assessment of the overall mortality due to the pandemic is precluded by the fragmentary nature of the available

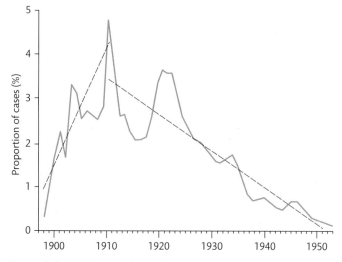

Figure 4.4 Global curve of annual plague incidence, 1899–1953. Annual counts of plague cases are expressed as a percentage proportion of all cases in the 55-year observation period. Underpinning trends are indicated for the periods 1899–1911 and 1911–53 by the broken lines.

Reproduced from Raettig, H. (1954–61). 'The plague pandemic of the 20th century.' In: E. Rodenwaldt and H.J. Jusatz (eds.), *Welt-Seuchen-Atlas: World-Atlas of Epidemic Diseases*. Parts II and III. Hamburg: Falk-Verlag, III/33.

evidence, although a global figure of greater than 10 million deaths—mainly in Asia—is cited by Khan (2004).

4.3 Pandemic Cholera

Classic Asiatic cholera (International Classification of Diseases, tenth revision (ICD-10) diagnostic code A00) is a severe, often rapidly fatal, diarrhoeal disease produced by the bacterium *Vibrio cholerae*. Transmission of the bacterium usually occurs via the ingestion of faecally contaminated water and, less commonly, food. As regards its clinical course, an incubation period of 2–5 days is usually followed by the sudden onset of diarrhoea and vomiting, giving rise to massive fluid loss and dehydration. Consequent symptoms include cramps, a reduction in body temperature and blood pressure leading to shock, and, ultimately, death within a few hours or days of symptom onset. Mortality is typically witnessed in 40–60 per cent of untreated cases (Heymann, 2015, pp. 102–8).

The alkaline soils and water of the Ganges–Brahmaputra delta region of northeastern India form the natural locus of *Vibrio cholerae*, an area whose fertility has ensured historically high population densities. As Tauxe (1998) observes, the bacterium is well adapted to the estuarine environment of the delta region and is likely to have been endemically established for many centuries prior to the sequence of pandemic upwellings in the nineteenth century.

4.3.1 Pre-Pandemic History: Asiatic Cholera Prior to 1817

The early (pre-pandemic) history of cholera is reviewed by Hirsch (1883–86, Vol. I), Pollitzer (1959), and Barua (1992), among others. While Sanskrit accounts of cholera or cholera-like illnesses can be deciphered in the writings of Hindu medicine, these and other ancient and medieval notices fail to mention the epidemic character of the disease. Beginning in the early sixteenth century, however, European visitors provide evidence of epidemic cholera over much of India. 'Incomplete or even fragmentary though the evidence … often is,' Pollitzer (1959, p. 16) observes, 'it leaves no room for doubt that cholera, present in India since ancient times, not only continued to exist but was apt to manifest itself periodically in widespread conflagrations.' Even then, the weight of evidence adduced by Hirsch (1883–86, Vol. I) and Pollitzer (1959) indicates that true Asiatic cholera remained largely confined to India and proximal countries prior to 1817.

4.3.2 The Nineteenth-Century Pandemics

The year 1817 marked 'a new epoch in the history of cholera' (Pollitzer, 1959, p. 17). In that year, cholera began to spread as the first in a series of six great pandemic waves that, during the nineteenth century, would extend across much of the inhabited world (Figure 4.5). The earliest reliable information relating to the spread of the first pandemic can be traced to the Ganges–Brahmaputra delta region of India, where the disease had attained epidemic proportions by the late summer of 1817. Cholera diffused over the 'greater part' of India in the course of the following year (MacNamara, 1876, p. 52) with onwards transmission, across the borders of indigenous territory, for Ceylon, Burma, Siam, Mauritius, and Réunion by 1819. Thereafter, the disease penetrated East Africa, Arabia, Persia, and, by way of the latter, Astrakhan in non-European Russia. The actions

of the authorities at Astrakhan served to halt the further advance of cholera towards European soil and, with the onset of the winter of 1823–24, the pandemic finally retreated from Central Asia and other extra-Indian locations. Thereafter, the disease spread in pandemic form on five further occasions in the nineteenth and early twentieth centuries (Table 4.1). These pandemics travelled on each occasion from India into Asia and Europe via the great trade routes to create the pandemic pathways plotted by the heavy vectors on the maps in Figure 4.5. On each occasion, certain common factors conspired to accelerate the progression of the pandemics over greater or lesser areas. The annual pilgrimages to Mecca (Hajj) were one such factor, as were major conflicts such as the Crimean War and the Austro-Prussian War.

4.3.3 The Seventh (El Tor) Cholera Pandemic (1961–)

The year 1961 marked the spread, apparently for the first time, of the El Tor biotype of *V. cholerae* serogroup O1 as a pandemic infection. While each of the preceding six pandemics of the nineteenth century had originated in the Indian subcontinent, the source of the El Tor pandemic can be traced to the Indonesian island of Sulawesi. Epidemics of El Tor cholera were first observed in southern Sulawesi in 1937–38 and, again, in 1939–40, 1944, and 1957–58. Beginning in 1960–61, outbreak activity began to extend to the north of the island and on to other parts of the Indonesian archipelago (Mukerjee, 1963; Hermann, 1973). From thereon, Figure 4.6 shows that the El Tor pandemic spread to mainland Asia (1960s) and subsequently to Africa (1970s) and Europe (1970s). The appearance of the disease in the Americas (1990s) marked the end of a cholera-free period of over 100 years and was associated with an explosive upsurge in cases. Major epidemics were also recorded in Africa in the 1990s, with the African continent emerging as the primary regional focus of reported cholera activity by the early twenty-first century. Kaper et al. (1995) cite the following factors that contributed to the extensive spread of El Tor cholera after 1961: (i) the enhanced capacity for El Tor vibrios to survive in environmental niches, (ii) the relatively mild nature of El Tor cholera and the high frequency of asymptomatic excretors, and (iii) the heightened opportunities for disease dispersal with air passenger traffic.

4.4 Pandemic Influenza

The emergence of novel subtypes of influenza A virus, to which the human population has little or no existing immunity, underpins the great pandemics of influenza that have periodically rolled around the world (Table 4.2). Historically, these events have been associated with large—sometimes massive—population losses. At an extreme, the 'Spanish' influenza pandemic of 1918–19 is estimated to have killed 20–50 million or more worldwide (Jordan, 1927; Johnson and Mueller, 2002). Other influenza pandemics have resulted in more modest death tolls, with the combined global excess mortality due to the so-called Asian (1957–58) and Hong Kong (1968–69) pandemics estimated at several million (World Health Organization, 2005b). Whatever the associated mortality, however, the broader social and economic impacts of pandemic influenza are always substantial. The overloading of health services, high levels of worker absenteeism, the disruption of essential services, and the interruption

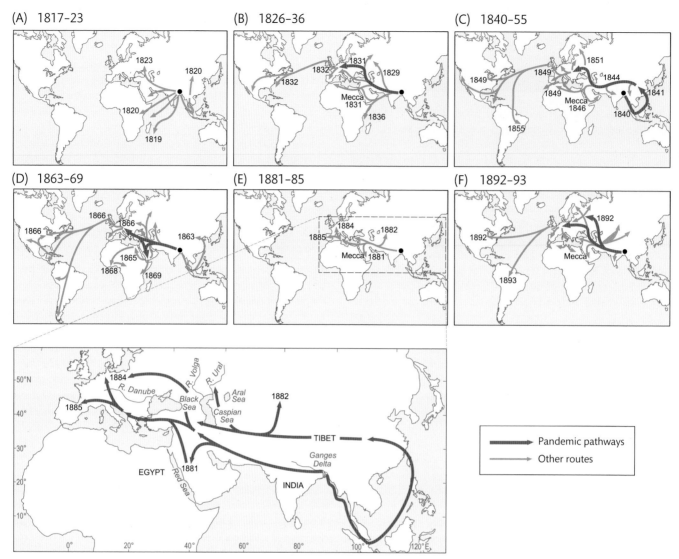

Figure 4.5 Cholera pandemics in the nineteenth century. Vectors show the diffusion of cholera associated with the first pandemic (1817–23; map (A)), and sample phases of diffusion associated with subsequent pandemics (B–F). The last map is an enlargement of the boxed area in (E). The regularly followed pandemic pathways are shown by the heavy vectors.

Reproduced from Cliff, A.D., Haggett, P., Smallman-Raynor, M.R. (2004). *World Atlas of Epidemic Diseases*. London: Arnold.

of trade and commerce underline the status of influenza pandemics as global public health emergencies (Gust et al., 2001).

4.4.1 Pandemic Origins

Influenza A viruses are defined by the expression of their surface proteins, haemagglutinin (H) (governing the ability of the virus to bind to, and enter, host cells) and neuraminidase (N) (governing the release of new virus particles from host cells). Antigenic changes in these proteins permit influenza A viruses to bypass existing immunity in the human host so that repeat infection and associated illness can occur. Antigenic changes are of two types: (i) frequent but minor *drifts* that result from the accumulation of mutations in the surface proteins and which yield influenza epidemics and (ii) infrequent but major *shifts* that result in the emergence of novel surface proteins and which yield influenza pandemics (Glezen and Couch, 1997). Virus subtypes associated with pandemics since the late nineteenth century are given in Table 4.2. One of the dramatic features

of these documented virus shifts is the rapidity with which the new subtype becomes dominant and replaces the old as the main virus in circulation.

The cause of antigenic shifts in influenza A virus is not fully understood. Among the competing hypotheses (Oxford, 2000), current evidence suggests that avian influenza viruses (influenza viruses for which birds are the natural reservoir; see, for example, section 3.4.1 in Chapter 3) might play a pivotal role in the evolutionary process. In short, a new pandemic strain might emerge when an influenza A virus, possessing novel viral genes from an avian source, appears in the human population (de Jong and Hien, 2006). Two principal mechanisms by which this might occur are generally recognized:

1. *Reassortment events*, in which genetic material is exchanged between avian and human influenza A viruses during co-infection in 'reassortment vessels' (e.g. pigs or humans). This process is believed to have underpinned the emergence of the virus subtypes

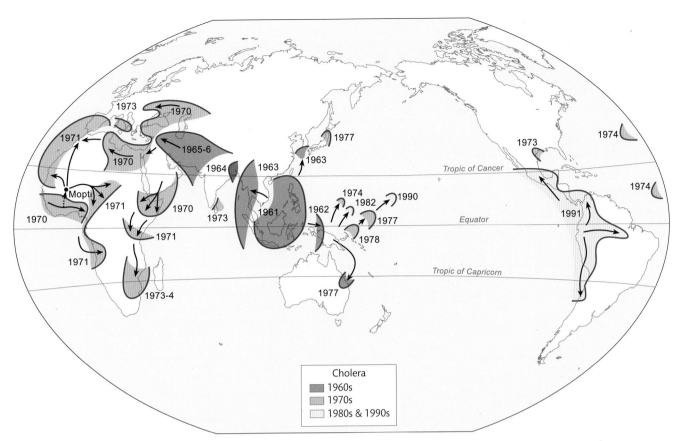

Figure 4.6 The Seventh Cholera Pandemic (El Tor biotype). The maps show the global spread of the seventh pandemic of cholera from an Indonesian source.

Reproduced with permission from Barua, D., Greenough, W.B. (1992). *Cholera*. New York: Plenum.

associated with the Asian (H2N2) and the Hong Kong (H3N2) pandemics.

2. *Adaptive mutation*, whereby an avian influenza A virus develops, through a process of genetic adaptation, an enhanced ability to bind to human cells. This process is believed to have underpinned the emergence of the virus subtype associated with the 'Spanish' (H1N1) pandemic of 1918–19.

The 'influenza epicentre' hypothesis

The hypothesis that Asia in general—and southern China in particular—might be a source of new pandemic strains of influenza A virus is outlined by Shortridge and Stuart-Harris (1982) and Shortridge (1992). Informed by the apparent emergence of the Asian (1957–58) and Hong Kong (1968–69) pandemics in Southeast Asia, the 'influenza epicentre' hypothesis is founded on (i) the high diversity of avian influenza viruses that circulate in aquatic and terrestrial birds in the region and (ii) the existence of intensive rice/duck/pig farming systems and live animal markets. Together these factors are viewed as providing ideal opportunities for the cross-species transfer and reassortment of influenza viruses and their genes—in a part of the world with massive, densely packed human populations in which any new strain might take hold. The influenza epicentre hypothesis has gained particular prominence with the emergence and spread of highly pathogenic avian influenza A (H5N1) in China and other countries of East Asia (see section 3.4.1 in Chapter 3). It remains the case, however, that some twentieth- and early

twenty-first-century pandemic strains of influenza A (including the 1918–19 and 2009–10 H1N1 viruses) appear to have first emerged in other parts of the world.

4.4.2 The Pandemic Record

Perspectives on the early history of influenza are provided by Hirsch (1883–86, Vol. I, pp. 7–54) and Clemow (1889–90). Consistent with the discussion in section 3.2 in Chapter 3, biological inference leads Crosby (1993) to suggest that the disease was unlikely to have been common in the period prior to the developments in agriculture, nucleated settlements, and human–animal relations that occurred some 5,000–10,000 years ago. Even then, Clemow (1889–90, p. 359) submits that it is 'almost impossible' to verify the occurrence of influenza in the pre-Christian era. Hippocrates records an epidemic in 400 BC or thereabouts ('Cough of Perinthus') that could have been influenza. Several years earlier, in 415 BC, the epidemic that struck the Athenian army during its campaign in Sicily has been adduced by some as influenza. In the Christian era, Clemow (1889–90) provides several instances of influenza-like epidemics in the sixth to eleventh centuries, although Hirsch (1883–86, Vol. I, p. 7) argues that many such early references 'bear a stamp too little characteristic' of the disease.

Pandemics since AD 1500

Table 4.2 is based, in part, on the combined evidence of Hirsch (1883–86, Vol. I) and Patterson (1986) and provides summary

Table 4.2 Pandemics and probable pandemics of influenza, 1500–2020

Year(s)	Source of information[a]		Interval since previous pandemic (years)	Influenza A subtype	England and Wales[b]	
	Hirsch (1883–86)[c,d]	Patterson (1986)[e]			Deaths (estimated)	Death rate (per 100,000)
1510	+		?	?	<400	<15
1557	+		47	?	500–1,000	15–30
1580	+		23	?	<600	<15
1593	+		13	?	<700	<15
1729–30		+	136	?	?	?
1732–33	+	+	2	?	?	?
1761–62	+		28	?	<1,100	<15
1767	+		5	?	<1,100	<15
1781–82	+	+	14	?	<1,200	<15
1788–89		+[f]	6	?	<1,200	<15
1802–03	+		13	?	<1,300	<15
1830–33	+	+[g]	27	?	3,900–5,800	30–45
1836–37	+	+[f]	3	?	2,100–4,200	15–30
1847–48	+		10	?	~13,000	30–45
1850–51	+		2	?	~3,500	<15
1855	+		4	?	~3,600	15–30
1857–58	+		2	?	~3,200	<15
1874–75	+		16	?	~700	<15
1889–90		+	14	H2?	~4,600	15–30
1899–1900		+	9	H3?	>14,400	>45
1918–19		+	18	H1N1	~180,000	~480
1957–58		+	38	H2N2	~20,000	~48
1968–69		+	10	H3N2	~30,000	~70
2009–10			40	H1N1/09	~140	~0.3

[a] Pandemics and probable pandemics are indicated '+' according to the source of information. Note that the 'Russian' influenza (H1N1) of 1977, which is occasionally classified as a pandemic event, has been excluded on account of the similarities of the causative agent to previously circulating A/H1N1 viruses. [b] For pandemics prior to the twentieth century, death rates are based on estimates from Eichel (1922). [c] Years 1500–1875. [d] Events listed by Hirsch (1883–86, Vol. I) as having spread in 'truly pandemic form' (p. 18) and excluding 'pandemics' that were apparently limited to the Western Hemisphere (1647, 1737–38, 1757–58, 1761–62, 1789–90, 1798, 1807, 1815–16, 1824–26, 1843, and 1873). [e] Years 1700–1977. [f] 'Probable' pandemic. [g] Patterson (1986) defines separate pandemic events in the years 1830–31 and 1833.

Source: Data from Cliff, A.D., Smallman-Raynor, M.R., Haggett, P., Stroup, D.F., Thacker, S.B. (2009). *Infectious Diseases. Emergence and Re-emergence: A Geographical Analysis.* Oxford: Oxford University Press.

details of influenza pandemics and probable pandemics in the period since AD 1500. According to Hirsch (1883–86, Vol. I, pp. 18–19):

> In truly pandemic form, we meet with authentic influenza in the years 1510, 1557, 1580, 1593, 1767, 1781–82, 1802–3, 1830–33, 1836–37, 1847–48, 1850–51, 1855, 1857–58, and 1874–75; in several of these pandemics, the disease extended not only over the Eastern Hemisphere, but it reached also to the Western; in others it remained limited to the former; while pandemics are known to have occurred exclusively in the Western Hemisphere in the years 1647, 1737–38, 1757–58, 1761–62, 1789–90, 1798, 1807, 1815–16, 1824–26, 1843, and 1873. (Hirsch, 1883–86, Vol. I, pp. 18–19)

Consistent with this summary, Morens, Taubenberger, et al. (2010) identify AD 1510 as marking the first recognition of influenza as a pandemic disease. In this year, eyewitness accounts attest to the influenza having 'spread to almost all the countries and the whole world [excepting the New World]' (Morens, North, and Taubenberger, 2010, p. 1895). From thereon, the available evidence

points to 24 pandemic and probable pandemic events in the last 500 or so years (Table 4.2). These events occurred on a highly irregular basis, with an average spacing of 21 years (range 2–136 years) and with a noteworthy absence of evidence of pandemic activity in the 1600s (Thompson, 1852). Finally, as evidenced by the sample information for England and Wales, a further noteworthy feature of Table 4.2 is the high degree of variability in the severity of the pandemic events. Thus, estimated death rates per 100,000 population varied from approximately 0.3 (2009–10 pandemic) to approximately 480 (1918–19 pandemic), but with a general tendency for relatively mild events (<15 deaths per 100,000 population) over the 500-year time span.

The maps in **Figure 4.7** are based on the analysis of Patterson (1986) and reconstruct the spatial diffusion of sample influenza pandemics in the European continent, 1700–1849. Each pandemic wave spread in a characteristic east → west direction, beginning in European Russia and diffusing across the continent as a well-defined wavefront, eventually to reach Iberia after an average

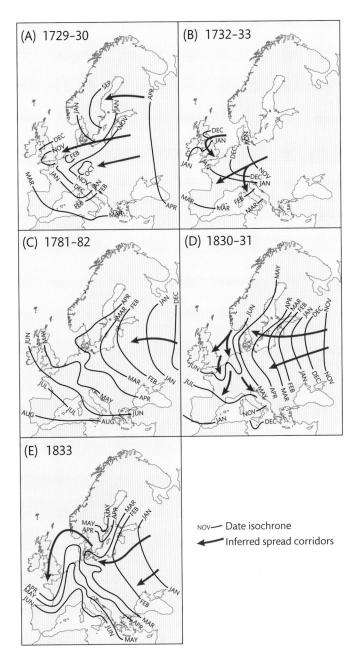

Figure 4.7 Diffusion of pandemic influenza in Europe, 1700–1849. Maps plot the diffusion of five pandemic waves of influenza identified by Patterson (1986) in the interval 1700–1849 (Table 4.2). (A) 1729–30. (B) 1732–33. (C) 1781–82. (D) 1830–31. (E) 1833. The pandemic waves of 1830–31 and 1833 form part of a single pandemic event (1830–33) for the purposes of Tables 4.1 and 4.2.

Reproduced with permission from Cliff, A.D., Smallman-Raynor, M.R., Haggett, P., Stroup, D.F., Thacker, S.B. (2009). *Infectious Diseases. Emergence and Re-emergence: A Geographical Analysis.* Oxford: Oxford University Press. Source: Data from Patterson (1986, Maps 2.1, 2.2, 2.4, 3.3, 3.4, pp. 14, 16, 21, 34, 37).

4.4.3 Spanish Influenza (H1N1), 1918–19

The 'Spanish' influenza pandemic of 1918–19 ranks as one of the greatest demographic shocks the human race has ever experienced. From uncertain origins in the spring of 1918, an apparently new variant of influenza A virus spread around the world as three successive waves, infecting over half a billion people and killing an estimated 20 million or more (Table 4.3). The pandemic spread in the closing stages and immediate aftermath of World War I (1914–18)—a war which had enveloped much of continental Europe and the Near East and which, through the combined agencies of battle, famine, and disease, had claimed over 20 million lives. As described by Patterson and Pyle (1991), the heightened population mixing engendered by the war was to provide ideal conditions for the rapid dissemination of the influenza virus. Not least, the continuous flux of troops in the European theatre—where the new, albeit mild, influenza had reputedly arrived with contingents from the United States in April 1918—ensured the early and widespread transmission of the disease on the European continent. In mid-November, however, with the disease having taken a much more severe turn, military demobilization served to spread the influenza virus far beyond its autumnal European focus to the rest of the world.

Origin and pandemic waves

The origin of the 1918–19 influenza pandemic cannot be ascertained with any certainty. As far as the historical record allows, outbreaks of influenza—generally assumed to be associated with the first wave of the pandemic—were first recognized in military training camps of the United States in March 1918 (Soper, 1918; Patterson and Pyle, 1991), with the disease appearing among United States and other troops on the Western Front during April (Stuart-Harris et al., 1985; Patterson and Pyle, 1991). Contemporary commentators, however, have pointed to the sporadic outbreaks of an unusually severe respiratory disease ('purulent bronchitis'), resembling Spanish influenza, among troops in France and troops and civilians in Britain as early as the mid-winter of 1916 (Ministry of Health, 1920, p. 69; Macpherson et al., 1922–23, I, pp. 212–4). The implication that the germs of the pandemic wave may have been circulating in Europe for up to 2 years prior to the massive outbreaks of 1918–19 is consistent with the suggestion that the ancestor virus entered the human species around 1912–15 (Reid et al., 1999; Webster, 1999; Oxford, 2000). Whatever its ultimate source, however, the pandemic

Table 4.3 Continent-level mortality estimates for wave II of the influenza pandemic, 1918–19

Continent	Deaths (millions)	Death rate (per 1,000)
Africa	1.9–2.3	14.2–17.7
Asia	19.0–33.0	19.7–34.2
Europe	c.2.3	c.4.8
Latin America	0.8–1.0	8.4–10.6
North America	0.6	5.3
Oceania	<0.1	–
Total	24.7–39.3	13.6–21.7

Source: Data from Patterson, K.D., Pyle, G.F. (1991). 'The geography and mortality of the 1918 influenza pandemic.' *Bulletin of the History of Medicine*, 65, 4–21.

interval of 6–8 months. As regards the geographical source of the novel influenza A viruses that underpinned these events, Patterson (1986) suggests that the broad area encompassed by southwestern Siberia, northern Kazakhstan, and the steppe country between the Volga and the Urals best fits the pre-twentieth-century evidence.

In the remainder of this section, we survey the four influenza pandemics of the twentieth and early twenty-first centuries.

occurred in three waves: spring and early summer 1918 (wave I), autumn 1918 (wave II), and winter 1918–19 (wave III). Here, we provide an overview of the global dispersal of the three influenza waves. Our account draws on the study of Patterson and Pyle (1991).

Wave I (spring and early summer 1918)

Wave I of the pandemic was attributed at the time to Spain by France and vice versa, and to eastern Europe by the Americans. But, whatever the truth, the disease acquired its popular name of *Spanish influenza* at this stage. Some of the first records of influenza activity can be traced to United States Army recruits at Camp Funston, Kansas, where an epidemic of influenza first manifested in early March 1918. By the end of the month, influenza had appeared in a number of military camps in the midwestern and southeastern United States, with the disease becoming widely diffused in April. The global spread of influenza from this putative beginning is traced in **Figure 4.8A**. Trans-Atlantic spread of the disease occurred with American troopships which reached France in April, with subsequent spread across the European continent. At about the same time, the map depicts the trans-Pacific spread of influenza from North America to Southeast Asia in April and May. The Caribbean Basin and Latin America were attacked in June. The disease finally reached the South Pacific in July (Patterson and Pyle, 1991).

Wave II (autumn 1918)

Wave I of the pandemic was comparatively mild. During the summer of 1918, the virus mutated into a more lethal strain and a

second, more severe, form of the disease emerged. Pneumonia often developed quickly, with death usually coming 2 days after the first indications of the influenza. The global dispersal of the new, more severe, wave II is traced in **Figure 4.8B**. As with wave I, the exact origins of wave II are also unknown, although western France is generally viewed as the source of the disease; the first reports can be traced to the French Atlantic port of Brest, a landing point for American troops, in late August. From here, ships appear to have carried the disease to coastal locations of North America, Africa, Latin America, South Asia, and the Far East by September. New Zealand was infected in October by ships from the United States; Australia remained largely free of the disease until January 1919 (Patterson and Pyle, 1991).

Wave III (winter 1918–19)

In the aftermath of wave II, a third influenza wave—of intermediate severity to the preceding waves—appeared in the winter of 1918–19. While relatively little is known of the origin and spread of this tertiary wave, the pandemic appears to have finally run its course by the spring of 1919.

Pandemic legacies? Encephalitis lethargica, 1918–26

The global pandemic of encephalitis lethargica (von Economo's disease) that spread with, and in the aftermath of, the Spanish influenza pandemic of 1918–19 ranks as one of the more mysterious disease events of the early twentieth century; see Ravenholt and Foege (1982) and Ravenholt (1993). While epidemics of encephalitic disease have historically occurred in conjunction with major waves of influenza activity, the 1918–26 pandemic of encephalitis lethargica was—like the influenza with which it appeared—characterized by an unusual virulence. The clinical course of the disease is reviewed by Ravenholt (1993) and reflected a diffuse involvement of the brain and the spinal cord. Disease onset was characterized by fever, with progressive lethargy, somnolence, and a range of other signs and symptoms including the disturbance of eye movements, headache, muscular weakness, delirium, and disablement. Lethargy varied in duration, from just a few days to weeks and months, terminating with death from comatose respiratory failure. The median interval from the onset of encephalitis to death was 14 days. The death rate associated with the acute stage of the disease was about 30 per cent, while a number of survivors developed parkinsonism in later years.

Although contemporary observers puzzled over the seemingly inconsistent temporal relationship between influenza and encephalitis lethargica (see, e.g. Parsons et al., 1922, pp. 22–4), an aetiological link between the two diseases has been proposed (Ravenholt and Foege, 1982; Ravenholt 1993). Among the lines of evidence, Ravenholt and Foege (1982, p. 862) note that:

- both pandemics were globally distributed, were closely related in time, and only one aetiological agent (swine influenza virus) has yet been identified
- at all geographical scales, epidemics of influenzal pneumonia typically preceded epidemics of encephalitis lethargica
- during the early part of the encephalitis lethargica pandemic, many cases reported a previous episode of clinical influenza.

The first reports of encephalitis lethargica in England and Wales can be traced to London and Sheffield in March and early April 1918 (Hall, 1918; Harris, 1918). Prior to June 1918, the disease was spatially

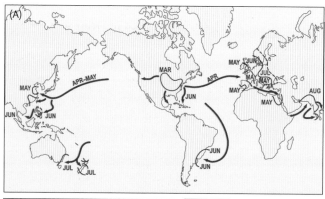

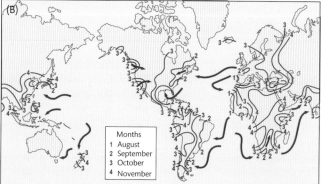

Figure 4.8 Global diffusion of pandemic influenza, March–November 1918. The transmission routes of influenza waves I (spring and early summer 1918) and II (autumn 1918) are plotted in (A) and (B), respectively.

Reproduced from Patterson, K.D., Pyle, G.F. (1991). 'The geography and mortality of the 1918 influenza pandemic.' *Bulletin of the History of Medicine*, 65, 4–21.

concentrated in the Eastern and Midlands counties. By the end of the year, the west of England had become involved. Describing the geographical spread of the disease at this time, Parsons et al. (1922, p. 12) observed:

> Not by any steady advance in one direction, … but in a seemingly haphazard way has encephalitis lethargica completed its invasion of this country, and the manner in which the disease here has skipped from place to place suggests in miniature some of its jumps from country to country which have been observed on the continent.

The temporal course of the epidemic in England and Wales is plotted for the period January 1919–January 1922 in **Figure 4.9B**; for reference, **Figure 4.9A** and **Figure 4.9C** plot the monthly incidence of two other diseases with nervous system involvement—cerebrospinal meningitis and acute poliomyelitis. As **Figure 4.9B** shows, encephalitis lethargica occurred throughout the seasons but with a general tendency to peak in the winter months (January and February) of the reporting years. Here, the upsurge in reported disease activity in the winter of 1920–21 is especially prominent. While this flare-up may be a reporting artefact associated with the anticipated publication of the Ministry of Health's *Memorandum on Encephalitis Lethargica*, a parallel increase in disease notifications was also observed for some other countries of Northern Europe (Parsons et al., 1922; Ravenholt and Foege, 1982).

4.4.4 Later Pandemics

Asian influenza (H2N2), 1957–58

In February 1957, a new strain of influenza A virus appeared for the first time in an epidemic in the Kweichow province of China. Eventually designated A/Asian/57 (H2N2), and popularly called 'Asian' influenza, this virus differed fundamentally from the H1N1 strain that had been in circulation, along with variants, certainly since 1947 and possibly for much longer. Wherever it was encountered, major attack rates ensued leading to a worldwide pandemic. From its initial hearth in China, the virus spread rapidly across the world in about 8 months, reaching Western Europe in the summer of 1957 (**Figure 4.10**).

The disease entered England and Wales in June 1957, with seaports (rather than airports) being the main points of entry. The epidemic flowered in September and, over the next 12 weeks, about 6 million cases of the disease occurred, an estimated incidence of 11.5 per cent. The corresponding percentage in a non-pandemic year is around 2 per cent. Distinct regional variations in attack rates were evident. Roughly 20 per cent of the population in the north was affected compared with 10 per cent or less in the south. Still lower rates were found in the Welsh hill counties and in the more isolated parts of northwest England.

The maps of weekly spread illustrated in **Figure 4.11** are based upon notifications of acute pneumonia cases (a recording surrogate for influenza) in the counties of England and Wales. As well as showing the initial outbreak of the disease in west Wales, the map for week 1 also plots the trajectory followed by the centre of gravity of the epidemic over the full 12-week period. Until early October, the centre was firmly located in northern England. Then, as the epidemic began to wane in the north, the centre began to shift rapidly southwards from week 4 and, by week 6, only three counties in southern England and five in central and west Wales were uninfected. Thus, much of southern England and Wales was invaded within a 3-week period.

Hong Kong influenza (H3N2), 1968–69

The onset of this pandemic first came to light in mid-July 1968, with accounts of a widespread outbreak of acute respiratory disease in south-eastern China. Within a week, authorities were reporting an increase in influenza-like illness and the isolation of novel influenza A viruses (H3N2). By the end of July, an estimated 0.5 million cases of influenza had occurred. In its onwards geographical spread from China, the pandemic initially resembled the events of 1957. It reached Singapore in early August, and Malaysia, Philippines, Taiwan, and Vietnam later in the month. Epidemics were reported in Thailand, India, Iran, and the Northern Territory of Australia in September. There were, however, some features of the spread that distinguished it from that of 1957; between the end of September and the end of December, there was very limited evidence of spread to new areas except in the United States where it reached the western seaboard in October. Thereafter, infection spread west to east across

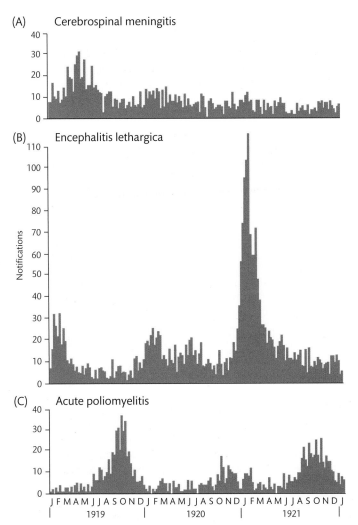

Figure 4.9 Weekly notifications of cerebrospinal meningitis, encephalitis lethargica, and acute poliomyelitis in England and Wales, 1919–21. Encephalitis lethargica was subject to notification in England and Wales from 1 January 1919.

Reproduced from Parsons, A.C., MacNalty, A.S., Perdrau, J.R. (1922). *Report on Encephalitis Lethargica*. Reports on Public Health and Medical Subjects, No. 11. London: HMSO.

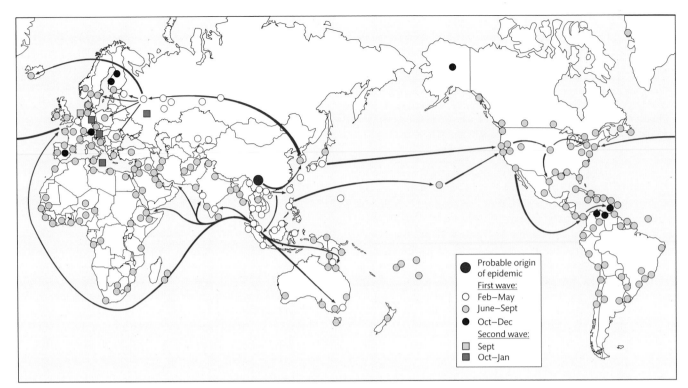

Figure 4.10 Origin and spread of the Asian influenza pandemic. Global sequence of spread of the 1957–58 pandemic is shown by vectors with figures indicating the month when the first cases appeared in each location. The pandemic appears to have originated in southern China and spread by two pathways: westwards via the trans-Siberian corridor into eastern Europe and by sea from Hong Kong to Singapore and Japan.

Reproduced with permission from Smallman-Raynor, M.R., Cliff, A.D. (2012). *Atlas of Epidemic Britain: A Twentieth Century Picture*. Oxford: Oxford University Press.

the country, resulting in an extensive epidemic that peaked towards the end of the year (Cockburn et al., 1969).

In the United Kingdom and elsewhere in Europe, the second season of the new strain (1969–70) was much more severe, giving rise to what Viboud et al. (2005) have called a 'smouldering pandemic' (see section 2.3.3 in Chapter 2). The 'smouldering' pattern in Europe—also evidenced for parts of Asia—was characterized by a second pandemic season that was two to five times more severe than the first. Viboud et al. (2005) hypothesized that the delayed onset in some areas may have arisen from a combination of pre-existing immunity from the preceding influenza A (H2N2) era, combined with genetic drift during the 1969–70 season.

To illustrate the delayed onset, **Figure 4.12** plots the monthly mortality rate per 100,000 population for pneumonia and influenza in the two pandemic seasons 1968–69 and 1969–70 for England and Wales and, for comparison, the United States. England and Wales displayed only a modest rise above baseline mortality in the first season but a major rise in the second. In the United States, the rise in the mortality rate was much higher in season one than two. Of the excess mortality due to pneumonia and influenza in 1968–69 and 1969–70, 23 per cent occurred in the 1968–69 season in England and Wales compared with 70 per cent in the United States (Viboud et al., 2005).

Swine flu (H1N1/09), 2009–10

Four decades on from the Hong Kong influenza of 1968–69, influenza re-emerged in pandemic form in 2009. Caused by a novel virus strain of swine lineage (H1N1/09), the first cases of the disease came to notice in Mexico in March 2009. The disease appeared in the United States in early April, spreading rapidly thereafter to Europe and the rest of the world. In recognition of these developments, under the contemporary six-phase system of influenza pandemic alert (**Figure 4.13**), the WHO raised the global alert level to Phase 4 (27 April), Phase 5 (29 April), and, eventually, the 'pandemic' Phase 6 (11 June).

As Doshi (2011) observes, the declaration of the pandemic reflected the widespread dissemination of the H1N1 virus and not the severity of the associated disease. In the event, the majority of clinical infections associated with the pandemic virus were characterized by mild symptoms, and the estimated global mortality (~0.3 million) was relatively low. More severe symptoms were occasionally seen in individuals with underlying illnesses (including asthma, diabetes, heart disease, and immunodeficiency) and pregnant women. Older people had some demonstrable immunity to the virus and, in Europe and North America, children and young adults were the principal groups affected by the disease.

The pandemic reached the United Kingdom in late April 2009. The earliest cases were identified among travellers who had recently returned from Mexico to Scotland, with the first evidence of indigenously acquired infections at the beginning of May. From thereon, the pandemic was associated with two pronounced waves of infection (**Figure 4.14**). In England, the first and most intense wave peaked at an estimated 110,000 cases in the week ending 26 July, followed by a rapid decline in August. The second wave was more protracted; it coincided with the early months of the regular influenza season and peaked in late October. In total, the two waves were associated

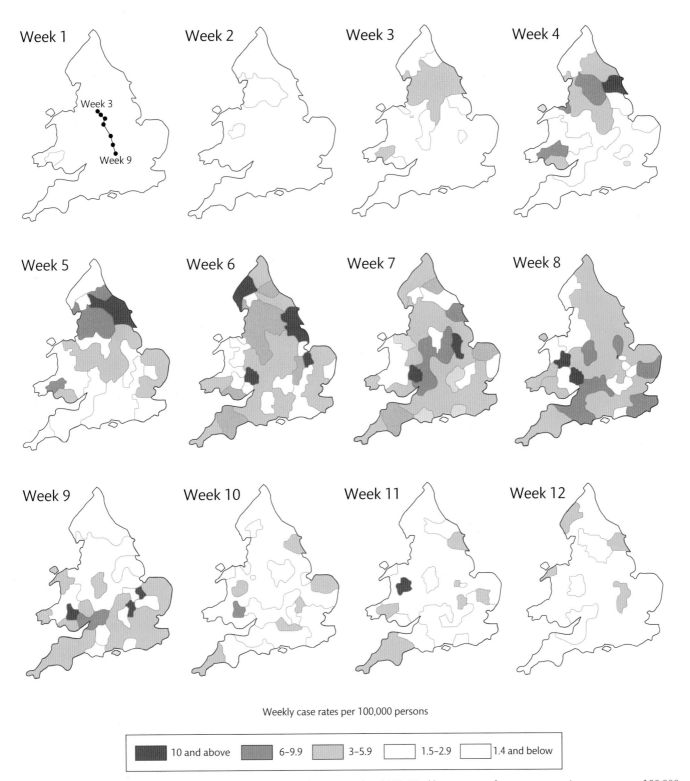

Weekly case rates per 100,000 persons

| 10 and above | 6–9.9 | 3–5.9 | 1.5–2.9 | 1.4 and below |

Figure 4.11 Asian influenza maps for England and Wales, September–November 1957. Weekly sequence of acute pneumonia case rates per 100,000 population reported in the counties of England and Wales. The first week is coded week 1 (ending 7 September), with subsequent weeks coded sequentially up to, and including, week 12 (ending 23 November). As well as showing the initial outbreak of the disease in west Wales, the map for week 1 also plots the trajectory followed by the centre of gravity of the epidemic.

Reproduced with permission from Smallman-Raynor, M.R., Cliff, A.D. (2012). *Atlas of Epidemic Britain: A Twentieth Century Picture.* Oxford: Oxford University Press. Source: Data from Hunter and Young (1971, Figures 5 and 6, pp. 643, 644).

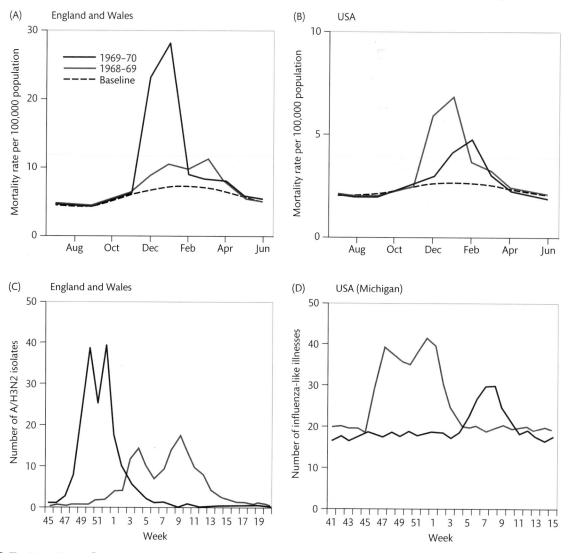

Figure 4.12 The Hong Kong influenza pandemic. For the pandemic seasons 1968–69 and 1969–70, graph (A) plots the monthly mortality rate per 100,000 population for pneumonia and influenza in England and Wales against a seasonal baseline; the United States is plotted in graph (B). Graphs (C) and (D) plot the weekly count of laboratory isolations of the pandemic virus (H3N2) in England and Wales and the weekly count of influenza-like illnesses in the state of Michigan, United States. In contrast to the evidence for the United States, in which morbidity and mortality was concentrated in the 1968–69 season, the graphs reveal evidence of a delayed pandemic in England and Wales in which morbidity and mortality was concentrated in the 1969–70 season.

Reproduced from Viboud, C., et al. 'Multinational impact of the 1968 Hong Kong influenza pandemic: evidence for a smoldering pandemic.' *Journal of Infectious Diseases*, (2005), 192 (2), 233–48, by permission of Oxford University Press.

with an estimated 848,000 cases (range: 444,000–1,661,000 cases) in England, with many thousands of additional cases in Scotland, Wales, and Northern Ireland.

A number of strategies were adopted to limit the severity of the pandemic in the United Kingdom. Public advice began to be broadcast on radio and television in late April and, in early May, the Department of Health distributed an influenza information leaflet to every household (**Figure 4.15**). Several school closures were also undertaken. While control of the disease was initially based on a containment principle to limit localized outbreaks, the rapid spread of the virus in late June and early July necessitated a change in approach that centred on clinical diagnosis and treatment. A National Flu Line telephone advice service was established in late July and antivirals (Tamiflu˚ and Relenza˚) were made available to the public on consultation. A vaccine became available for mass administration

in the United Kingdom in October 2009. Some 3.2 million doses of vaccine had been dispensed by the start of 2010.

Following debriefs and reflections on the first wave of the pandemic, the Health Protection Agency published its *Pandemic Influenza Contingency Plan* in October 2009 (Health Protection Agency, 2009). As described there, work undertaken within the remit of the Health Protection Agency indicated the following:

1. It may be possible to contain a new pandemic virus at source through the rapid application of stringent social distancing measures, area quarantine, and geographically targeted antiviral prophylaxis. Evidence indicates, however, that the H1N1 virus had been spreading for some time in Mexico before it was detected.

2. The containment measures in (1) are unlikely to prevent a pandemic virus spreading in the United Kingdom. Multiple and

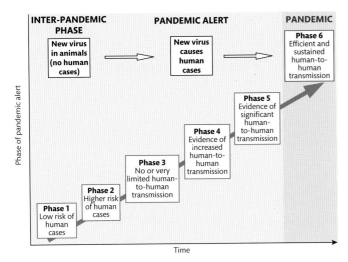

Figure 4.13 WHO phases of global pandemic alert for influenza at the time of the 2009–10 influenza pandemic. The contemporary *WHO Global Influenza Preparedness Plan* (World Health Organization, 2005d) identified six phases of pandemic alert. Each phase of alert was associated with a series of recommended responses and activities to be implemented by the WHO, the international community, governments, and industry. The epidemiological behaviour of the disease and the characteristics of circulating viruses, among other factors, determined changes from one phase to another.

Reproduced with permission from Cliff, A.D., Smallman-Raynor, M.R., Haggett, P., Stroup, D.F., Thacker, S.B. (2009). *Infectious Diseases. Emergence and Re-emergence: A Geographical Analysis*. Oxford: Oxford University Press. Source: Data from World Health Organization (2005). *Avian Influenza: Assessing the Pandemic Threat*. Geneva: WHO (WHO/CDS/2005:29).

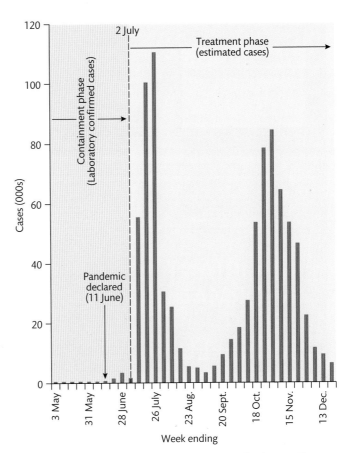

Figure 4.14 Weekly series of swine flu cases in England, 2009. The first cases in the United Kingdom were identified on 27 April. The initial response of the Health Protection Agency was to attempt to contain local outbreaks of the disease, with laboratory testing of all suspected cases. From 2 July, the containment phase was replaced by a treatment phase and the abandonment of routine laboratory testing of all cases. The associated change in surveillance strategy is reflected in the time series which plots laboratory-confirmed (May–July) and Health Protection Agency-estimated (July–December) cases of the disease.

Reproduced with permission from Smallman-Raynor, M.R., Cliff, A.D. (2012). *Atlas of Epidemic Britain: A Twentieth Century Picture*. Oxford: Oxford University Press. Source: Data from the Health Protection Agency (HPA).

simultaneous importations are to be expected and antiviral stocks would soon become depleted. Treatment, prophylaxis, and school closure did not contain the 2009 pandemic, although these measures may have served to delay spread.

3. International travel restrictions are likely to have only a short-term delaying effect on the spread of a pandemic virus; imposing a 90 per cent restriction on travel to the United Kingdom might delay an epidemic peak by only 1–2 weeks. Entrance screening at airports is unlikely to be effective as many arriving passengers are likely to be incubating the disease on entry.

4. Treatment of confirmed cases and prophylaxis of contacts in the early stages of the pandemic in the United Kingdom is estimated to have reduced transmission by some 16 per cent. Prompt treatment with antivirals can reduce the severity of clinical disease and, if used widely and rapidly enough, may reduce the overall clinical attack rate.

5. Children may be a more effective target for disease prevention and control measures than other age groups. School closure may reduce clinical attack rates and slow spread. The school holidays in the summer of 2009 may have reduced rates of virus transmission, although school holidays may not have the same effect as school closures.

4.4.5 Post-Pandemic Debates: Designating an Influenza Pandemic

The events of 2009–10 prompted controversy over the WHO's designation of a pandemic and, more particularly, the absence of a severity criterion in the definition of such an event (Doshi,

2011). After all, many national governments had mounted costly responses to what was, for the most part, a mild disease. In response, in 2017 the WHO published new guidelines on pandemic influenza risk management. These guidelines include a focus on national-level risk assessments, a revised approach to global phases of pandemic alert, and enhanced flexibility though the uncoupling of national actions from global phases (World Health Organization, 2017).

4.5 HIV/AIDS (1981–)

The acquired immunodeficiency syndrome (AIDS) is a severe, life-threatening, disease which was first recognized as a distinct clinical syndrome in 1981. The syndrome is a manifestation of advanced infection with the human immunodeficiency virus (HIV). The general term 'HIV/AIDS' is used by the Joint United Nations Programme on HIV/AIDS (UNAIDS) and other official bodies to refer to the

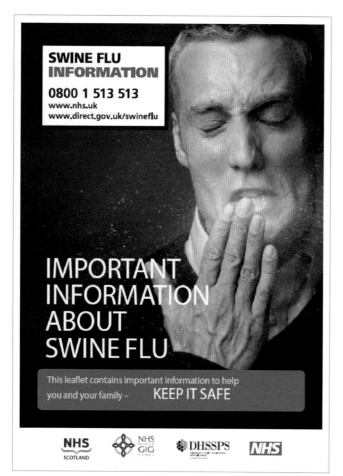

Figure 4.15 Public information leaflet on swine flu in the United Kingdom. A nationwide public information campaign on pandemic influenza was launched in the United Kingdom in May 2009. Beginning on Tuesday 5 May, all households in the United Kingdom received a copy of the illustrated leaflet. It provided advice on the prevention of influenza transmission (encapsulated in the slogan 'catch it, bin it, kill it') and, in the event of illness, guidance on the establishment of networks of neighbours, friends, and relatives ('flu friends') to assist in the provision of medicines and other supplies.

© Crown copyright.

pandemic of HIV infection and disease and we adopt that term in the present discussion.

4.5.1 Nature of HIV/AIDS

The immune system usually serves to safeguard the body against the invasion of disease-causing microorganisms such as bacteria, protozoa, and viruses. In HIV/AIDS, however, the immune system collapses and leaves the body open to potentially life-threatening opportunistic infections, the development of rare and unusually aggressive cancers, dementia, wasting, and other severe conditions. The immune dysfunction that eventually gives rise to AIDS is a continuous process over a variable, but usually protracted, period of several years or more. During this time, an HIV-infected person will typically pass through a series of stages ranging from an acute retroviral syndrome (a short-lived glandular fever-type disease) in the very early stages of infection with HIV, through a prolonged period of asymptomatic infection associated with a progressive subclinical

immune dysfunction, eventually progressing to advanced or late-stage disease (AIDS). During the typically long course of infection, the disease manifestations range from none, through non-specific illnesses and opportunistic infections, to autoimmune and neurological disorders and various types of malignancy (Heymann, 2015, pp. 287–94).

Two major types of HIV were recognized in the early years of the HIV/AIDS pandemic: HIV-1 and HIV-2. HIV-1 achieved the status of a global infection in the 1980s, having spread to virtually every country of the world by the latter years of the decade. In contrast, HIV-2 is primarily concentrated in West Africa and, although there has been limited spread to other parts of the world, the virus has not established itself as a pandemic infection of HIV-1 proportions. Human beings are the reservoir of HIV, and three primary routes of virus transfer can be identified: sexual, parenteral, and perinatal. Susceptibility to HIV infection and associated immune deficiency appears to be general. The incubation period for AIDS is highly variable, with the observed time from primary infection with HIV to the diagnosis of AIDS ranging from less than 1 year to longer than 15 years. The roll-out of effective antiretroviral therapies has served to reduce the development of clinical AIDS since the mid-1990s (Heymann, 2015, pp. 287–94).

4.5.2 Origins and Global Dispersals

The geographical origins of the global HIV/AIDS pandemic have been the subject of intense speculation, although a number of scientists now consider that the origins of HIVs rest with multiple cross-species transmissions of related viruses of non-human primates (simian immunodeficiency viruses, or SIVs) in sub-Saharan Africa (Van Heuverswyn and Peeters, 2007; Sharp and Hahn, 2011). HIVs are known to have been infecting humans in the 1950s and 1960s (Smallman-Raynor et al., 1992, pp. 120–8), with current evidence pointing to human infection with the common ancestral virus of the pandemic HIV-1 group M prior to the 1940s (Sharp et al., 2001).

Global diffusion patterns, I: HIV-1

A number of models have attempted to reconstruct the geographical corridors by which HIV-1 has spread from its postulated origin in central Africa to establish itself as a global pandemic infection (Shannon et al., 1991, pp. 40–50; Smallman-Raynor et al., 1992, pp. 143–6). Foremost among the models proposed is that of Robert C. Gallo, co-discoverer of the virus. Figure 4.16A is underpinned by the Gallo model and shows one possible scenario for the time-sequenced global spread of HIV-1. Gallo hypothesized that, from a hearth in sub-Saharan Africa, HIV-1 was carried to Haiti by Haitian technicians and professionals who had been working in the erstwhile Zaire (now the Democratic Republic of the Congo) under the auspices of the United Nations during the 1960s and 1970s. These workers, who had replaced the expelled Belgian administrators following Zairean independence in 1960, began to return at a time when Haiti was becoming a vacation destination for North American homosexual men. Haiti was then seen as a stepping stone for HIV spread into North America, from whence the virus diffused to the rest of the world (Gallo, 1987; Smallman-Raynor et al., 1992, pp. 144–6). Although the estimated timings of events vary, the initial spread sequence invoked by the model (Central Africa → Haiti →

United States) is consistent with the early phylogenetic analysis of Li et al. (1988) and, more recently, Gilbert et al. (2007).

Global diffusion patterns, II: HIV-2

The global extent of HIV-2 differs fundamentally from that of HIV-1. At the time of its first isolation in 1983–84, HIV-1 was already firmly established in much of the Americas, Europe, and Central Africa. In contrast, HIV-2, originally isolated from West African patients in the mid-1980s, is still primarily concentrated in sub-Saharan Africa. Although there has been limited spread to other regions, and this evidence has been used by Smallman-Raynor et al. (1992, pp. 174–82) to construct the general model of global transmission in **Figure 4.16B**, HIV-2 has not established itself as a pandemic infection of HIV-1 proportions. Indeed, since the available evidence points to West Africa as the source of the virus, it appears that HIV-2 has remained largely concentrated in its original heartland.

4.5.3 Global Morbidity and Mortality Patterns

An estimated 33 million people have died of HIV/AIDS in the four decades since the first recognition of the disease in 1981 (**Table 4.1**). Some impression of the current size and geography of the pandemic can be gained from **Table 4.4** and **Figure 4.17**. As global estimates for the year 2019, UNAIDS reported that 38.0 million people were living with HIV, 1.7 million people were newly infected with HIV, and 690,000 people had died of AIDS. Some two-thirds of recorded HIV infections and AIDS deaths are estimated to have occurred in sub-Saharan Africa. With the distant prospect of a marketable HIV vaccine (Hsu and O'Connell, 2017), the prevention of HIV/AIDS continues to depend on education, condom promotion, and the treatment and control of other sexually transmitted diseases. Once HIV infection has been acquired, antiretroviral therapy has the potential to lengthen life, as well as to reduce the risk of interpersonal HIV transmission and transmission from mother to child. Notwithstanding these therapeutic advances, however, HIV/AIDS continues to rank as one of the most important infectious health threats in the early twenty-first century (UNAIDS, 2020).

(A) HIV-1

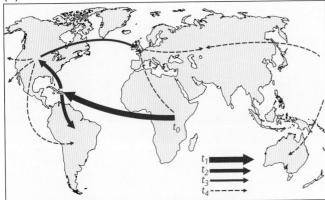

(B) HIV-2

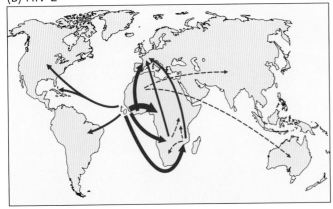

Figure 4.16 Global transmission routes of HIV-1 and HIV-2. (A) Global spread of HIV-1, illustrating the Gallo hypothesis of an initial series of linkages between Central Africa, the Caribbean, and North America. (B) Global spread of HIV-2, based on the case histories of patients reported in the 1980s and the early 1990s. Vector weights indicate the inferred time sequences ($t_1, ..., t_4$) of virus transmission.

Reproduced with permission from Cliff, A.D., Smallman-Raynor, M.R., Haggett, P., Stroup, D.F., Thacker, S.B. (2009). *Infectious Diseases. Emergence and Re-emergence: A Geographical Analysis.* Oxford: Oxford University Press.

Table 4.4 Regional estimates of HIV infections and AIDS deaths for 2019

UNAIDS Region[a]	Adults and children living with HIV	Adults and children newly infected with HIV	Adult and child deaths due to AIDS
Eastern and Southern Africa	20.7 million	730,000	300,000
Western and Central Africa	4.9 million	240,000	140,000
Middle East and North Africa	240,000	20,000	8,000
Asia and the Pacific	5.8 million	300,000	160,000
Latin America	2.1 million	120,000	37,000
Caribbean	330,000	13,000	6,900
Eastern Europe and Central Asia	1.7 million	170,000	35,000
Western and Central Europe and North America	2.2 million	65,000	12,000
Total	38.0 million	1,658,000	698,900

[a] UNAIDS regions are mapped in Figure 4.17A.

Reproduced from UNAIDS (2020). UNAIDS Data 2020. Geneva: UNAIDS. https://www.unaids.org/en/resources/documents/2020/unaids-data

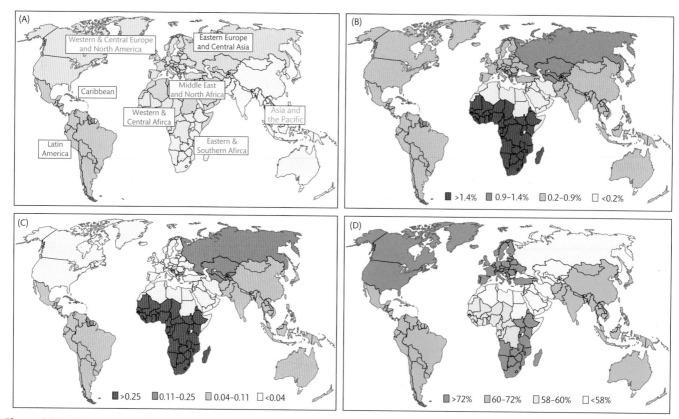

Figure 4.17 Global patterns of HIV/AIDS by UNAIDS region, 2019. (A) Location map of UNAIDS regions. (B) Percentage proportion of adults (aged 15–49 years) living with HIV. (C) AIDS deaths per 1,000 population. (D) Percentage proportion of people living with HIV who were in receipt of antiretroviral therapy.

Source: data from UNAIDS AIDSinfo, https://aidsinfo.unaids.org/, accessed 23 January 2021.

4.6 Conclusion

This chapter has examined long-term trends in four major human infectious diseases that have undergone phases of pandemic expansion over the last 1,500 years. While the pandemic surges of recent centuries have been greatly facilitated by the exponential increases in inter-locational connectivity resulting from the transport changes described in section 3.3.3 in Chapter 3, microbial changes have also played a central role in the pandemic stories of cholera and influenza. In the instance of HIV/AIDS, previously unrecognized pathogens have entered the human population by zoonotic transmission to start a new pandemic. The same process of zoonotic transmission brings us to the present day and the current pandemic of COVID-19. It is to COVID-19 that we now turn.

5

Pandemics, II
COVID-19

CONTENTS

newly recognized virus was officially named 'severe acute respiratory syndrome coronavirus 2' (SARS-CoV-2) by the International Committee on Taxonomy of Viruses. On the same day, the WHO named the associated disease as 'coronavirus disease 2019' or COVID-19 (World Health Organization, 2020i).

In this chapter, the global geography of the COVID-19 pandemic is described and analysed. At the time of writing (March 2021), the pandemic is still ongoing, and it is likely to continue to do so for many months to come. We have therefore taken the decision to take *c.*31 December 2020 as the closing date of our account. This date is broadly coincident with the beginning of vaccine roll out to control the causative virus in many advanced economies.

The WHO officially declared the COVID-19 situation to be a Public Health Emergency of International Concern on 31 January 2020 (World Health Organization, 2020j) and then, on 11 March, a global pandemic was declared on the basis of 'alarming levels of spread, severity, and inaction' (cited in Bedford et al., 2020, p. 1015). By late March 2021, the pandemic toll had reached approximately 125.8 million reported cases with approximately 2.8 million reported deaths (see Table 4.1 in Chapter 4). While global dispersal appears to have occurred in the spring of 2020, subsequent retrospective work by the Istituto Superiore di Sanità (ISS), Italy, detected the causative agent in waste water collected in the northern cities of Milan and Turin on 18 December 2019, and in Bologna on 29 January 2020. The data were in line with results obtained from retrospective analysis of samples of patients hospitalized in France, which found cases positive for SARS-CoV-2 dating back to the end of December. Given a putative origin in China, this evidence suggests that the virus had probably achieved undetected community circulation by the latter days of 2019 in many widely dispersed geographical locations.

5.1 Introduction

On 31 December 2019, the WHO was alerted to an unusual cluster of pneumonia patients in the city of Wuhan, Hubei Province, China. Clinical signs and symptoms included fever and breathing difficulties; chest radiographs revealed invasive lesions of both lungs. The causative agent of the disease was identified as a coronavirus distantly related to the virus that had caused the SARS outbreak in 2003–04 (see section 3.4.2 in Chapter 3). On 11 February 2020, the

5.2 Epidemiological Properties of the Virus

SARS-CoV-2 is a highly transmissible and pathogenic virus. Genomic analysis has revealed that it is phylogenetically related to SARS-like bat viruses, so that bats could be the primary reservoir. The intermediate source and mode of transfer to humans is not known but rapid human-to-human transfer has been widely confirmed. The epidemic hearth of the outbreak appears to have been the seafood market in Wuhan City, China; live animals are frequently illegally sold at the market, including bats, frogs, snakes, birds, marmots, and rabbits (Shereen et al., 2020).

5.2.1 Incubation Period

Based upon evidence from 181 confirmed cases in China with identifiable exposure and symptom onset windows, Lauer et al. (2020) estimated the median incubation period of COVID-19 as 5.1 days (95% confidence interval (CI), 4.5–5.8 days), and that 97.5 per cent of those who developed symptoms did so within 11.5 days (95% CI, 8.2–15.6 days) of infection.

5.2.2 Serial Interval

Du et al. (2020) and Nishiura et al. (2020) have attempted to estimate the serial interval of COVID-19, defined as the time from illness onset in a primary case (infector) to illness onset in a secondary case (infectee) (see section 1.2.1 in Chapter 1). This information is needed to understand the turnover of case generations and the transmissibility of the disease. The median appears to be approximately 4–5 days with very little variation (~1 day) around these values.

The fact that the serial interval is so close to or shorter than its median incubation period suggests that a substantial proportion of secondary transmission may occur prior to illness onset (**Figure 5.1**). It is also possible that presymptomatic transmission

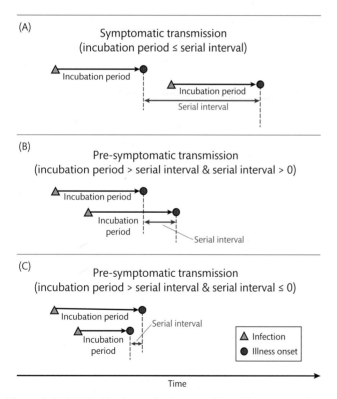

Figure 5.1 COVID-19: relationship between the incubation period and the serial interval. (A) If transmission takes place during the symptomatic period of the primary case, the serial interval is longer than the incubation period. However, this relationship can be reversed when presymptomatic transmission takes place (B). Furthermore, it is possible that the secondary case may experience illness onset prior to onset in their infector (C).

Reproduced from Nishiura, H., Linton, N.M., Akhmetzhanov, A.R. (2020). 'Serial interval of novel coronavirus (COVID-19) infections.' *International Journal of Infectious Diseases*, 93, 284–6.

may even occur more frequently than symptomatic transmission. As discussed later in this chapter, the rapid global diffusion of COVID-19 from its Chinese hearth may be partly attributed to these properties. Nishiura et al. (2020) also note an important public health implication of presymptomatic transmission—namely, transmissions cannot be prevented solely through isolation or quarantine of symptomatic cases. By the time contacts are traced, they may have already become infectious themselves and generated secondary cases. Thus, containment via the isolation of clinically recognized cases alone is likely to be a vain hope.

5.2.3 Case-Fatality Rate

The case-fatality rate has been estimated as 5.3–8.4 per cent for COVID-19 (Jung et al., 2020), which is lower than for SARS or MERS (Heymann, 2015, pp. 539–49). As discussed later, a striking feature of the pandemic in many countries has been the skewed age distribution of mortality. Over time, the average age of infected people has declined and this has resulted in a lowering of the case-fatality rate.

5.2.4 Infectivity

As discussed in section 1.3.2 in Chapter 1, the most commonly used measure of the infectivity of a communicable disease agent is the *basic reproduction number*, denoted R_0, defined there as the number of secondary cases which one infected individual would produce unchecked in a completely susceptible population (Dietz, 1993). As Dietz notes, the value of R_0 depends on the duration of the infectious period, the probability of infecting a susceptible during a single contact, and the number of new susceptible individuals contacted per unit time. This implies that R_0 can vary not only for different infectious diseases but also for the same disease in different populations. Epidemic theory associates outbreaks of epidemic disease and the persistence of endemicity with $R_0 > 1$. Values less than one indicate that a single infective is not replacing itself and the epidemic will extinguish itself over time; when $R_0 > 1$, each infective causes more than one new infective, thus more than replacing itself so that any epidemic will grow over time. The magnitude of R_0 therefore indicates the amount of effort which must be expended to contain an epidemic.

Table 5.1 gives examples of the R_0 values which have been calculated for several infectious diseases. The R_0 for COVID-19 appears to be in the range 2.0–6.5 (Liu, Gayle, et al., 2020)—comparable to, or a little higher than, that for SARS (R_0 of 2.0–5.0) (Lipsitch et al., 2003), but much higher than R_0 for influenza and equally much lower than R_0 for measles.

In the spatial domain, our ability to control the spread of an epidemic disease will be affected by the rate at which the infection moves from one geographical area to another, and so in section 1.6.2 in Chapter 1 we defined a spatial equivalent, R_{0A}, of the aspatial R_0. R_{0A} measures the speed of spatial propagation, or the spatial epidemic velocity of a disease wave. Waves that move rapidly through a system of areas are harder to control than slowly moving waves.

5.2.5 Predisposing Factors for Poor COVID-19 Outcomes

Systematic reviews of ethnically homogeneous cohorts from China suggest that the key risk factors for hospital admission and poor clinical outcomes include age, male sex, and comorbidities such as certain cancers and treatments which cause immunosuppression,

Table 5.1 Estimates of the basic reproduction number, R_0, for sample infectious diseases

Disease	Transmission	R0	Source
Measles	Aerosol	12.0–18.0	Guerra et al. (2017)
Chickenpox (varicella)	Aerosol	3.0–17.0	Medić et al. (2018)
Mumps	Respiratory droplets	10.0	Béraud et al. (2018)
COVID-19	**Respiratory droplets**	**2.0–6.5**	Liu, Gayle, et al. (2020)
SARS	Respiratory droplets	2.0–5.0	Chowell et al. (2004)
Pertussis	Respiratory droplets	5.5	Kretzschmar et al. (2010)
Smallpox	Respiratory droplets	3.5–6.0	Gani and Leach (2001)
Diphtheria	Saliva	1.7–4.3	Truelove et al. (2020)
Influenza (1918 pandemic strain)	Respiratory droplets	1.4–2.8	Ferguson et al. (2006)
Ebola (2014 Ebola outbreak)	Body fluids	1.5–1.9	Khan et al. (2015)
Influenza (2009 pandemic strain)	Respiratory droplets	1.4–1.6	Fraser et al. (2009)
Influenza (seasonal strains)	Respiratory droplets	0.9–2.1	Coburn et al. (2009)
MERS	Respiratory droplets	0.3–0.8	Kucharski and Althaus (2015)

cardiovascular disease, hypertension, and diabetes (Khunti et al., 2020). Of particular note has been the much higher mortality among older people and members of ethnic minority groups.

The United Kingdom was one of the first countries with an ethnically very diverse population to record high levels of COVID-19 activity. Analysis of United Kingdom data suggests the disease has a differential impact upon diverse ethnic groups, with noticeably poorer outcomes among infectees of BAME (Black, Asian, and Minority Ethnic) heritage and, so far as the United Kingdom is concerned, these were more marked in the first disease wave than in the second (Khunti et al., 2020). The causes of this disparity remain to be investigated.

In a similar study in the United States, designed to quantify the increased risk of hospitalization by various comorbidities, Killerby et al. (2020) calculated odds ratios for a sample of 506 COVID-19 patients in metropolitan Atlanta during March 2020 (**Figure 5.2A**). Again, race and ethnicity were associated with an increased risk of hospitalization—in some instances by as much as 10 per cent. The CDC in the United States identified the same pattern of racial and ethnic bias in COVID-NET data for age-adjusted COVID-19-associated hospitalization rates by race and ethnicity, collected between March and June 2020 (**Figure 5.2B**). The CDC attributed the ethnic biases to long-standing systemic health and social inequities that included poorer living conditions and poorer work and health circumstances. As of 12 June 2020, age-adjusted hospitalization rates (**Figure 5.2C**) were highest among non-Hispanic American Indian or Alaska Native and non-Hispanic black persons, followed by Hispanic or Latino persons.

Differences in COVID-19 mortality by sex in 23 European countries have been studied by Pérez-López et al. (2020). Their sample comprised 484,919 men and 605,229 women who tested positive for SARS-CoV-2. The mortality rate was significantly higher in men than in women (risk ratio, 1.60; 95% CI, 1.53–1.68) (**Figure 5.3**).

5.2.6 Multiple Waves

Very little is yet known about the rate of evolution of the COVID-19 virus or, for those who have contracted the disease and recovered, the duration of immunity afforded by prior exposure. As we have seen in section 4.4 in Chapter 4, influenza A virus, for example, is genetically very unstable and mutates rapidly, by-passing any acquired population immunity from other strains—hence the need for an annual influenza vaccine tailored to protect against the influenza strains expected to be in circulation in a given winter. Conversely, the measles virus is genetically stable so that one attack or vaccine sequence will confer, for all practical purposes, lifelong immunity.

In the case of COVID-19, by 1 July 2020, only about 5 per cent of the United Kingdom population had caught the virus, well below the percentage needed to produce herd immunity (~60–90 per cent); globally, the COVID-immune population is approximately 0.1 per cent. These results are supported by a seroprevalence study (Pollán et al., 2020) of over 60,000 participants living in Spain, one of the European countries most seriously affected in the early stages of the COVID-19 pandemic. The authors estimated that the seroprevalence of SARS-CoV-2 infection in Spain at both national and regional levels was approximately 5 per cent, with no differences by sex and with a lower seroprevalence in children aged younger than 10 years. There was substantial geographical variability, with higher prevalence around Madrid (>10 per cent) and lower in coastal areas (<3 per cent). Thus, the majority of the Spanish population was seronegative for SARS-CoV-2 infection at the time of the investigation (27 April–11 May 2020), even in hotspot areas.

The public health implications of these findings are serious. Although several vaccines are now available, there remains a large susceptible population everywhere to sustain community circulation of COVID-19. Further, new and more transmissible strains of the virus are emerging. Extreme vigilance will be needed to mitigate the risk of multiple waves and small outbreaks at all geographical scales—national, regional, and local. There have already been second outbreaks in many locations—for example, in Beijing (China), Seoul (South Korea), Iran, and across Europe (**Figure 5.4**). At the time of writing (March 2021), the United Kingdom has just begun to ease its third phase of national lockdown. At the same time, other European countries (including France, Germany, and Italy) are just entering new phases of lockdown restrictions.

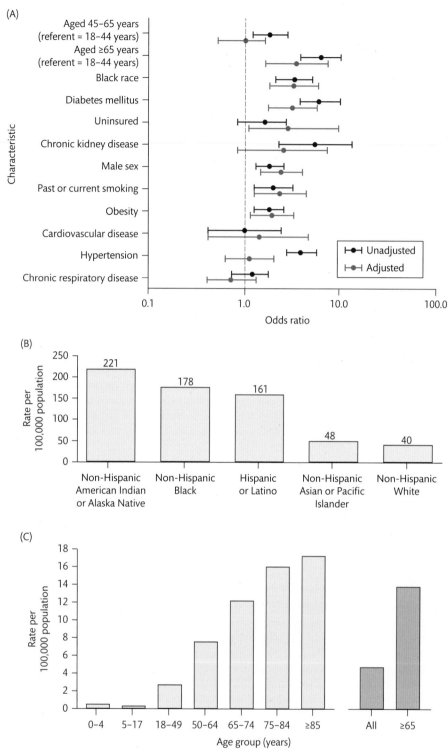

Figure 5.2 Metropolitan Atlanta, Georgia: cofactors of hospitalization with COVID-19. (A) Odds ratios and 95% CI for hospitalizations in COVID-19 patients (*n* = 506), unadjusted and adjusted for age, sex, race, obesity, past or current smoking, insurance status, and other underlying conditions. Data from six acute care hospitals and associated outpatient clinics by selected characteristics, 1 March–7 April 2020. Graphs (B) and (C) reinforce the impact of race and age upon the incidence of laboratory-confirmed COVID-19-associated hospitalization rates, COVID-NET data, 14 states, 1–28 March, 2020.

(A) Reproduced from Killerby ME, Link-Gelles R, Haight SC, et al. Characteristics Associated with Hospitalization Among Patients with COVID-19 — Metropolitan Atlanta, Georgia, March–April 2020. *MMWR Morb Mortal Wkly Rep* 2020;69:790–794; (B) CDC, https://www.cdc.gov/coronavirus/2019-ncov/need-extra-precautions/racial-ethnic-minorities.html, accessed 23 January 2021; (C) Garg S, Kim L, Whitaker M, et al. Hospitalization Rates and Characteristics of Patients Hospitalized with Laboratory-Confirmed Coronavirus Disease 2019 — COVID-NET, 14 States, March 1–30, 2020. *MMWR Morb Mortal Wkly Rep* 2020;69:458–464.

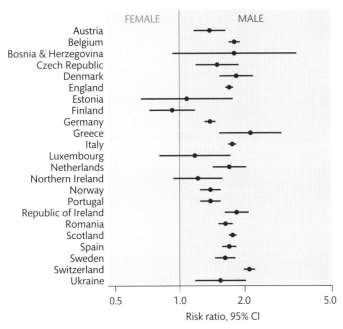

Figure 5.3 Differences in COVID-19 mortality by sex, Europe. Risk ratio and 95% CI for COVID-19-related deaths in 23 European countries.

Reproduced with permission from Pérez-López, F.R., Tajada, M., Savirón-Cornudella, R., Sánchez-Prieto, M., Chedraui, P., Terán, E. (2020). 'Coronavirus disease 2019 and gender-related mortality in European countries: A meta-analysis.' *Maturitas*, 141, 59–62.

5.3 Origins and Global Dispersal

5.3.1 The Wuhan Outbreak

As noted previously, it was an outbreak of COVID-19 in the Chinese city of Wuhan in late 2019 that first brought the disease to international attention. Sun et al. (2020) divide this original outbreak into three phases on the basis of the epidemic curve plotted in **Figure 5.5A**:

1. *Phase I, seafood market hearth.* The outbreak remained localized, caused by exposure to SARS-CoV-2 in the wet seafood market. A total of 41 cases were confirmed between the first recorded case (December 2019) and the emergence of new cases beyond the city (13 January 2020).

2. *Phase II, China-wide and international spread.* The second phase started on 13 January. In Wuhan, this phase was marked by rapid expansion and spread of the virus within hospitals (nosocomial infection) and by within-family close contact transmission. Disease diffusion became widespread in the provinces of eastern China (**Figure 5.5B**). By 19 January, cases were being reported outside Hubei province, from Beijing City to the north, and from Guangdong Province (bordering Hong Kong and Macau) to the south. The first international case was reported outside China on 13 January from Thailand and was associated with a Wuhan resident travelling to that country. By 23 January, extensive internal and external spread of COVID-19 had occurred to 29 of China's 34 provinces and similar areas and six other countries; 846 confirmed cases had been reported (**Figure 5.5B**). A lockdown was implemented in Wuhan city but, unfortunately, this period coincided with the traditional mass movement of people

immediately prior to the Chinese New Year, so more than 5 million people had already left Wuhan by this time.

3. *Phase III, growth of disease clusters in China and continued international spread.* Rapid growth of disease clusters within China took place from 26 January, accounting for 50–80 per cent of all confirmed cases in Beijing, Shanghai, Jiangsu, and Shandong by mid-February. By the end of January, China had 9,826 confirmed cases, and the WHO declared this epidemic a Public Health Emergency of International Concern. By 11 February, the epidemic had exploded to 44,730 confirmed cases and 16,067 suspected cases spread across some 1,400 counties and districts in China. Internationally, although there were only 441 confirmed cases, 24 countries were involved (**Figure 5.5C**). Note that interpreting the Chinese figures up to mid-February is complicated by a case definition change on 12 February to include both laboratory-confirmed and clinically diagnosed cases. Prior to this date, only laboratory-confirmed cases were recorded. The definition change in Hubei province led to newly confirmed cases jumping to 14,840, of which 13,332 cases were based only on a clinical diagnosis. By that time, 25 countries had reported 60,329 infections (**Figure 5.5A**). The Chinese epidemic appears to have peaked in early February after which cases in Hubei began to fall consistently. Whether that reflected the success of the Wuhan lockdown and other public health measures, or virus transmission reduced for other reasons, remains to be confirmed.

5.3.2 Geographical Dispersal

Geographical spread of COVID-19 from the Wuhan hearth and China in subsequent months was broadly east to west, with southern sweeps into Africa and Latin America from the Middle East and North America respectively. The sequence shown in **Figure 5.6** uses choropleth mapping to track the moving disease epicentre by plotting the number of new cases by country as a 5-day moving average, calculated for each day by averaging the values of that day, the 2 days before, and the next 2 days. This helps to prevent events, such as a change in reporting methods or data variability, from skewing the case count. Visualizing new cases demonstrates where the coronavirus actively spread during the past 1–2 weeks.

Figure 5.6A shows the Chinese origin at 1 February, while **Figure 5.6B** illustrates the importance of international air travel in spreading communicable diseases. New centres of COVID-19 became established in Italy and Iran. Italy's first confirmed cases were on 31 January when two Chinese tourists in Rome tested positive for the virus. A week later, an Italian man who had been repatriated back to Italy from Wuhan was hospitalized and confirmed as the third case. A cluster of cases was later detected, beginning with 16 confirmed cases in Lombardy on 21 February, and with local spread (contagious geographical diffusion) throughout much of northern Italy. Iran followed a similar pattern. The first confirmed cases were reported there on 19 February from the city of Qom (population ~1.2 million), thought to have been brought to the country by a merchant who had travelled to China. Iran's government initially rejected lockdown as a control measure, and heavy traffic between cities continued ahead of the spring equinox which marks the beginning of the Iranian New Year. Country-wide spread of COVID-19 occurred; this was then followed by a clamp down on travel. Government restrictions were gradually eased in April so that cases

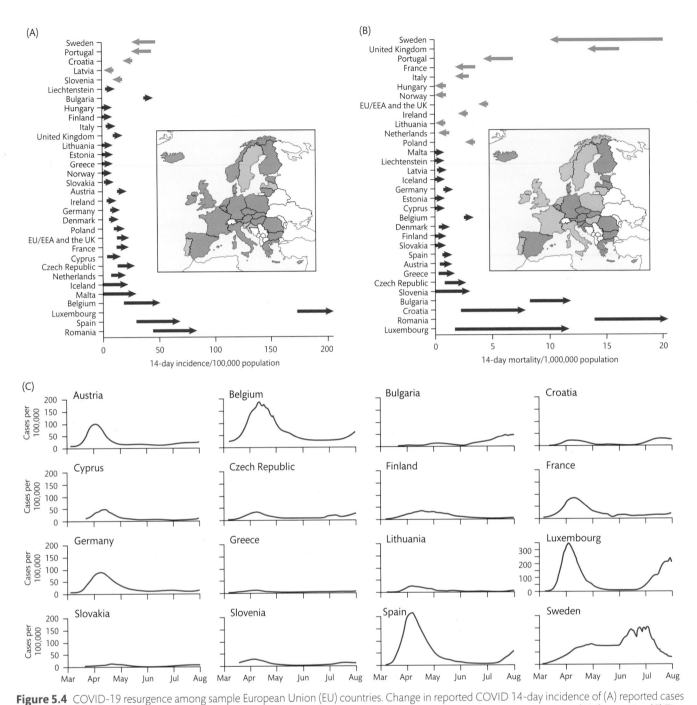

Figure 5.4 COVID-19 resurgence among sample European Union (EU) countries. Change in reported COVID 14-day incidence of (A) reported cases per 100,000 population and (B) deaths per 1,000,000 population, 19 July–2 August 2020 among EU/European Economic Area (EEA) countries. (C) Time series for sample European countries of 14-day incidence of reported COVID-19 cases per 100,000 population, March–August 2020.

Reproduced from European Centre for Disease Prevention and Control (2020). Coronavirus Disease 2019 (COVID-19) in the EU/EEA and the UK – Eleventh Update, 10 August 2020. Stockholm: ECDC.

began to climb again to a second peak in early June. Iran acted as a diffusion pole for the disease in the Middle East, as did Italy, along with France and Spain, in Europe.

By the second half of March, generalized global diffusion of the virus had occurred with Europe and, subsequently, the United States becoming epicentres of the disease (**Figure 5.6C**). In the WHO European Region, COVID-19 surveillance was implemented on 27 January 2020. The origin of the first European cases other than in the United Kingdom is shown in **Figure 5.7**. By 21 February, nine

European countries had reported 47 cases. Of the 38 cases for whom the source of infection was established, 21 were linked to two clusters in Germany and France, while 14 were infected in China. The source of the French cluster was Wuhan. The first three cases (two in Paris and one in Bordeaux) were confirmed on 24 January. All had a recent stay in Wuhan (Bernard-Stoecklin et al., 2020).

Initial German clusters developed in January and, as in Italy, show the importance of (i) long-distance international travel links and (ii) local social gatherings in spreading infectious diseases:

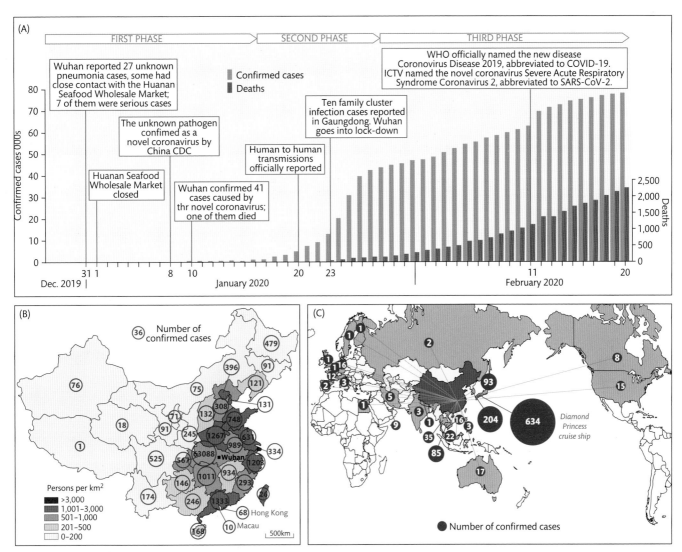

Figure 5.5 Global spread of COVID-19. (A) Timeline of events during the early stages of the pandemic. (B) Human confirmed cases of COVID-19 infection in China by 20 February 2020. (C) Human confirmed cases of COVID-19 infection in the world up to 20 February 2020. CDC, Centers for Disease Control and Prevention; ICTV, International Committee on Taxonomy of Viruses.

Reproduced with permission from Sun, J., He, W.T., Wang, L., Lai, A., Ji, X., Zhai, X., Li, G., Suchard, M.A., Tian, J., Zhou, J., Veit, M., Su, S. (2020). 'COVID-19: Epidemiology, evolution, and cross-disciplinary perspectives.' *Trends in Molecular Medicine*, 26, 483–95.

1. On 27 January, the first German case was confirmed at an automobile parts manufacturer near Munich in a Chinese woman (patient 0) from Shanghai. Most of the other German cases in January and early February can be traced to this source. Patient 0 had been visited by her parents from Wuhan before she flew to Germany on 19 January for a business meeting in the auto parts company. Patient 0 returned to Shanghai on 22 January (Böhmer et al., 2020). Between 27 January and 11 February, 16 cases of COVID-19 were identified in this cluster. On 25 and 26 February, multiple cases caused by bi-directional travel links with COVID-infected parts of Italy were detected in Baden-Württemberg.

2. A large cluster linked to a superspreading carnival event was formed in Heinsberg, near Dusseldorf (metropolitan region of Rhein-Ruhr, North Rhine-Westphalia), in mid-February (Streeck et al., 2020). New clusters in other regions owed their origin both to visitors to the Heinsberg event and also to people arriving from China, Iran, and Italy, from where non-Germans could arrive by plane until 17–18 March (Walker et al., 2020).

Spain, like Italy, was especially hard hit in the early stages of the COVID-19 epidemic in Europe. Post hoc genetic analysis has shown that at least 15 strains of the COVID-19 virus were imported into Spain early on, and community transmission began by mid-February. The virus was first confirmed in Spain on 31 January 2020, when a German tourist tested positive for SARS-CoV-2 in La Gomera, Canary Islands (Böhmer et al., 2020). The infected person had close contact with a business woman of Chinese origin in Germany before he travelled to La Gomera. The second confirmed case of the disease in the islands was found on 24 February, following the outbreak in Italy, when a medical doctor from Lombardy, Italy, who was vacationing in Tenerife tested positive for the disease. Afterwards, multiple cases were detected in Tenerife that involved people who had come into contact with the doctor. By 13 March, cases had been confirmed in all 50 provinces of the country.

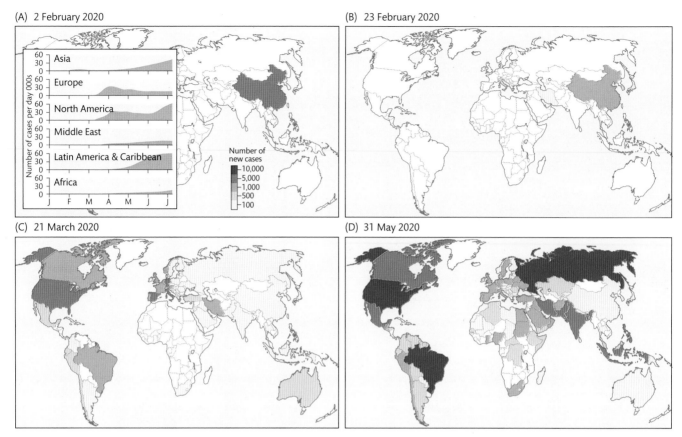

Figure 5.6 Global geographical diffusion of COVID-19 from China, February–May 2020. The map sequence uses choropleth shading to show the number of new cases by country as a 5-day moving average centred on each map date.

Reproduced from Johns Hopkins University Coronavirus Resource Center, https://coronavirus.jhu.edu/data/animated-world-map, maps downloaded 27 June 2020. This work is licensed under a Creative Commons Attribution 4.0 International License.

Figure 5.6D clearly shows the shift of the pandemic epicentre away from Europe and into the Americas, especially the United States and Brazil, by the end of May 2020. Thereafter, India and parts of Africa began to experience intensified outbreaks of COVID-19.

5.4 The United Kingdom: A Time–Space Analysis

The pandemic of COVID-19 reached the United Kingdom in late January 2020. As of Saturday 27 March 2021, there were 4.33 million confirmed cases and 126,573 deaths of confirmed cases, one of the world's highest death rates per capita among major countries (GOV.UK, https://coronavirus.data.gov.uk/). More than 90 per cent of those dying had underlying illnesses or were over 60 years old. There has been substantial regional variation in the severity of the pandemic, and we examine this later in this section. **Figure 5.8** shows the reported daily number of COVID-19 cases and deaths for the United Kingdom, March 2020–January 2021.

Pybus et al. (2020) generated greater than 20,000 SARS-CoV-2 genome sequences from infections in the United Kingdom by the beginning of June. The authors used phylogenetic analysis of these genomes, and those from other countries, to identify individual United Kingdom transmission lineages. The key geographical conclusions of their analysis were as follows:

1. The United Kingdom epidemic comprised a large number of importations due to inbound international travel, represented in the analysis by 1,356 independently introduced transmission lineages. The rate and source of introduction of lineages changed greatly and rapidly through time (**Figure 5.9**). The rate peaked in mid-March, collapsing after the introduction of the first United Kingdom lockdown (announced 23 March, and enforced in emergency legislation on 26 March) and the introduction of restrictions on air travel. Restrictions were further extended on 16 April, and on 7 and 28 May.

2. An estimated approximately 34 per cent of detected transmission lineages arrived via inbound travel from Spain, approximately 29 per cent from France, approximately 14 per cent from Italy, and approximately 23 per cent from other countries. The relative contribution of individual locations at any point in time was highly variable, but the general trend in **Figure 5.9** is clear (Italy → Spain → France), thus echoing the shift of the pandemic epicentre around southern Europe.

3. The increasing rates and shifting source locations of SARS-CoV-2 importations were not fully captured by early contact tracing.

To place the United Kingdom's experience of the first COVID-19 wave into a European context, **Figure 5.10** shows weekly excess

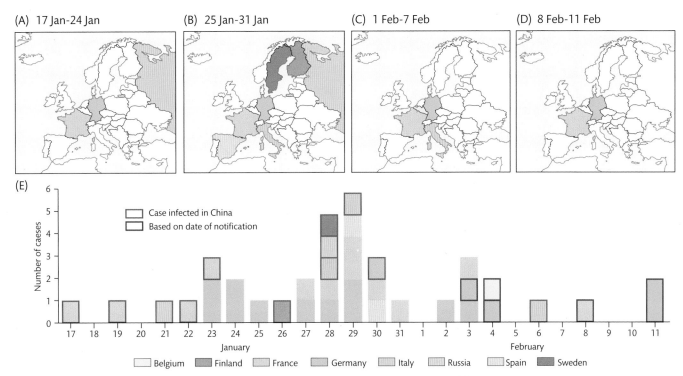

Figure 5.7 First reports of COVID-19 in European countries excluding the United Kingdom. Graph (E) plots the epidemic curve of reported COVID-19 cases by date of symptom onset, or date of notification, WHO European Region, as of 21 February 2020 (*n* = 38). Four cases were reported by Germany with unknown date of onset and unknown symptomatology. Belgium and France reported one asymptomatic case each. These cases are plotted by their date of notification. Maps (A)–(D) show those countries to which the cases relate in each of four time periods.
Reproduced from Spiteri, G., Fielding, J., Diercke, M., et al. (2020). 'First cases of coronavirus disease 2019 (COVID-19) in the WHO European Region, 24 January to 21 February 2020.' *Eurosurveillance*, 25(9):2000178. This work is licensed under a Creative Commons Attribution 4.0 International License.

deaths for selected European countries. In each case the pandemic profile forms a wave with the number of excess deaths rising to a peak and then declining to zero when the first wave of the pandemic receded. It is clear from the height and breadth of the curves that different countries were affected very differently:

- Spain had the highest peak, with deaths in the peak week being 155 per cent more than usual.
- The United Kingdom also had a high peak (109 per cent) and had a slow descent.
- Until the first week of April, France and the United Kingdom seemed on the same trajectory, but this was actually the peak week in France and the curve flattened quickly thereafter while the United Kingdom's deaths continued to grow.
- Germany is notable for the flatness of its wave.

5.4.1 Care Homes

Of particular concern has been the COVID-19 death rate in the United Kingdom's care homes. Up to the middle of June 2020, the death rate was the second worst in Europe (**Figure 5.11A**). Relative to the start of the COVID-19 outbreak in England and Wales, care homes saw the biggest increase in deaths over time compared to deaths in other settings. At the beginning of May, deaths in care homes from all causes were beginning to stabilize but remained 159 per cent higher than at the start of the COVID-19 outbreak. This was largely because, in the early months of the pandemic, government distribution schemes for personal protective equipment were insufficient to reach the fragmented care home sector. This was

compounded by the absence of routine regular COVID-19 testing for both staff and patients, especially when patients from hospital were discharged into care homes or returned into the community. Infection was also widely transmitted at first by those who visited relatives in care homes. Despite the fact that vaccines have now been offered to all care home residents, the sector remains a concern with many residents unable or unwilling to be vaccinated for one reason or another.

5.4.2 Temporal Evolution: The Instantaneous Reproduction Number, R_t

Many of the political decisions made by the United Kingdom government to control the geographical spread of COVID-19 have been grounded in advice received from its Scientific Advisory Group for Emergencies. Extensive use has been made of estimates of R_0 and of R_t, the instantaneous real-time value of R_0 calculated at regular intervals during the temporal evolution of the pandemic. Real-time tracking of a pandemic, as data accumulate over time, is seen as an essential component of a public health response to a new outbreak. A team of statistical modellers at the Medical Research Council Biostatistics Unit have regularly nowcast and forecast COVID-19 infections and deaths over the course of the pandemic and fed the information directly to the Scientific Advisory Group for Emergencies subgroup, the Scientific Pandemic Influenza subgroup on Modelling (SPI-M), and to regional Public Health England teams. The work has used a transmission model, data on daily COVID-19 confirmed deaths from Public Health England, and published information on the risk of dying and the time from infection to death, to

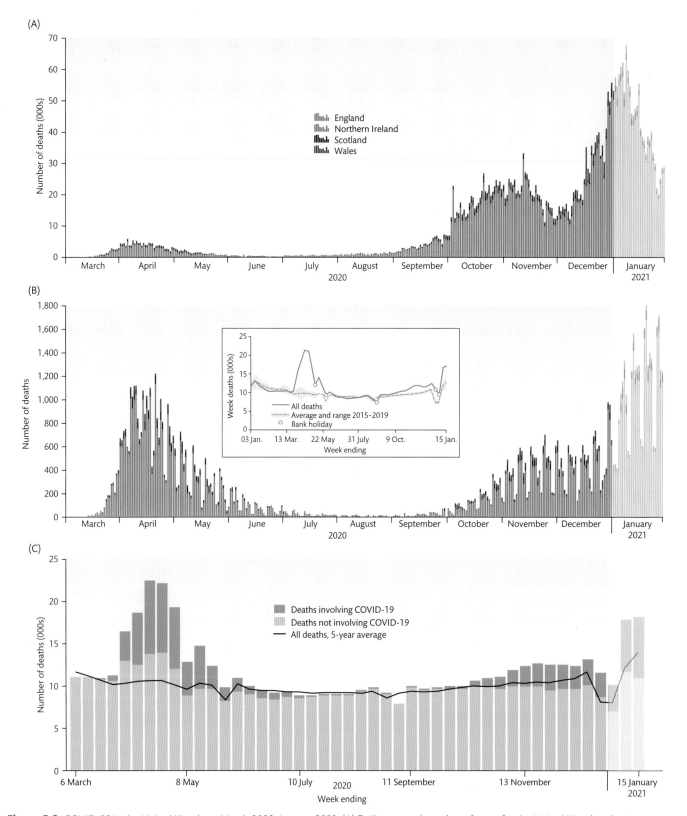

Figure 5.8 COVID-19 in the United Kingdom, March 2020–January 2021. (A) Daily reported number of cases for the United Kingdom by administration. (B) Daily reported number of deaths in England within 28 days of a positive test. (C) Weekly excess mortality attributable to COVID-19, England and Wales, March 2020–January 2021.

Source: data from ONS coronavirus website, https://coronavirus.data.gov.uk/, downloaded 30 January 2021.

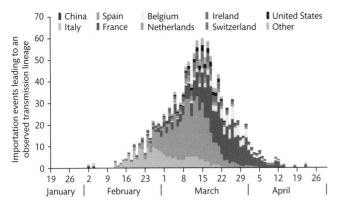

Figure 5.9 Country of origin of COVID-19 lineages in the United Kingdom, January–May 2020. Estimated fraction of importation events attributable to inbound travellers from different countries by date. The impact of the United Kingdom lockdown in late March upon importations is striking.

Reproduced under a Creative Commons Attribution 4.0 International (CC BY 4.0) Licence from du Plessis, L., McCrone, J.T., Zarebski, A.E., et al. (2021). 'Establishment and lineage dynamics of the SARS-CoV-2 epidemic in the UK.' *Science*, 371, 708–12. doi: 10.1126/science.abf2946

(i) reconstruct the number of new COVID-19 infections over time, (ii) estimate a measure of ongoing transmission at time t (R_t), and (iii) predict the number of new COVID-19 deaths in different regions and age groups.

Figure 5.12 shows the estimated time trajectories of R_t for the National Health Service (NHS) regions of England from mid-February 2020 to the year end, along with the 95% CI. The immediate impact of the first lockdown in reducing R_t in all regions of England is striking. Prior to lockdown, community circulation of the SARS-CoV-2 was widespread, with R_t values in the range 2.5–3.0. During the lockdown, R_t was maintained below the critical value of 1 in all regions, although it drifted unevenly upwards towards 1 over the course of the lockdown as people settled into new routines and periodically stretched the lockdown rules. This pattern became more evident after lockdown began to be eased from mid-May. R_t exceeded 1 in some areas (**Figure 5.13**), especially in the South West

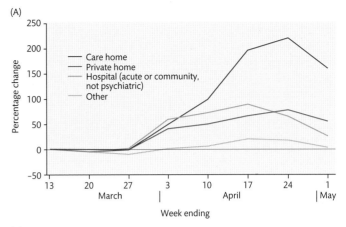

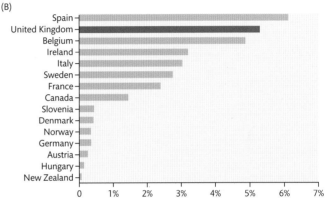

Figure 5.11 United Kingdom care home mortality from COVID-19. (A) Relative to the week ending 13 March 2020, percentage change in deaths from any cause by place of death in England and Wales to the end of April 2020. (B) Deaths attributed to COVID-19 in care homes, from the start of the pandemic to mid-June 2020, as a percentage of all care home residents/beds in sample countries.

(A) Reproduced from Health Foundation, https://www.health.org.uk/news-and-comment/charts-and-infographics/deaths-from-any-cause-in-care-homes-have-increased, accessed 23 January 2021; (B) Source: data from Comas-Herrera et al. (2020, Table 2, p. 21).

and North West regions as the holiday season got underway, while lockdown guidance was increasingly ignored in several major urban areas as people began to return to work. Local and regional lockdowns were imposed in parts of the Greater Manchester and West Yorkshire conurbations. Other COVID-19 hotspots began to appear in such cities as Leicester and Luton (**Figure 5.13B**).

The Medical Research Council Biostatistics Unit estimated that it was very likely that R_t was close to 1 in most regions of England at mid-August, with the holiday area of South West as the region in which it was most likely that R_t exceeded 1 (probability 60 per cent). At the same time, and in stark contrast, the probability that R_t exceeded 1 was less than 20 per cent for London and the South East and less than 5 per cent in the East of England. As **Figure 5.8A** shows, new cases were consistently low and plateauing at less than 1,000 new confirmed cases per day from the beginning of June. This is suggestive of established low-level community transmission rather than epidemic conditions. Associated with a median estimate for R_t which was generally less than 1 in most regions, it appeared that, by early August, the first wave of the pandemic was under control in the United Kingdom. The situation changed, however, as

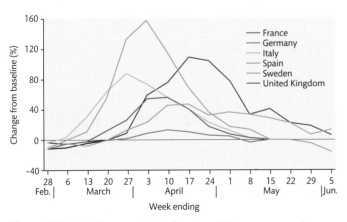

Figure 5.10 Weekly excess deaths for selected European countries, February–June 2020. Change from baseline weekly deaths, by week, shows the impact of COVID-19 on mortality.

Reproduced from The Health Foundation, https://www.health.org.uk/news-and-comment/charts-and-infographics/comparing-covid-19-impact-in-the-uk-to-european-countries, accessed 23 January 2021.

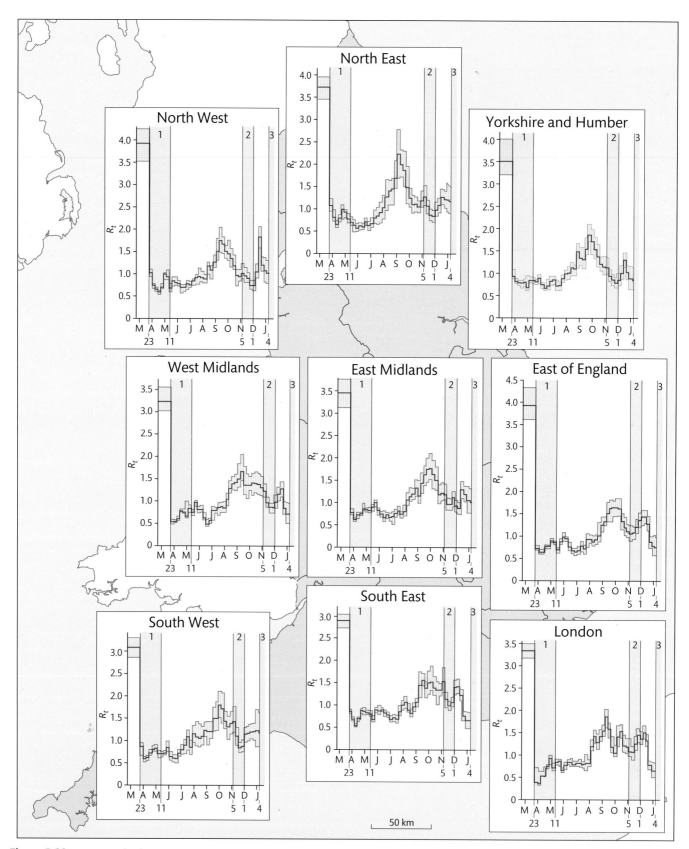

Figure 5.12 Estimates of R_t for PHE regions. The line traces give the median estimated real-time trajectories of R_t by week from mid-February 2020 to mid-January 2021. The 95% CIs are also shown. The grey zones mark the times of the three national lockdowns (labelled '1', '2', and '3'); the specific days of the month on which lockdowns began and ended are marked on the horizontal axes. During the time interval between the second and third lockdowns, a four-level system of regional tiers was employed in an attempt to control the spread of the COVID virus.

Reproduced from Medical Research Council (MRC) Biostatistics Unit, https://www.mrc-bsu.cam.ac.uk/now-casting/report-on-nowcasting-and-forecasting-6th-august-2020/, accessed 23 January 2021.

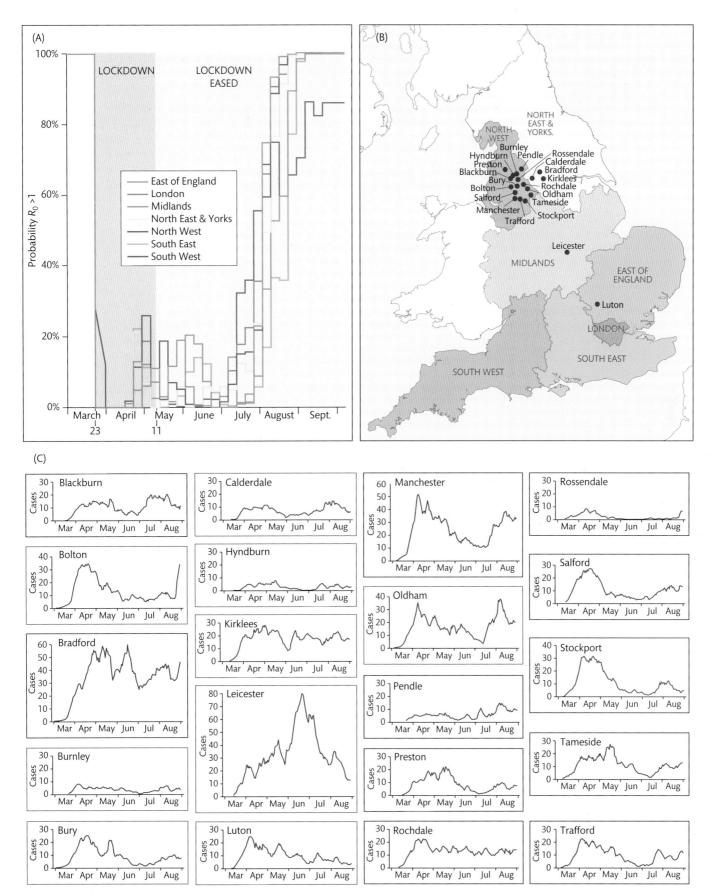

Figure 5.13 Weekly estimated probability that R_t >1 in the NHS regions of England, 23 March–October 2020. (A) The line traces show the probability that R_t >1 in the English NHS regions over the lockdown period (23 March–11 May 2020) and after the lockdown was relaxed. Once population mixing recommenced after restrictions were eased, R_t grew rapidly up to the second COVID wave in the autumn. (B) Location of 20 hotspots on Public Health England's virus watch list at risk of local lockdown, mid-August 2020. (C) Daily reported COVID-19 cases in the hotspots identified in (B), March–August 2020.

(A) Reproduced from Medical Research Council (MRC) Biostatistics Unit, https://www.mrc-bsu.cam.ac.uk/now-casting/report-on-nowcasting-and-forecasting-6th-august-2020/, accessed 23 January 2021; (B) Source: data from Public Health England (2020b).

schools and institutions of higher education reopened in September and October, with their influx of domestic and overseas students reinforced by holidaymakers returning from other parts of the world. As **Figure 5.12** shows, R_t ballooned through the fourth quarter of 2020 as a second COVID-19 wave took hold across the United Kingdom.

5.4.3 Geographical Anatomy of the First Pandemic Wave (January–July 2020)

The swash model, described in section 1.6.2 in Chapter 1, was applied to daily confirmed COVID-19 cases for 149 spatial units. The units comprise the upper tier of local government in England— that is, all unitary authorities, London boroughs, metropolitan boroughs, and combined districts of non-metropolitan counties classified as unitary authorities. The start and end dates of the dataset (30 January–24 July) spanned the duration of the first pandemic wave in the United Kingdom. Figures 5.14–5.16 summarize the results of the modelling procedure. As shown by **Figure 5.14A**, the pandemic flooded the English regions in the last week of February and the first 2 weeks of March. The graph in **Figure 5.14B** plots the percentage of areas in each NHS region infected by various dates over this 3-week period. It clearly indicates that

London and the South East led the spread of infection which then diffused generally northwest along the dense population axis, London–Midlands–North West. The North East and Yorkshire was the last region to be swept by the pandemic.

Consistent with **Figure 5.14**, the integrals in **Figure 5.15** showed erratic behaviour until the end of February. Then, a sharp rise in I_A and a concomitant fall in S_A occurred; there was a similar sharp rise in R_{OA}. Lockdown slowed the spatial spread (flattening of the line trace for R_{OA}) of the pandemic, and this continued into the period of eased restrictions until late July when R_{OA} began to increase again. This probably reflected the appearance of localized COVID-19 flare-ups, for example, in Leicester and towns of the southern northwest; see **Figure 5.13B**.

Figure 5.16 illustrates the changing values per day of the average leading edge and velocity parameters ($\bar{t}_{LE}$ and V_{LE} respectively) over the build-up phase of the pandemic, January–March. Until mid-February, spread occurred in a limited number of geographical areas in the London area and the South East. Generalized and rapid spread across England took place during the last week of February and the first 2 weeks of March, and this is reflected in the almost vertical rise in the line trace for $\bar{t}_{LE}$. The trace for V_{LE} slowly declined over this period as the initial wave energy from a point source morphed into a large polygon.

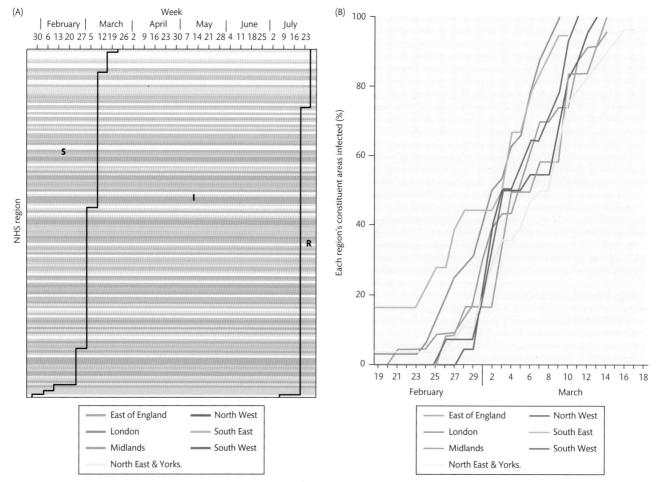

Figure 5.14 COVID-19 pandemic in England, January–July 2020: swash model results, I. (A) *SIR* space–time integrals map for England. The vertical axis uses colour coding to indicate which areas comprise each NHS region. (B) Percentage of areas in each region first reached during the swash stage of the pandemic, last week of February–second week of March 2020.

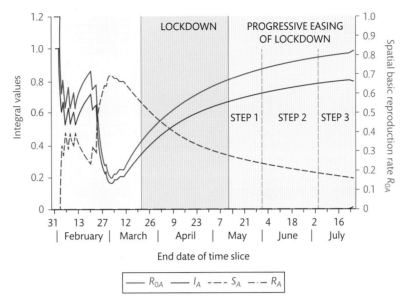

Figure 5.15 COVID-19 pandemic in England, January–July 2020: swash model results, II. Time trajectories of epidemic integrals, S_A, I_A, R_A (left-hand axis), and of the spatial basic reproduction number, R_{0A} (right-hand axis). On 11 May, the United Kingdom government published its 'COVID-19 recovery strategy' consisting of three phases for easing lockdown measures in England. Step 1 began on 11 May. It included encouraging people back to their workplaces if they could not work from home. The public were allowed 'unlimited exercise' and could rest and sit outside or play sports with members of their household. Step 2 commenced on 1 June. People were allowed to leave the house for any reason. Up to six people from different households were allowed to meet outside, in both parks and private gardens, provided they observed social distancing rules. Some school years returned on this date, and outdoor markets and car showrooms reopened. All shops which were still subject to closure were permitted to reopen from 15 June. Step 3 began on 4 July. Public houses, restaurants, and hairdressers were permitted to open with social distancing measures in place. Two households were permitted to meet indoors with social distancing in place. Hotels, camping, and other accommodation sites also reopened.

5.5 The United States, I: Urban–Rural Contrasts

If the United Kingdom's experience of the first year of the COVID-19 pandemic was poor, that of the United States was, in some respects, even worse. **Figure 5.17A** shows the daily time series of confirmed COVID-19 cases and deaths between 20 January and 25 August 2020. Over this period, 5.7 million cases occurred with deaths totalling 176,000—a mortality rate of approximately 3 per cent. **Figure 5.17B** plots the excess mortality from COVID-19 on a weekly basis over the course of the pandemic to September 2020.

5.5.1 County-Level Analyses

Figures 5.18 and **5.19** summarize a critical feature of the COVID-19 pandemic in the United States which is discussed in Oster et al. (2020). By mapping the geographical distribution of COVID-19 hotspots at the county level in the period 8 March–15 July, Oster

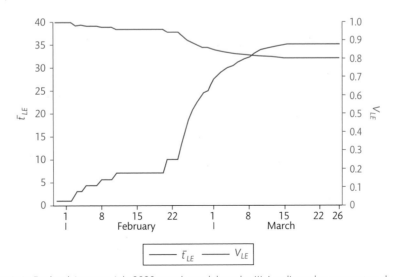

Figure 5.16 COVID-19 pandemic in England, January–July 2020: swash model results, III. Leading edge parameters during the build-up phase of the pandemic, 1 February–26 March 2020. Line traces of the daily values of the average leading edge, $\bar{t}_{LE}$ (left-hand axis), and the leading edge velocity, V_{LE} (right-hand axis), parameters.

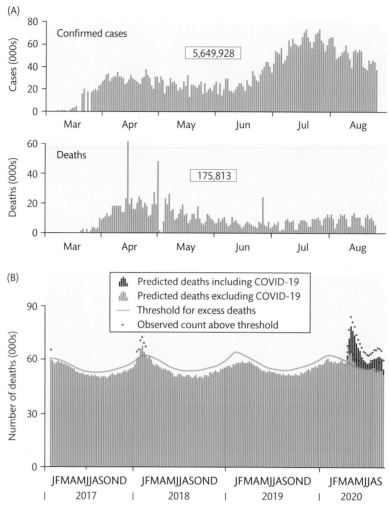

Figure 5.17 COVID-19 pandemic in the United States, I. (A) Daily time series of confirmed cases and deaths, March–August 2020. (B) Estimated weekly excess mortality attributable to COVID-19 as judged against a 3-year estimate of expected deaths in a non-COVID year. (A) WHO COVID-19 Dashboard, https://covid19.who.int/region/amro/country/us, accessed 23 January 2021; (B) CDC, https://www.cdc.gov/nchs/nvss/vsrr/covid19/excess_deaths.htm, accessed 23 January 2021.

and colleagues identified an urban–rural dichotomy in the observed levels of disease activity. Over the study period, 818 (26 per cent) of the 3,142 United States counties met hotspot criteria for 1 or more days (**Figure 5.18**). These 818 counties encompassed approximately 80 per cent of the population in the United States. Counties met the hotspot criteria for a median of 10 days over the entire observation period. The daily number of counties meeting hotspot criteria peaked at 175 in early April, decreased to less than 75 per day during mid-April to early June, before increasing again to 179 in early July.

According to Oster et al. (2020, p. 1128), the percentage of counties meeting hotspot criteria changed over time: "During March–April, 40% of northeastern counties … met hotspot criteria for ≥1 day, whereas hotspot criteria were met by 8–13% of counties in other regions. During May, 8–11% of counties in all four U.S. census regions met hotspot criteria" (**Figure 5.18A, B**). However, during "June and July, 28% of southern counties, representing 67% of the population in the South census region, and 22% of western counties, representing 86% of the population in the West census region, met hotspot criteria, whereas 9–10% of counties in the Northwest

and Midwest … met the hotspot criteria" (**Figure 5.18C**). Thus, a picture emerges of an initial concentration of disease in the northeastern US (March–April), which developed into a generalized geographical distribution of contagion in May. After a summer lull, the pandemic concentrated spatially again, but this time in the south and west of the United States.

Oster et al. (2020) also examined the association of COVID-19 hotspots with the degree of urbanization of counties (**Figure 5.19**). They found that the

percentage of large central metropolitan counties meeting hotspot criteria was 97% during March–April, 46 per cent in May, and 78% during June–July; the proportions were lower for large fringe metropolitan counties (31%, 16%, and 39%, respectively). The proportion of counties in medium metropolitan areas meeting hotspot criteria during June–July was higher (46%) than the percentage during March–April (26%), as was true for counties in small metropolitan areas (32% versus 13%) and micropolitan areas (16% versus 5%). Few counties in non-core areas met hotspot criteria (1–3%) (Oster et al., 2020, p. 1128).

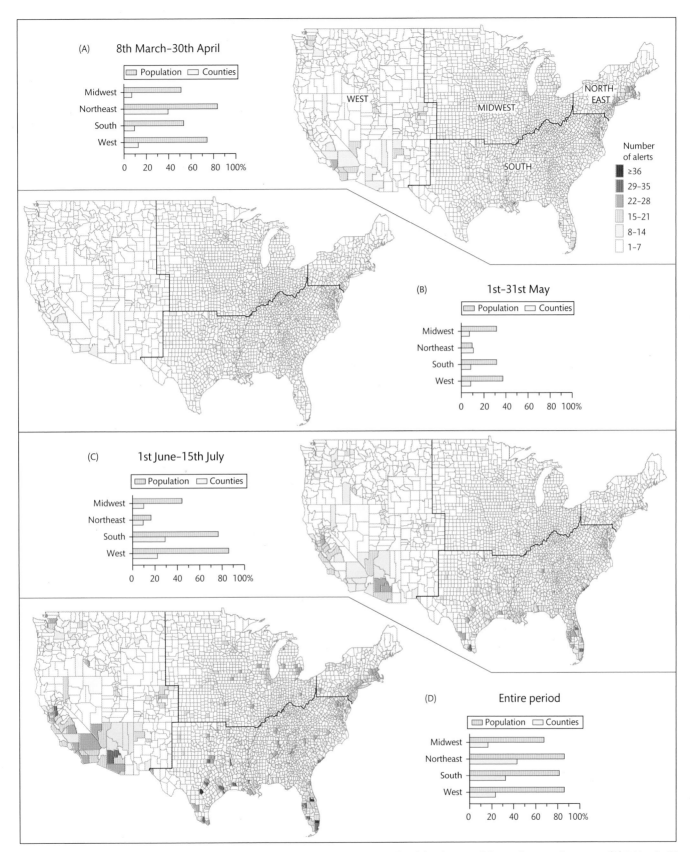

Figure 5.18 COVID-19 pandemic in the United States, March–July 2020, II. Geographical distribution of disease hotspots by county. (A) 8 March–30 April. (B) 1–31 May. (C) 1 June–15 July. (D) Entire period, 8 March–15 July. The definition of hotspot counties is given in Oster et al. (2020). Each county is shaded according to the number of days that the county met hotspot criteria. For each time period, the bar charts give the percentage of counties, and the corresponding percentage of the population, that were classified as hotspot counties in the four census regions.

Reproduced from Oster, A.M., Kang, G.J., Cha, A.E., et al. (2020). 'Trends in number and distribution of COVID-19 hotspot counties – United States, March 8–July 15, 2020.' *Morbidity and Mortality Weekly Report*, 69, 1127–1132.

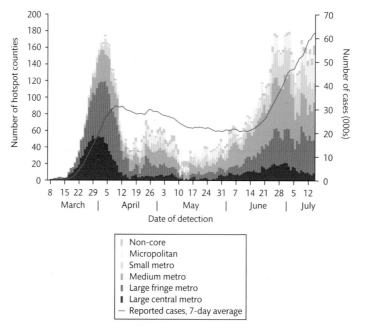

Figure 5.19 COVID-19 pandemic in the United States, III. Daily time series of number of COVID-19 hotspot alerts at the county level by degree of county urbanization, 8 March–15 July 2020. The line trace is a 7-day moving average of newly reported COVID-19 cases. The degree of urbanization of a county follows CDC's National Center for Health Statistics urban–rural classification scheme: *large central metro counties*, in metropolitan statistical areas (MSAs) of ≥1 million population that contain all or part of the area's principal city; *large fringe metro counties*, in MSAs of ≥1 million population and do not qualify as large central; *medium metro counties*, in MSAs of 250,000–999,999 population; *small metro counties*, in MSAs of <250,000 population; *micropolitan counties*, in micropolitan statistical areas; *non-core counties*, not in metropolitan or micropolitan statistical areas.

Reproduced from Oster, A.M., Kang, G.J., Cha, A.E., et al. (2020). 'Trends in number and distribution of COVID-19 hotspot counties – United States, March 8–July 15, 2020.' *Morbidity and Mortality Weekly Report*, 69, 1127–1132.

Overall, it appears that the urbanized, densely populated fringes of the Atlantic and Pacific seaboards and the Gulf coast suffered disproportionately compared with rural America between the Rockies and the Appalachians during the first 7 months of the pandemic. These states experienced more cases and deaths than rural areas.

Urban centres also tended to act as diffusion poles for the spread of COVID-19 into less urbanized locations. **Figure 5.20** confirms this picture. Using United States Bureau of the Census data on the degree of urbanization of states, the trend line in **Figure 5.20A** identifies an inverse association between urbanization and the week of report of

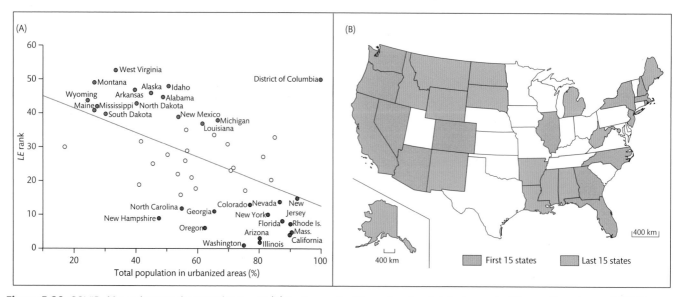

Figure 5.20 COVID-19 pandemic in the United States, IV. (A) Scatter graph of the rank order of states by week of first confirmed case of COVID-19 (representing the leading edge, *LE*, of the infection wave; vertical axis) against percentage of the total population of the state in urbanized areas (horizontal axis). The inverse relationship is highlighted by the linear trend line. Points have been colour coded and then mapped in (B) if they were in the first or last 15 states to report their first COVID case.

the first COVID-19 case (the leading edge of the pandemic in the swash model) for the set of states. Consistent with this observation, Otterstrom and Hochberg (2021, p. 27) reported a 'sizeable degree of rural diffusion' of COVID-19 in the United States in the latter part of 2020.

5.6 The United States, II: Forecasting the Progress of Epidemics

Throughout this book we have seen how scientific understanding has increased and provided ways to ameliorate the impact of epidemics. However, during an epidemic, shorter-term operational issues become dominant, such as the provision of medical supplies and the planning of hospital capacity. These operational considerations require forecasts of the progress of an epidemic, both in the short term and for longer-term capacity planning.

As we saw in Chapter 1, there are two general approaches to disease forecasting: (i) classical *SIR* compartmental models that consider the flow of cases over time and (ii) more empirically based statistical time series approaches that may focus on only some components (or 'compartments'), such as the number of new cases. Recent examples of the latter approach include Smallman-Raynor et al. (2015) on cholera in Haiti, and Rivers et al. (2014) and Ord and Getis (2018) on Ebola virus disease in West Africa. It is in this spirit that we examine some approaches to forecasting the progress of the COVID-19 pandemic. In so doing, it is emphasized that the models we describe are limited in scope and are intended primarily as illustrations of what is possible.

Any forecasting study needs to begin with the question—Why? In the context of a pandemic, one obvious need is for short-term forecasts that enable the planning of, for example, intensive care unit beds and medical equipment. Such forecasts may extend 1 or 2 weeks into the future. There is also a need for forecasts to project the likely course of the epidemic over the longer term. The short-term forecasts may be developed using dynamic linear time series models but, in the longer term, it is necessary to account for the growth and decline of the epidemic wave using some form of growth curve analysis (see section 1.4 in Chapter 1). Such longer-term models provide a way of monitoring the epidemic process, checking for changes in transmission rates or other factors.

In this section, simple models are used to explore each situation separately, although it should be noted that some more advanced models are available that combine both these features; see, for example, Harvey and Kattuman (2020). To illustrate our approaches, we draw on daily records of COVID-19 in sample areas of the United States, March–December 2020.

5.6.1 Sample Areas and Data Sources

Four states (California, Florida, New York, and Wyoming) were selected for the present analysis. New York City was the initial epicentre of the COVID-19 pandemic in the United States, and strict control measures were introduced throughout the state after the initial severe outbreak. California and Florida were selected on account of their contrasting geographical locations on the west and east costs, their high absolute case counts, and the major surges of disease activity that both states experienced in the wake of Memorial

Day (25 May 2020). Finally, and in contrast, Wyoming was selected as a rural state with a relatively small population and a much lower case count. We also note here the well-documented role that political affiliations played in determining the responses of state authorities to the outbreaks in locations under Republican (Florida and Wyoming) and Democratic (California and New York) control (Akovali and Yilmaz, 2020).

Daily counts of newly reported and cumulative COVID-19 cases for each of the four sample areas were accessed from the Johns Hopkins Coronavirus Resource Center (https://coronavirus.jhu.edu/) and the Bing COVID-19 Tracker (http://www.bing.com/covid) for a 306-day study period, 1 March–31 December 2020. This period extended from the approximate start of the epidemic in the United States and included several major public holidays: Memorial Day (25 May), Independence Day (4 July), Labor Day (7 September), and Thanksgiving (26 November). These holidays are deemed to have been potentially significant dates on the COVID-19 calendar for two reasons. First, owing to the heightened population mixing, they signify the sources of a potential surge in COVID-19 activity in succeeding days and weeks. Second, they mark a potential change in the age composition of new cases, from an initial focus in older age groups (with relatively high death rates) to a focus in younger age groups (with relatively low death rates). Based upon these considerations, the data were analysed for three time periods: up to 31 May, up to 31 August, and up to 30 November. Here, the end-of-month dates were selected to permit analysis of the post-holiday surges. To allow for daily reporting effects, all analysis was conducted on time series that had been pre-whitened using a smoothing (7-day moving average) operator.

5.6.2 Short-Term Forecasting

The first step is an exploratory analysis of the raw daily data. This reveals a series of rather weak short-term trends and a strong weekly cycle with lower numbers of cases reported on Sundays. The general pattern of new cases may be described as a series of surges, each of which tends to be positively skewed (a rapid build-up and a much slower decay). Based on these observations, we may consider a simple approach that tracks only the number of infected cases. For a given state, the number of new cases may be represented by a model of the form:

$$y_t = m_{t-1} + s_{t-7} + \varepsilon_t,$$
$$m_t = m_{t-1} + \alpha\varepsilon_t,$$
$$s_t = s_{t-1} + \gamma\varepsilon_t \tag{5.1}$$

The notation is defined as follows:

y_t: the number of reported cases.

m_t: the local mean level.

s_t: the day of the week effect (seven terms).

ε_t: the error term.

The number of newly reported deaths may be represented by a linear regression-autoregressive scheme. The appropriate number of lags for new cases will be resolved empirically; a single lag is shown for convenience in the equation:

$$z_t = \beta_0 + \beta_1 z_{t-1} + \beta_2 y_{t-L} + \delta_t \tag{5.2}$$

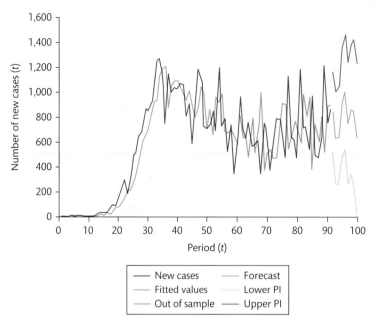

Figure 5.21 Short-term forecasts of COVID-19 cases in Florida, March–June 2020. The state-space model was fitted using data from 2 March to 30 April (60 observations). One-step-ahead forecasts were then generated for May. The model was then used to provide forecasts for the first 10 days of June without any additional data.

Here, the terms are as follows:

z_t: the number of reported deaths.

δ_t: the error term.

L: a suitable lag (may be more than one such term).

$\beta_0, \beta_1, \ldots$: regression coefficients.

Short-term results for Florida

We illustrate the results of our analysis for Florida. The model was fitted using data from 2 March to 30 April 2020 (60 observations) (**Figure 5.21**). One-step-ahead forecasts were then generated for May 2020. As **Figure 5.21** shows, the fitted values and forecasts track the series reasonably well. The model was then used to provide forecasts for the first 10 days of June without any additional data. The rapidly diverging (95 per cent) prediction intervals indicate how the forecasts deteriorate as the lead time increases. From these results, we conclude that such models can provide adequate short-term forecasts for facilities planning but provide no real guide to the longer term.

The reporting of deaths is somewhat irregular. To reduce the noise in the data, we worked with a 7-day moving average of new deaths (NDA). A best subsets model, based upon the 7-day lag of ND (NDA_7) and selected lags of new cases (all lags were considered from lag 1 to lag 20, NC_1 to NC_20), yielded the fitted model:

$$NDA = 5.05 + 0.565 \, NDA\_7 + 0.004 \, NC\_2 + 0.010 \, NC\_16. \quad (5.3)$$

As might be expected, NDA_7 was the most important variable, followed by NC_16. Dropping NC_2 had only a marginal effect. The model had an adjusted R^2 value of 87.7 per cent. The 2-week lag reflected in NC_16 is in line with expectations; adjacent lagged values are highly autocorrelated, so lag 16 should be interpreted as 'about 2 weeks'.

As the pandemic progressed and treatments improved, so the coefficients for NC_2 and NC_16 would be expected to decline and a variable coefficients model should be used to account for these improvements.

5.6.3 Longer-Term Forecasting

In the longer term, we must paint in broad brushstrokes and the analysis has two general aims. The first is to create a simple, yet robust, structure that provides a reasonable description of the ebb and flow of the number of cases. To these ends, we employ a trend curve analysis so that the general behaviour of the epidemic can be understood. The second objective is to provide a framework for analysing shocks to the system, as when large groups gather but ignore public health guidelines. Such circumstances represent a substantial increase in the number of susceptible–infective (S–I) interactions and are precursors to a surge of cases.

Trend curves

A major aim of the analysis is to examine the effects of a major 'spreader' event, such as the high level of social interaction over the Memorial Day (25 May 2020) weekend. One way of examining the effects of a Memorial Day surge is to use trend curves of the form:

$$g(t) = K_1 f(t, P_1, T_1), \, T_1 < t \leq T_2$$
$$= K_1 f(t, P_1, T_1) + K_2 f(t, P_2, T_2), \, T_2 < t \leq T_3 \quad (5.4)$$

In this expression, terms are defined as follows:

$g(t)$: the number of cases in period (day) t.

f: a suitably chosen probability density function (used as a trend curve when multiplied by an appropriate constant).

(K_1, K_2): scaling constants.

(P_1, P_2): sets of unknown parameters of the density functions.

(T_1, T_2, T_3): times corresponding to the start of the outbreak, an intermediate time (such as the Memorial Day weekend), and the end of the series (or the start of the next surge) respectively.

In the absence of a surge associated with Memorial Day, the second term of the trend curve would be negligible. However, if a surge occurs, it will be described by the second term after allowing for the residual effects of the initial outbreak. Clearly, additional terms of a similar form could be added when later surges occur.

Recognizing that the distribution of COVID-19 cases over time tends to be positively skewed, a symmetric distribution such as the logistic (see section 1.4.2 in Chapter 1) is unlikely to provide an effective description. While the Gompertz curve is widely used in epidemiological studies and displays positive skewness, its application in the current analysis fails to describe either the slow start of the epidemic or the extended slow decay. A more flexible alternative that overcomes these limitations is the incomplete gamma function. In brief, the gamma (or Erlang) distribution is used to describe arrival times in models of queuing processes. While the 'arrivals' of COVID-19 cases are not independent, the counts observed over time may be interpreted in the manner of a histogram albeit with dependent observations. Thus, the incomplete gamma function, scaled to reflect the number of cases, is a reasonable description of the flow of cases and takes the form:

$$f(t) = K(t - T_1)^{a-1} \exp(-b(t - T_1)) \qquad (5.5)$$

When expressed as a density function, the expected value is $E(t) = a/b$, the mode (peak of the outbreak) occurs at $(a-1)/b, 1/b$ is related to the rate of transmission, and a is a shape parameter. The parameter K is related to the time origin and has no direct interpretation. As the data refer to counts, the trend curves were fitted using a chi-squared error criterion (EC):

$$EC = \sum((observed - expected)^2 / expected) \qquad (5.6)$$

Other criteria, such as the sum of squared errors, were also considered; occasionally, the results differ but they are usually quite close. Each surge is fitted consecutively so the parameters of a given surge are set and not modified by data from a subsequent surge. This approach has several advantages: the estimation procedure is simplified, the results reflect the 'real-time' information about a given surge, and a given surge provides initial parameter estimates for the next surge.

A detailed analysis is presented next for Florida, with brief summaries for the other three states. Further analytic results are available from one of the authors (KO).

Forecasts, I: Florida

The first recorded case of COVID-19 in Florida was dated 2 March (coded Day 1), with the number of cases accelerating from 9 March (Day 8). On this basis, the daily series of cases was analysed with the settings $T_1 = 8$, $T_2 = 91$ (31 May), $T_3 = 185$ (31 August), and $T_3 = 276$ (30 November). The curves were fitted with start dates of 9 March, 3 June, and 1 September, thereby allowing a week after the 'onset' before new cases were likely to emerge. As indicated in the description of the trend curves, the results for the period ending 31 May were held fixed throughout the later analyses. The results are summarized in **Figure 5.22**; again, detailed numerical results are available from one of the authors (KO).

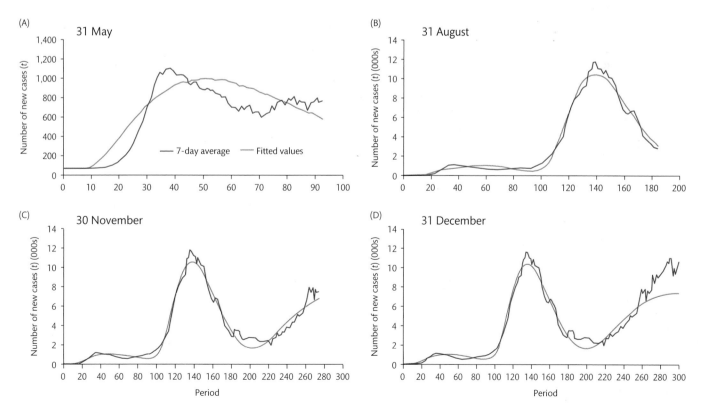

Figure 5.22 Observed and fitted values for the number of newly reported cases of COVID-19 in Florida to December 2020. (A) To 31 May. (B) 31 August. (C) 30 November. (D) 30 November fit, with forecasts to 31 December. Observed values, formed as a 7-day average, are represented by the red line traces.

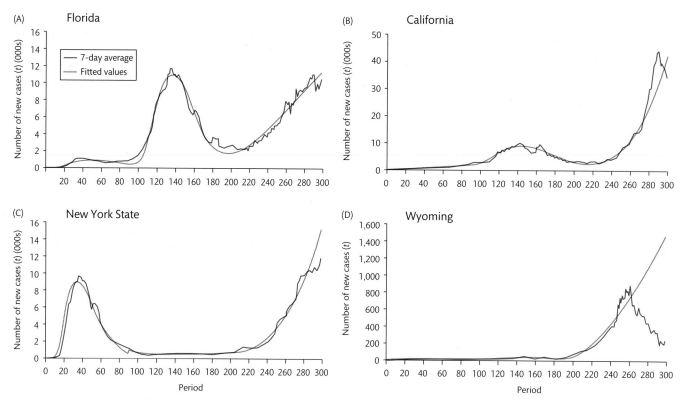

Figure 5.23 Forecasts of the numbers of new COVID-19 cases to December 2020. (A) Florida. (B) California. (C) New York. (D) Wyoming. For each area, the graphs plot (i) observed values to 31 December 2020 (represented by the red line traces) and (ii) fitted values to 30 November, followed by the forecasts for the month of December with 30 November as the forecast origin.

Figure 5.22A shows that the initial outbreak in Florida was largely contained by late May, only to explode after the Memorial Day celebrations (**Figure 5.22B**). This surge was waning by late summer, but a more serious wave arose in the autumn after Labor Day (**Figure 5.22C**). **Figure 5.22D** represents long-term forecasts for the month of December, with 30 November as the forecast origin. The forecasts systematically undershoot the actual values but serve to show that the epidemic continued to increase in severity. This would have served as an early warning sign of the heightened pressure as hospitals were overwhelmed by the increased need for intensive care facilities.

Forecasts, II: other areas

When compared with Florida, the longer-term forecasts for other areas (California, New York, and Wyoming) reveal several interesting features. First, the pattern for California was similar to that for Florida, although the later surge was much more serious. Strong actions to protect public health at the state level had enabled New York City to avoid the Memorial Day surge, but the subsequent relaxation of those policies contributed to the later surge after Labor Day. Wyoming maintained a low level of infections until mid-September; the series peaked in mid-November and then declined, a feature not picked up by the fitted growth curve.

The forecasting performance and potential problems are illustrated in **Figure 5.23**, which shows the observed values through to 31 December 2020 and the fitted values to 30 November, followed by the forecasts for the month of December with 30 November as the forecast origin.

For all four states, the forecasts are monotone increasing, although they track the data quite closely, except for Wyoming. When the models are fitted using the entire series, the fitted values turn down, although the change for Wyoming comes far too late. The reasons behind the sudden change in the Wyoming series are unclear, but could reflect a combination of cold weather, the end of the tourist season, and stricter control measures that served to reduce virus transmission. Whatever the reasons, changes in the frequency of *S–I* contacts resulted in a change in the parameters of the growth curve.

5.6.4 Summary

Forecasting the progress of an epidemic requires a variety of sources of information. The transmission mechanisms and the length of time for which an infected person can infect others are obviously critical to any attempts to understand the overall process. However, forecasts must often be based upon imperfect scientific knowledge and the data available may be less accurate than desired, due to reporting delays or the lack of testing. That said, progress is still possible. First, we must identify the purpose behind the forecasting exercise. If it is a matter of a few days ahead for resource planning, a time series model will often suffice. However, if the planning horizon is longer term, then growth curves offer a way forward. The models presented in this section are basic, but clearly more sophisticated versions are possible. As in any forecasting exercise, the need is to develop models that are tailored to the problem in hand.

5.7 Conclusion

In the light of the discussion in Chapter 1, it can readily be seen why the COVID-19 pandemic has wrought such global devastation on the human population. It is a novel virus spreading through a virgin soil population with little or no immunity to the contagion. Neither is it surprising to find that community circulation is being maintained in the high-density populations of the world's cities which then act as diffusion poles for the later spread of infection into less densely populated rural areas. In towns and cities, human interaction is greater than in rural areas, driven by packed housing units, so that social distancing is difficult to maintain. Towns and cities are also the principal centres of employment and trade in the world economy. As with the 1918 influenza pandemic, we should expect periodic hotspots of COVID-19 both geographically and temporally while community circulation of the virus persists. Until something approaching herd immunity is achieved by a combination of natural exposure to the virus and mass vaccination, there will remain the possibility of repeated waves of COVID-19 infection.

6

Infectious Disease Control

CONTENTS

6.1 Introduction

This chapter begins at a local spatial scale, seven centuries ago, among the plague-ridden lazarettos of Venice. It ends at the global scale with twenty-first-century developments in the Internet-based monitoring and surveillance of infectious diseases. It was in medieval Europe that the first significant attempts at infectious disease control began. In the twenty-first century, the world is still working at disease control, elimination, and eradication. New words and phrases have entered the disease lexicon: *lockdown*, *self-isolation*, and *social distancing*. These intrinsically geographical ideas have become common currency, and they evoke the global effort mounted to control the ongoing pandemic of COVID-19 (see Chapter 5). Confronted with a disease agent to which the human population has little or no immunity, three approaches to control may be employed: (i) allow the agent to spread so that natural herd immunity is established among the survivors, (ii) separate the susceptible and infected components of the population by isolation or quarantine, and (iii) develop and deploy safe and effective vaccines and treatments. This chapter examines how approaches (ii) and (iii) have evolved historically, and how methods that were first developed and implemented in medieval times have been adapted to fit twenty-first-century epidemic and pandemic control. For potentially severe diseases, adoption of the 'do nothing' route to herd immunity, (i), may result in such high levels of morbidity and mortality as to be politically and socially unacceptable in a modern society. But, as we shall see, herd immunity can be achieved through vaccination.

6.2 The Underpinnings of Disease Control

In Figure 1.8 in Chapter 1, a simple model of the spread of an infectious disease in a human population was outlined. The population was divided into three subpopulations: those at risk of infection (susceptibles, S), those who are infected (infectives, I), and those who have recovered from the infection (recovereds, R). Propagation of an epidemic occurs by mixing between the S and I subpopulations. This generates new cases by the transition $S{\rightarrow}I$. Once an epidemic has begun, its continuation is dependent upon the presence of a sufficiently large S subpopulation for transitions of the type $S{\rightarrow}I$ to be uninterrupted and, hence, for community transmission to be maintained. The size of the I subpopulation will fall as those infected either recover, R, or die, while the S subpopulation is renewed by births.

In order to control the geographical spread of an infection, it is necessary to halt the transition, $S{\rightarrow}I$. **Figure 6.1** focuses upon ways in which this can be done. The first approach, labelled (i) in **Figure 6.1**, is inherently geographical and involves the breaking of chains of transmission by preventing the mixing of the I and S subpopulations through the establishment of protective spatial barriers. Such barriers range from the highly local (social distancing and individual isolation), through community isolation and quarantine, to the imposition of regional or national restrictions on movement via 'buffer zones' or *cordons sanitaires*. Such methods were finely developed and honed during medieval times, especially in Italy, to control the spread of bubonic plague from the thirteenth to the early eighteenth centuries (the so-called Plague Centuries). The second method of interrupting the chains of infection,

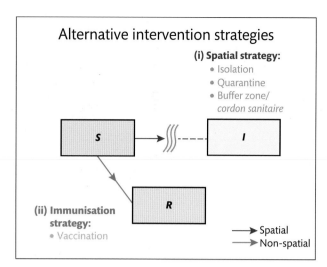

Figure 6.1 Interrupting chains of infection. Alternative intervention strategies based on: (i) a *spatial strategy*, blocking links by isolation and quarantine between susceptibles and infectives; and (ii) a generally *aspatial strategy*, opening of new direct pathways from susceptible to recovered status through immunization. This outflanks the infectives (I) box.
Reproduced from Cliff, A.D., Haggett, P. (1989). 'Spatial aspects of epidemic control.' *Progress in Human Geography*, 13, 315–47.

labelled (ii) in **Figure 6.1**, is to short-circuit the route from the *S* to *R* states by creating population immunity through immunization. Immunization is commonly achieved today through the use of vaccines and may, prima facie, be viewed as an aspatial control strategy. However, as a means of epidemic control, immunization is usually geographically directed to achieve optimum results. This strategy evolved from the late eighteenth century and is discussed in section 6.4.

6.3 Spatial Strategies—Blocking Spread

In **Figure 6.2B** and **C**, ways of blocking spread are summarized. In the diagrams, infected areas are shown in blue, while disease-free areas are shown in pale yellow. In **Figure 6.2B**, the disease-free area needs to be protected by isolation. Such defensive isolation entails the building of a spatial barrier to restrict movement between the diseased and disease-free areas, the aim being to prevent infectious cases in any diseased area from gaining access to susceptibles in a disease-free area. *Cordons sanitaires* are one of the principal tools used to achieve this. Offensive containment (**Figure 6.2C**) is the flipside of this, where a containment barrier is interposed between known diseased and disease-free areas to prevent spread from the former to the latter. The diseased area is then cleared of infection. We consider each of these approaches in turn using examples of their development in medieval Italy. We then show how each approach has been applied in the present century.

6.3.1 Defensive Isolation

The basic tenets of defensive isolation are well illustrated by developments in plague control in medieval and early modern Italy. To implement defensive isolation, Italy's states and principalities north of Rome, led by Venice, Milan, and Genoa, used a system of *bans* and *suspensions*. When infectious disease was uncovered anywhere

by a particular Magistracy, a proclamation of *ban* (when the presence of communicable disease was positively ascertained) or *suspension* (precaution because there was legitimate suspicion of disease) was issued. Bans were long term, suspensions short term. Bans and suspensions were used to denote the interruption of regular trade and communication. With banishment and suspension, no person, boat, merchandise, or letter could enter the state issuing the order except at a few well-specified ports or places of entrance where quarantine stations, discussed later, were set up. At the stations, incoming people, boats, and merchandise were subject to quarantine and disinfection even if they carried health certificates issued at the point of departure (**Figure 6.3**). The health certificates were the seventeenth- and eighteenth-century equivalents of the present-day international vaccination certificates, certifying that travellers and boats were free of disease. The authorities also reserved the right to refuse access (even, if necessary, to the quarantine stations) to anything or anybody from banished areas. People attempting to violate the ban or enter the territory of the banishing state were commonly executed.

The *cordon sanitaire* was a much-used tool for enforcing bans. At one time or another, the entire coastline of Italy had such cordons to try to prevent entry of the plague carried by people and goods from Asia. Here, we look at just one example (Sicily and the Plague of Messina in 1743) to show how the cordons were managed when fully developed. See Cliff and Smallman-Raynor (2013, pp. 1–20) for a full account of this and other examples.

Sicily 1743: the Plague of Messina

Defensive isolation was used in the heel of Italy (Puglia) and in Sicily in 1743 to thwart the generalized spread of what turned out to be the last major outbreak of plague in Europe—the Plague of Messina. The regulations under which plague control operated in the Kingdom of the Two Sicilies is best summarized in the *Regolamento generale di servizio sanitario marittimo, sanzionato da S.M. il 1 gennajo 1820, in*

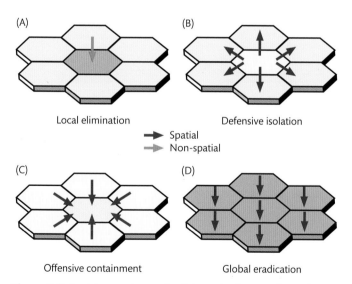

Figure 6.2 Spatial control strategies. Schematic diagram of spatial control strategies to prevent epidemic spread. (A) Local elimination. (B) Defensive isolation. (C) Offensive containment. (D) Global eradication. Geographical areas are shown schematically as hexagons. Infected areas are shown in blue; disease-free areas are pale yellow.
Reproduced from Cliff, A.D., Haggett, P. (1989). 'Spatial aspects of epidemic control.' *Progress in Human Geography*, 13, 315–47.

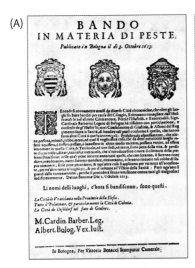
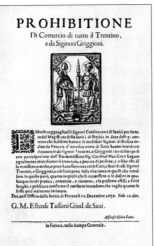
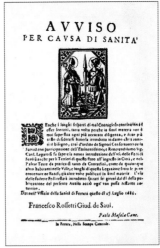

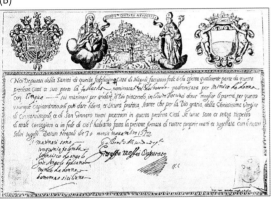
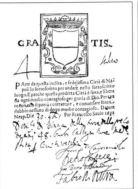
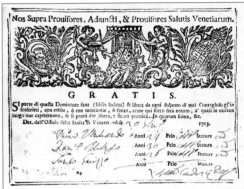

Figure 6.3 Certificates issued at times of plague. (A) From left to right: Bologna, 1613, poster proclaiming no contact, on pain of death, with people or animals from Cologne, Düsseldorf, or Vratislavia where there was plague; Ferrara, 1679, poster proclaiming restrictions on trade to help combat the transmission of plague; Ferrara, 1682, poster stating health passes to be introduced in 6 days. (B) Travel documents issued by Naples (*left*) and Venice (*right*). The document to the left, dated 1632 and measuring 35 × 25 cm, is embossed with coats of arms and a panorama of Naples. It was issued to the captain of the fellucha (a type of boat) named *Santa Maria del Rosario*, which was sailing from Naples to Civitavecchia, the port of Rome, with five sailors on board. Their names are listed at the end of the certificate. It declares Naples to be free of all infectious disease, and asks for unrestricted and secure *pratique* (*prattica*: a licence to deal with a port after quarantine or on producing a clean bill of health). Nearly one hundred years later (1713) and the health passport for Venice (*right*) appears essentially the same as that for Naples. The document in the centre, measuring 16 × 12 cm and embossed with the arms of the city of Naples, was given in plague periods to each traveller from the port of Naples at embarkation. It declares the city to be healthy and free of all morbid contagions. It also declares that it is safe to trade and negotiate with the bearer without fear of infection. The almost illegible handwriting gives the date (30 June or July 1632), the name and a description of the bearer, his destination, and the signatures of the four representatives of the city authorities. The anonymous source author (p. 32), interprets the script as Giovanni Angelo Baucano, of the Greek Tower (*de la Torre dello Greco* barely recognizable at the end of line 1), age 48 (de anni 48, line 2), with a dark chestnut moustache (*castagno*, middle of line 2) and a mole on the upper left cheek, travelling to Civitavecchia (line 3). The signatories are Francesco Caracciolo, Delio Capece, Giov. Battista d'Alessandro, and Fabio di Ruvo. Such certificates were issued to try to guarantee free passage and continuance of travel in the face of bans and suspensions.
Sources: (B), left and centre, Ministero dell'Interno, Direzione Generale Della Sanità Pubblica, Napoli, 1910, Plates II and III, following p. 32.

esecuzione dell'articolo 20 legge de' 20 ottobre 1819. Inter alia, paragraphs 219–235 of the general service regulations specify the geographical structure of a defensive isolation *cordon sanitaire* to be applied around coastlines, its manning, operation, and reporting system. The critical elements are listed in Table 6.1 and included (i) the siting of guard posts within viewing distance of each other; (ii) a complement of three soldiers per guard post; and (iii) a hierarchical reporting structure from the heads of local guard posts, via intermediate officers, to the provincial military commander and the sanitary superintendent.

Messina had been free from plague since 1624, and the Sicilians prided themselves on the rigour of their quarantine laws that they

thought had preserved them. A protective *cordon* of observation posts existed around the entire coastline of Sicily as part of this enforcement. In May 1743, a Genoese vessel arrived in Messina (Figure 6.4) from Morea (near Patras in the Little Dardanelles), on board of which had occurred some suspicious deaths (plague was present in the Levant at this time). The ship and cargo were burnt but, soon after, cases of a suspicious form of disease were observed in the hospital and in the poorest parts of the town. *The Supremo Magistrato di Commercio* preferred commercial expediency to rigorous enforcement of the sanitary laws and a major epidemic of plague developed which killed an estimated 40,000–50,000 persons. It was this plague that led to the establishment of

Table 6.1 Kingdom of the Two Sicilies: geographical structure of the *cordon sanitaire* specified in the general service regulations of 1820

Paragraph	Regulation	Cordon structure
Geographical features		
221	La distanza tra un posto e l'altro dev' esser tale, che l'uno sia sempre a vista dell' altro	Each guard post to be within sighting distance of its neighbours
222	Quando in una provincia o valle vi sieno delle coste inaccessibili, per le quali vi ha bisogno di poca o niuna custodia, l'Intendente deve impiegare questo risparmio di forze de cordone per assicurare le spiagge aperte, ed i siti più esposti a degli sbarchi furtive	Any economies in manpower from not having to patrol inaccessible coastal sections to be used to guard open beaches and places most available for clandestine landings
Integrity of the cordon		
229	Gli obblighi di tutti gl'individui destinati a formare il cordone, si riducono generalmente ad impedir nel le spiagge l'approdo di qualsivoglia legno, qualunque ne sia la provenienza, obbligandolo a dirigersi ne'punti più vicini, ove risiede una deputazione de salute	All individuals in the cordon must act to prevent, through a general reduction of manpower, unauthorized beach landings by boat by funnelling those concerned towards the nearest points manned by sanitary officers
230	Ne' casi di burrasca, i legni amici o nemici possono, quando il naufragio è quasi sicuro, farsi approdare nelle spiagge, impiegando all' uopo tutte le cautele di custodia, ed un rigoroso cordone *parziale*, sino a che non accorrano i deputati di salute corrispondenti per applicarvi l'analogo trattamento sanitaria	Shipwrecks to be quarantined by a local *cordon sanitaire* until sanitary officers can attend
231	Se qualche posto fosse minacciato da gente, che volesse sbarcare a viva forza, ed alla quale non potesse resistere, il capo posto deve innalzare un bandiera di convenzione, ed a questo segnale deve accorrere subito la forza de' posti limitrofi. Avvenendo questo caso in tempo di notte, il segnale per aver soccorso sarà di due fuochi consecutive	Post heads must signal for support from neighbouring posts if a forced landing is threatened. Two consecutive fire signals used at night
232	In ogni posto devono farsi, durante la notte, de'fuochi convenuti di corrispondenza, a fin di assicurarsi della vigilanza de'posti limitrofi	Fire signals to be agreed between adjacent posts for night communication
233	Nei tempi di cordone l'esercizio della pesca non è più libero. Le barche pescarecce possono uscire dal levare al tra montar del sole; ed in questo periodo è anche proibito loro di allontanarsi dal lido oltre le quattro miglia. I padroni di queste barche devono essere allora muniti di una *bolletta*, che i deputati di salute corrispondenti devono loro vistare giorno per giorno	A charge is made for fishing during times of cordon, collected daily by the sanitary inspectors from the boat captain. Fishing is permitted only during daylight hours and not more than 4 miles from the beach
235	I cordone sanitari marittimi possono anche stabilirsi per mezzo di altrettante crociere di barche armate, applicandosi a queste, sotto certe tali necessarie modificazioni, le norme di sopra indicate per la distribuzione, il servigio e la dipendenza de' posti situati a terra su i littorali	Armed boats (*felucca*) patrol the coastline
Manning		
223	In ogni posto devono montar di guardia tre individui ed un basse uffiziale, che farà le funzioni di capo posto. Quando le spiagge sieno aperte ed esposte in modo che non bastion a custodirle in quattro individui destinati per ciascun posto, può allora aumentarsene il numero a seconda del bisogno e delle circostanze	Normally three guards per post with a low-level official as head of post; four on open beaches difficult to guard, augmented if necessary to suit the conditions
224	La guardia dee recarsi al suo posto la mattina, ed esserne rilevata il domane alla stess'ora, durante il qual tempo è vietato agl'individui che la compongono, il potersi appartare dal posto sotto qualunque pretesto. Il capo-posto dee rimaner fisso per un'inera settimana, ad oggetto di conoscer bene le consegne e trasmetterle, e di conoscere i segnali e le pratiche da osservarsi. Egli ha l'obbligo particolare d'invigilar sulla condotta de'suoi subalterni	Guards must be on station from daylight and relieved the following morning. The head guard has a 1-week tour of duty; he has recording, reporting, and supervisory duties
225	Per ogni sei posti vi sarà un'Uffizial comandante, che dee rimaner distaccato per un'intera settimana, e tener presso di se una o più persone a cavallo per la sollecita diramazione degli ordini. La posizione da assegnarsi al suddetto Comandante sarà, per quanto è possibile, la centrale. Egli avrà specialmente l'incarico d'invigilare all'adempimento dgli obblighi ingiunti a(i) I capi-posti	A sanitary official every six posts, centrally located, on a weekly tour of duty. The official is responsible for distributing orders rapidly using horsemen
226	Per ogni tre distaccamenti di sei posti l'uno, vi sarà un sottoispettore, che anche deve avere una situazione centrale. Il suo incarico è quello d'invigilare alla regolarità del servisio de'tre distaccameni che compongono la sua sotto-ispezione	Three detachments per six posts under the supervision of an under-inspector in a central position
Reporting system		
228	Tra tutt' i capi del cordone vi deve essere una corrispondenza giornaliera ed esatta, onde si rilevi il modo con cui si attende al servizio, e le novità che possono avervi luogo. Affinchè la corrispondenza suddetta proceda colla massima regolarità, e nel modo più celere, i capi-posti devono corrispondere coi rispettivi Comandanti di distaccamento, questi col sotto-ispettore, il sotto-ispettore col' Ispettore, l'Ispettore contemporaneamente coll' Intendente, e col Comandante militare della provincia o valle. Da siffatta regola sono eccettuati i casi di seria considerazione ne' quali, oltre del rapporto regolare da passarsi col cennato metodo, i Comandanti di distaccamento sono autorizzati di far rapporto straordinario, e spedirlo con espresso all' Intendente ed al Comandante della provincia o valle	Cordon commanding officers must communicate daily with each other. The normal upwards reporting system is from local guard post heads via intermediate officers to the provincial military commander and the sanitary superintendent; the intermediate officers can be by-passed in an emergency

Source: Data from Petitti, P. (1852). *Repertorio Administrativo ossia collezione di leggi, decreti, reali rescritti, ministeriali di massima regolamenti, ed istruzioni sull'amministrazione civile de Regno delle Due Sicilie*. Volume 3 (fifth edition). Naples: Tipografia di Gaetano Sautto.

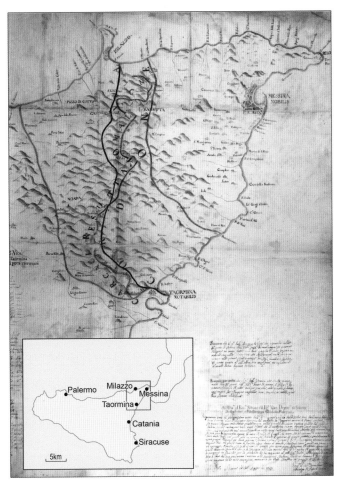

Figure 6.4 Plague of Messina, 1743: plague containment. Location of the three defensive isolation *cordon sanitaire* lines used to separate the plague-free parts of Sicily from Messina.

Vicari Generali (Messina, 1743). *Relazione topografica dell' intèro cordone, commandato dalli 3: Vicaj Generi il quale hà li suoi termini nelli due mari di Milazzo, e Taormina che per linea retta saria miglia so mà per tortuosa come al pres ritrouasi si estende a miglia.* Dim mm 910 × 920; disegno a inchiostro acquerellato. Piante e disegni, busta XXXIII, 8. Archivio di Stato di Napoli.

the island-wide permanent sanitary magistracy with jurisdiction over the pre-existing local health deputations which had existed for decades to control the importation of infectious diseases.

To prevent spread from Messina to the rest of plague-free Sicily, defensive isolation was established in August 1743 for most of the island by the health officials in Palermo. Three internal *cordon* lines were constructed, stretching across the neck of land from Milazzo on the north coast to Taormina on the south (**Figure 6.4**). From east to west, the *cordon* lines were (east) 26 miles (42 km) long, number of posts and men unrecorded; 23 miles (37 km), 152 posts, 700 men; and 21 miles (34 km), 130 posts, 633 men (west). This defensive isolation appears to have worked for there is no surviving evidence that plague ever reached other parts of the island.

6.3.2 Offensive Containment: Quarantine

Spatial approaches to the offensive containment of infection (**Figure 6.2C**) can be traced back to the fourteenth century and the great pandemic of Black Death in Europe; see section 4.2.3 in Chapter 4. The first landmark moves against the disease were taken

by the republic of Ragusa (modern-day Dubrovnik, Croatia). On 27 July 1377, the city's Major Council passed a law which stipulated that 'those who come from plague-infested areas shall not enter [Ragusa] or its district unless they spend a month on the islet of Mrkan or in the town of Cavtat, for the purpose of disinfection' (Tomić and Blažina, 2015, pp. 106–7). The Republic was also the location of the world's first permanent health office. Thereafter, the fight against plague was led by the states of Venice, Milan, and Genoa. The northern Italian focus of this evolution was driven by the position of Italy at the interface of Europe and Asia, its location on arms of the Silk Road, and the dependence of the great republics like Venice and Genoa upon trade with Asia for their prosperity, factors which combined to ensure that the importation of plague, especially by ships returning from the Levant, was an ever-present threat. Similar developments to those in northern Italy took place north of the Alps but remained at a much more primitive level—as they did in Italy south of the Dukedom of Tuscany (Cipolla, 1981, pp. 4–5).

Venice

Venice itself became the focus of developments, establishing in 1423 an island hospital (*Lazzaretto Vecchio*) in the centre of the lagoon—the first in the world—for the treatment of plague-infected people and later goods. A second lazaretto, *Lazzaretto Nuovo*, was added in 1468 at the entrance to the Venetian lagoon from the Adriatic (**Figure 6.5**). Islands became a favoured location for quarantine because of their physical separation by water from contiguous geographical areas. The Venetian plague hospitals were designed so that each patient had a separate cell; adjacent gardens were used for food production to ensure, as far as possible, self-sufficiency. The system became overwhelmed during major epidemics, but the basic idea of quarantining disease-infected areas to protect the disease-free population from a contagion has its echo today in the approach of many countries to the COVID-19 pandemic. In the United Kingdom, for example, isolation has its parallel in shielding and 14-day self-isolation.

Lazzaretto Vecchio (Old Lazaretto) was 525 feet by 425 feet, *Lazzaretto Nuovo* (New Lazaretto) 560 feet by 460 feet. Each was capable of holding 6730 bales of merchandise. The Old could properly house about 300 passengers, the New 200 (Palmer, 1978, pp. 183–210). The lazarettos were not only externally isolated but constructed to provide internal isolation of goods and passengers at the individual level. Conditions were frequently appalling. It was not uncommon for people to die at the rate of 500 per day in *Lazzaretto Vecchio* during plague outbreaks in the sixteenth century, while *Lazzaretto Nuovo* was recorded as holding 8,000 inmates on one occasion, far beyond the capacities of either lazaretto to do anything worthwhile (see, e.g. Palmer, 1978, p. 195).

Trying to prevent plague arriving by sea is described in a mid-eighteenth-century booklet by Venice's *Magistrato della sanità*:

> Experience has shewn [*sic*], that in the *Ottoman* Dominions, the Plague is never utterly extinct: Hence it is an immutable Law with the Magistrate of the Office of Health, to consider the whole Extent of the *Ottoman* Dominions and every State dependent on it, as always to be suspected to be in an infected Condition, to such a Degree, as not to receive, in any Part of the Dominions of the Republick [Venice], either confining to or commercing with them, any Persons, Merchandizes,

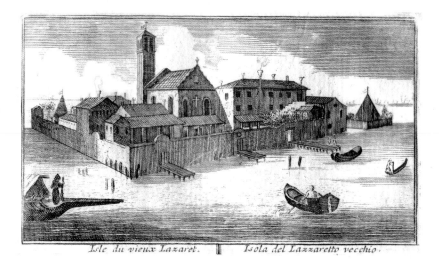

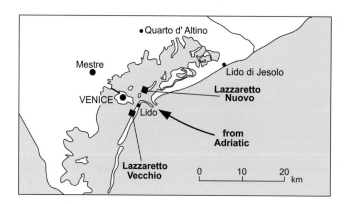

Figure 6.5 Lazarettos of Venice. Location map of the Old (*Lazzaretto Vecchio*) and New (*Lazzaretto Nuovo*) Lazarettos of Venice. The engravings show the ground floor plan of *Lazzaretto Vecchio* and a prospect of the lazaretto from the northwest corner. *Lazzaretto Vecchio* was established in 1423 about 2 km from Venice on a small island then known as Santa Maria di Nazareth, close to the modern Lido. *Lazzaretto Nuovo* was established in 1468 on the island historically known as Vigna Murada, separated by a navigable channel from the southern tip of the island of Sant' Erasmo, about 3 km from Venice. It occupied a strategic location at the entrance to the Venetian lagoon from the Adriatic and, when visited by John Howard in 1786, was used primarily to quarantine Turks, soldiers, and the crews of plague-infected ships (Howard, 1791, p. 11). By decree, ships, passengers, and goods were isolated for a limited period to allow for the manifestation of any disease and to dissipate imported infection. Originally the period was 30 days, *trentina*, but this was later extended to 40 days, *quarantina*. The choice of this period is said to be based on the period that Christ and Moses spent in isolation in the desert.

Ground floor plan of *Lazzaretto Vecchio* from Howard (1791, Plate 12); prospect is a mid-eighteenth-century copper engraving by the Venetian artist, Giuseppe Filosi. The ground floor plan has been distorted to conform with the prospect.

Animals, or any other Thing coming from thence, without the necessary Inspection of the Office of Health, and the previous purifications. (*Magistrato della sanità*, Venice, 1752, p. 4)

Although the Ottoman Dominions were perceived as the prime risk, the same procedures were followed for 'every Vessel, coming from any Part of the World, that is either infected, or suspected to be so' (*Magistrato della sanità*, Venice, 1752, p. 4). Vessels were normally expected to stop at Istria to take on board a pilot, or were towed up to Venice. Spies were maintained on the high tower of San Marco to watch for approaching vessels. The Magistrate sent one of his 60 Guardians to meet the ship which was moored in distant canals up to 25 km from the city according to the level of perceived risk. The captain of the vessel was taken ashore by a guarded way to a point of examination. The examination turned upon whence the vessel had come, the duration of the journey, places visited and their health, visits ashore, contact with other vessels at sea, the health of the ship's crew and passengers, and the nature of the cargo. Account had to be rendered of any crew or passengers who had died on board or who had left the ship en route 'and particularly the Condition of that Person who is wanting' (*Magistrato della sanità*, Venice, 1752, p. 8). If the examining officer was satisfied 'if the Vessel really came from a place that is free, it [the vessel] is declared free; if from a suspected one [place], the ship was place in quarantine [*sic*]'.

Ships were guarded throughout the quarantine period. They were unloaded of goods and passengers and both were dispatched to one of the city's two lazarettos. Generally, unless they were displaying clinical symptoms of plague, new arrivals were confined in *Lazzaretto Nuovo*. The unfortunate creatures who were determined to be suffering from plague either on arrival or during quarantine were dispatched to *Lazzaretto Vecchio*. Only when the ship had been fully unloaded did the statutory 40-day quarantine period begin. The principles of quarantine for goods were frequent handling, airing, and smoke fumigation with aromatic herbs. Cloth and untreated animal hides were regarded as especially risky. Although the procedure varied in detail by product, bales were generally opened, aired, rummaged, and cleaned up to twice a day, and moved from one location to another once a week. For people, social interaction was prevented (cf. the rules for COVID-19, centuries later), and each individual had his/her own cell, garden plot, and cooking facilities. Individuals who died in quarantine were checked for plague marks before being buried in lime in holes at least 12 feet deep. In the event that any disease broke out during a quarantine period, the process was repeated so that second and third quarantines were not unheard of for individual ships.

6.3.3 Modern Parallels

The concept of health organization as developed in the Renaissance Italian states eventually found systematic expression and elaboration from the late 1770s in the *System einer vollständigen Medizinischen Polizey* by Johann Peter Frank (1745–1821) (Cipolla, 1976, pp. 65–6). By the end of the eighteenth century, however, the philosophical mood of the times favoured the individual, and the state was viewed as a centralized oppressor. Plague had retreated from Europe, and with its retreat, opposition to health controls and regulations became progressively more vociferous. Laissez-faire prevailed and Italian ideas on control were regarded as obsolete and abandoned. Then it took the vision and energy of people like Benjamin Disraeli and Sir

John Simon to embrace the ideas and to develop a system of public health. There was rediscovery rather than continuity of methods of disease control and this time the British and the French led the way, uncovering once more many of the Italian ideas now used in current disease control systems. In this subsection, we take the opportunity to look briefly at the twentieth- and twenty-first-century adaptations of Italian ideas into their modern guises.

Quarantine and self-isolation

Provision for preventing the community circulation of a series of infectious diseases by isolation became a preoccupation of health movements across the developed world from the middle of the nineteenth century. In the United Kingdom, the Isolation Hospitals Act (1893) enabled county councils either to provide isolation hospitals or compel local authorities within the county to do so. By World War I, more than 750 isolation hospitals (or so-called fever hospitals) had been constructed by local councils and charities, containing over 30,000 beds for infectious patients, most of whom were children (Eyler, 1987; Mooney, 2009). As Mooney (2009, p. 147) comments:

The fundamental rationales for the institutional exclusion of the infected—namely the protection of the wider population, the prevention or stamping out of an epidemic outbreak—are practically self-evident. Yet scrutiny in a variety of metropolitan and colonial contexts also reveals a set of practices that, over the course of the nineteenth century, seemingly were ever more laden with undertones of coercion, moral and physical rehabilitation and normalisation.

The National Archives' *Hospital Records Database* lists some 385 fever hospitals in the period prior to 1948, probably about 40 per cent of those built. Nearly all were closed with the coming of the National Health Service in 1948. The remainder disappeared soon thereafter with the coming of mass vaccinations and therapies such as antibiotics that facilitated the control of the vast majority of fever hospital infections by methods other than isolation. Most of the hospitals had been built to serve urban areas. Wherever possible, locations remote from dense population clusters were sought—coastal locations, parks, and other open spaces. Their modern equivalent are the NHS Nightingale and other field hospitals that were established to take COVID-19 patients into isolation for treatment away from the standard hospital system. Hospital isolation still finds a place in communicable disease control in the twenty-first century when all else fails.

Eyler (1987) and Mooney (2009) discuss the ways in which the systems that evolved during Victorian and Edwardian times raised a host of issues that, we note, have subsequently become familiar during the ubiquitous attempts to control the geographical diffusion of COVID-19 by self-isolation and lockdowns. These include, inter alia, the mental health of those confined, the role of visiting (or not) in spreading infection back into the community, the passage of responsibility from governments to the individual to exercise control, and institutionalized mentalities among those detained for any length of time. Eyler (1987) goes even further and asks whether isolation worked at all in the long run, or whether seemingly cured patients still carried infection back into the community on their release. In similar fashion, some media reports in the United Kingdom linked outbreaks of COVID-19 in care homes (see section 5.4.1 in Chapter 5) with the discharge of patients who had contracted the infection in hospitals. See Emmerson et al. (2021) for an examination of the evidence.

There are still occasions today, at airports and seaports, when quarantine and isolation may appropriately be used to prevent the importation of infections by travellers or immigrants into a country, and to control the within-country spread of infectious diseases between people and places. For example, the United States has quarantine stations at 20 ports of entry and land-border crossings where most international travellers arrive. The stations are managed by the CDC's Division of Global Migration and Quarantine with the stated purpose of limiting the introduction of contagious diseases into the country. These diseases currently include cholera, diphtheria, infectious tuberculosis (TB), plague, smallpox, yellow fever, viral haemorrhagic fevers, severe acute respiratory syndromes, and new types of influenza that could cause a pandemic (Centers for Disease Control and Prevention, 2021).

Personal protective equipment

The idea of personal protective equipment to help doctors and other health workers remain free of infection when treating patients with communicable diseases is not new. During the Plague Centuries, to assist in surveillance at the local level and to examine suspected patients, there emerged the ubiquitous plague doctor who, COVID-like, wore his own personal protective equipment. Introduced in Italy in 1630, the protective suit consisted of a light, waxed fabric overcoat, a mask with glass eye openings, and a beak-shaped nose, typically stuffed with herbs, straw, and spices. Social distancing between doctor and patient was facilitated by a cane that permitted the plague doctor to examine patients without the need for direct contact. The doctor maintained records of plague-infected individuals, their dwellings, and their contacts in a medieval version of 'track and trace'.

Surveillance

Surveillance has played a long-standing and central role in the design of strategies to prevent the spread of infections between people and places. As far as the Italian approach to plague control during the Plague Centuries is concerned, it utilized surveillance at the local level via plague doctors and additionally by the church.[1] Above the local level, inter-state sharing of information on health matters became common using border controls, medical passports for goods and people, and quarantine. During the sixteenth and seventeenth centuries, the Health Magistracies of the capital cities of the republics and principalities of Italy north of Rome established the custom of regularly informing each other of all news they gathered on health conditions prevailing in various parts of Italy, the rest of Europe, North Africa, and the Middle East (Cipolla, 1981, p. 21).

These early moves in disease intelligence are the forebears of the modern disease surveillance systems we describe in section 6.6. In the context of COVID-19, they find local expression in the form of England's NHS Test and Trace contact tracing system that was established in May 2020. The service provides temporary sites where samples are taken from individuals that are then processed at a network of laboratories, and the results communicated to testees. Infected people are instructed to isolate themselves from others and are asked to provide details of their recent close contacts, who are

also required to isolate. In light of the early criticism of the NHS Test and Trace system, a web-based performance tracker is maintained for public information and scrutiny (The Health Foundation, 2021).

6.4 Vaccines and Vaccination

Vaccination—the process of conferring immunity to diseases through the administration of a vaccine—is now considered to be among the most effective of health interventions. It has been used as a means of controlling an expanding list of infectious diseases since the late eighteenth century. In this section, we briefly review the history of vaccination and the principles that underpin the use of vaccination as a disease control strategy. We then examine the vaccine control of common childhood and other infections at the global level through the WHO's Expanded Programme on Immunization (EPI) and subsequent programmes. Finally, we look at the risks posed by vaccine scares and the consequent spatially heterogeneous uptake of vaccines.

While practices analogous to the process of conferring increased resistance to infection ('immunization') can be traced to antiquity, the modern history of vaccines dates to the late eighteenth century and local knowledge from the southwest of England that dairy farm workers who contracted cowpox were immune to smallpox. It was the English physician, Edward Jenner, who studied and promoted the prophylactic powers of cowpox. On 14 May 1796, Jenner vaccinated James Phipps with material obtained from a pustule on the hand of a milkmaid. Six weeks later he attempted, without success, to infect Phipps with pus from a smallpox patient. After 12 more successful vaccinations, he privately published a report of his findings and a new epoch in disease control dawned. Jenner's ideas were triumphant. In England, more than 100,000 people were vaccinated against smallpox in 1801 alone. Within 3 years, Jenner's *Inquiry* had been translated into six languages. Between 1804 and 1814, 2 million were vaccinated in Russia, and so on across the industrializing world.

The early work on smallpox vaccine was empirical and undertaken with no knowledge of the aetiology of the disease. The development of what Parish (1968, p. 21) terms 'scientific immunization' awaited advances on several fronts. These included the identification of the causes of major diseases (bacteria especially in the 1880s and viruses after 1930), and the development of tools for clinical examination and laboratory analysis (Cliff and Smallman-Raynor, 2013, pp. 99–103). Theory also played a critical role. Rokitansky's text on systematic pathology was published between 1842 and 1846, while Virchow announced the cell theory in 1855. By the middle of the nineteenth century, a small number of diseases had been shown to be caused by living organisms and Henle had given his closely reasoned account of the hypothesis that infectious diseases were not the result of unspecified 'miasmas' but transmitted by living organisms. The second half of the nineteenth century saw the heyday of bacteriological theory and practice with Louis Pasteur (1822–95), Ferdinand Cohn (1828–98), and Robert Koch (1843–1910) using the new laboratory tools to establish hypotheses of infection and contagion, often against entrenched opposition.

6.4.1 The Early Laboratory Vaccines

The successful development of laboratory vaccines began with the pioneering work of the nineteenth-century French chemist, Louis

---

[1] At an earlier date, English parallels on the role of the church emerge in Hatcher's (2008) fascinating account of the Black Death in a Suffolk parish, 1345–50.

Pasteur. Initially concerned with the development of attenuated veterinary vaccines for fowl cholera (1879), anthrax (1881), and, somewhat less successfully, swine erysipelas (1883), Pasteur's rabies vaccine (1885) was the first laboratory vaccine to make an impact on human disease. Pasteur developed both the theory and the experimental practice for attenuating the (then unknown) rabies virus in the spinal cords of rabbits. Having initially demonstrated the protective effect of the vaccine on dogs, the first human test of the vaccine came in July 1885 when a 9-year-old boy who had been bitten by a rabid dog 2 days earlier was brought to Pasteur's laboratory.

The successful development of vaccines against a series of major human bacterial diseases followed in short order. By 1896, the German scientist Wilhelm Kolle—an assistant to Robert Koch—had developed a heat-inactivated cholera vaccine that would serve as a model for cholera vaccines in the next century. In the same year, the British bacteriologist Almroth E. Wright developed a killed vaccine against typhoid fever that would subsequently be used by the British Army during the Second Boer War (1899–1902), while Waldemar Haffkine's plague vaccine was developed and introduced in India in 1896–97 (Parish, 1968).

Post-1900 developments

While antitoxins and vaccines were developed for a range of bacterial diseases (including anthrax, cholera, diphtheria, plague, tetanus, typhoid, and TB) in the early decades of the twentieth century, the rapid development of virus vaccines awaited the advent of the electron microscope, from the 1930s, and methods for the laboratory culture of viruses. Vaccines for poliomyelitis and other common childhood diseases such as measles, mumps, and rubella (MMR) followed in quick succession. In the late twentieth and early twenty-first centuries, new methods and techniques have been adopted in vaccine development (notably recombinant DNA technology). To illustrate the pace and dimensions of these developments, **Figure 6.6** gives a timeline for the introduction of sample vaccines in the United Kingdom.

6.4.2 Vaccination and Disease Control

As discussed in the context of Figure 1.8 in Chapter 1, once an epidemic has begun, its continuation depends upon the presence of a sufficiently large S subpopulation for transitions of the type $S \rightarrow I$ to be uninterrupted. This gives rise to the notion of herd immunity—the proportion of the population which must be immune to a disease for community transmission to cease; see section 1.3.2 in Chapter 1. Individuals who are immune act as a barrier to spread, slowing or preventing the transmission of disease to others. Immunity may be acquired after infection with a disease agent or by vaccination. Once the herd immunity level is reached, community circulation of the disease agent stops, the disease ceases to be present, and can only recur by reintroduction from other reservoir areas. It follows that vaccines can be used to reduce the S subpopulation, raise the

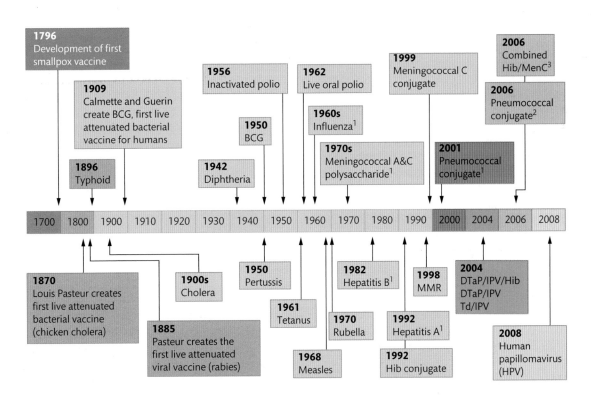

[1]For the immunisation of at-risk groups. [2]For routine use in children under 2. [3]As a booster in the second year of life.

Figure 6.6 Timeline of vaccine developments in the United Kingdom, 1796–2010. BCG (Bacillus Calmette–Guérin) tuberculosis vaccine. Hib (*Haemophilus influenzae* type b) vaccine. MMR (measles, mumps, and rubella) combined vaccine. DTaP (diphtheria and tetanus toxoids, and acellular pertussis) vaccine. IPV (inactivated poliovirus vaccine). Td (tetanus and diphtheria toxoids) vaccine for adults. DTaP/IPV, DTaP/IPV/Hib, and Td/IPV are combined preparations.

R subpopulation, and effectively force an infectious disease out of a community or geographical area.

Vaccine-preventable diseases and the Expanded Programme on Immunization

The global eradication of smallpox, formally announced by the WHO in December 1979, was one of the outstanding successes in the control of vaccine-preventable diseases. Then, policy advisors to the WHO looked for a successor to the smallpox eradication campaign. Representatives from industrialized countries, particularly those from Europe, were now seeing the results from their own immunization programmes against a variety of vaccine-preventable childhood diseases and urged that these diseases be made the new WHO target area. The resolution creating the Expanded Programme on Immunization (EPI) was adopted by the World Health Assembly in 1974, with the initial aim of targeting six vaccine-preventable diseases (diphtheria, measles, pertussis, poliomyelitis, tetanus, and TB) for a substantial reduction in global incidence. Programme policies of the EPI were formalized by the World Health Assembly in 1977. It was at this time that the twin goals were set of (i) providing immunization services for all children of the world by 1990 and (ii) giving priority to developing countries.

When the EPI began, global vaccine coverage for the initial six target diseases was around 5 per cent. From this low baseline, immunization services in developing countries were extended to almost 80 per cent of children (aged <1 year) by the mid-1990s and, with the exception of TB, there was a rapid, commensurate decrease in the incidence of the diseases (**Figure 6.7**). The TB epidemic continues in spite of an available, cost-effective, and broadly implemented vaccine for infants—Bacillus Calmette–Guérin (BCG)—and the carefully managed use of drugs through directly observed therapy for those who become infected. This is because BCG vaccination is only partially effective: it provides some protection against severe forms of paediatric non-pulmonary TB (such as TB meningitis) but is unreliable against adult pulmonary TB, which accounts for most of the TB disease burden worldwide. In addition, resistance to previously effective TB drug regimens is increasing, while infection with HIV can increase the likelihood of TB acquisition by up to 25-fold.

Despite the EPI initiative, millions of children continued to be born each year in the poorest areas of the world that lacked adequate immunization programmes. In response, additional programmes have been developed to increase vaccine coverage—including the Global Alliance for Vaccines and Immunization (GAVI) (2000) and the Global Immunization Vision and Strategy (GIVS) (2006)—as

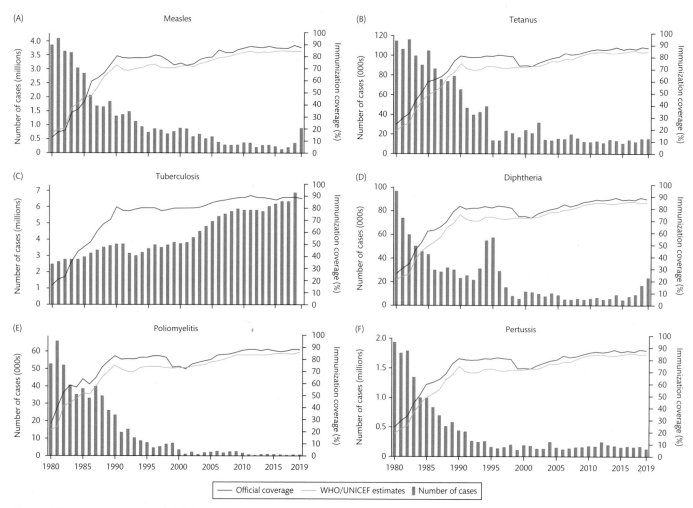

Figure 6.7 Vaccine coverage and global annual reported cases, 1980–2019, for the six initial EPI diseases. (A) Measles. (B) Tetanus. (C) Tuberculosis. (D) Diphtheria. (E) Poliomyelitis. (F) Whooping cough (pertussis).

Source: data from WHO Global Health Observatory. https://www.who.int/data/gho/, accessed 18 February 2021.

a contribution to achieving the United Nations' goal of reducing childhood mortality. A number of remarkable developments have followed, including the substantial global retreat of wild polioviruses under the Global Polio Eradication Initiative (GPEI) (section 6.5.3) and the elimination of indigenous measles in the Americas (Doherty et al., 2016).

Opposition to vaccination

While the control of many infections by mass vaccination has been a global success story, social and political opposition to vaccination (and immunization more generally) emerged soon after the development and standardization of smallpox vaccination practices in Jenner's time. James Gillray's 1802 caricature of the consequences of being vaccinated against smallpox by Edward Jenner is legendary (**Figure 6.8**), and illustrates a strand of opposition against vaccination that has persisted ever since. In England and Wales, the Vaccination Act of 1853 and associated legislation mandated the compulsory vaccination of children against smallpox. This prompted the rise of opposition movements such as the Anti-Compulsory Vaccination League (later, the National Anti-Vaccination League) that objected to vaccination on political, medical, and religious grounds. Although the laws on compulsory vaccination in England and Wales were relaxed at the end of the nineteenth century, anti-vaccinationist sentiment continued to cast a shadow over smallpox control in the decades that followed (Rafferty et al., 2018).

Unfounded or unproven health concerns have sometimes prompted public anxiety over vaccines, with the associated reduction in vaccine uptake having potentially disastrous public health consequences. The controversy over the combined MMR vaccine in recent decades illustrates the point. In a controversial paper published in *The Lancet* in 1998, Andrew Wakefield and colleagues described a series of children with developmental disorders who had been referred to the Royal Free Hospital, London, and which, they suggested, pointed to an apparent association between the MMR vaccine and autism. Although subsequent studies in the United States and the United Kingdom failed to identify a link, and Wakefield's original paper was fully retracted by *The Lancet* in 2010, public fears over the safety of the MMR vaccine resulted in reduced vaccinations to levels well below those required for herd immunity for the target diseases. From a high of 92 per cent in the mid-1990s, MMR vaccine coverage among 2-year-olds in England and Wales fell to just 80 per cent in 2003–04—a full 15 per cent below the WHO-recommended level for herd immunity (Asaria and MacMahon, 2006). Amid increased calls for a change in national immunization policy to permit parents to choose between the triple MMR and single vaccines, measles and mumps re-emerged in epidemic form in the early twenty-first century. We consider each disease in turn.

Measles

In the United Kingdom, levels of susceptibility to measles grew rapidly. Starting from a position in which indigenous measles virus transmission had been effectively eliminated, in England 1.9 million school children and 0.3 million preschool children were estimated to be incompletely vaccinated against measles by 2004–05. Of these, approximately 1.3 million children aged 2–17 years were deemed susceptible to the disease. Fourteen of the 99 districts and strategic health authorities of England, including 11 London districts, had levels of susceptibility that were sufficiently high to support sustained measles virus transmission, while mathematical modelling pointed to the potential for a measles epidemic of up to 100,000 cases

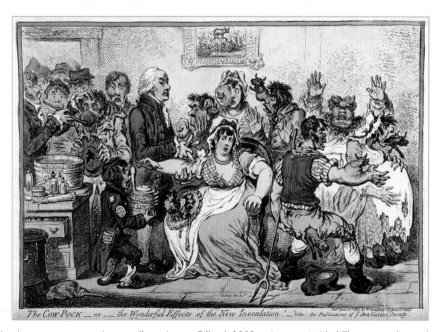

Figure 6.8 The anti-vaccination movement against smallpox. James Gillray's 1802 caricature, entitled *The cow-pock – or the wonderful effects of the new inoculation! – vide the publications of the Anti-Vaccine Society*, shows Jenner vaccinating patients against smallpox. Vaccinated patients sprout cows from various parts of their bodies. Gillray's assistant (in a green jacket) is spooning *opening mixture* into patients to prepare them for vaccination. An urchin stands close to Jenner holding out a tub of *vaccine pock not from the cow*, while a newspaper with the headline *benefits of the vaccine excellent* protrudes from his pocket.

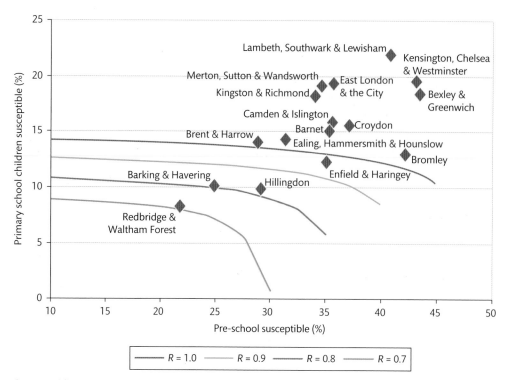

Figure 6.9 Estimated potential for measles virus transmission in districts of London, 2004. The potential for measles virus transmission (assessed according to levels of susceptibility in the population) is summarized by the effective reproduction number, R. Unlike the basic reproduction number R_0 (see section 1.3.2 in Chapter 1), which assumes an entirely susceptible population, the effective reproduction number R relates to a population with some level of immunity. When $R > 1.0$, each measles case generates an average of more than one secondary case, thereby resulting in an increase in cases and sustained transmission of measles virus. Conversely, when $R < 1.0$, the measles transmission chain will be broken. For the majority of London districts $R > 1.0$, sufficient to generate a London-wide epidemic of measles.

Reproduced from Health Protection Agency (2006). *Communicable Disease in London 2002–05. A Review by the Health Protection Agency in London.* London: HPA. Contains public sector information licensed under the Open Government Licence v3.0.

(Hong Choi et al., 2008). Informed by these estimates, the Health Protection Agency announced in June 2008 that the number of susceptible children was sufficient to support the continuous transmission of measles virus and that the disease was once again endemic in the United Kingdom (Health Protection Agency, 2008).

Despite all efforts, measles continued to spread widely, with London especially badly affected. An outbreak of measles—the largest since the mid-1990s—was recorded in preschool children in south inner London in 2001–2 while, by 2004–5, levels of susceptibility among schoolchildren were sufficiently high to support a London-wide epidemic (**Figure 6.9**). In response, the MMR Capital Catch-up Campaign of 2004–05 was launched with the aim of delivering one dose of MMR vaccine to children of primary school age with an incomplete vaccination history. To promote coverage, special vaccination sessions were arranged in schools and general practices (Asaria and MacMahon, 2006; Health Protection Agency, 2006). A range of socioeconomic factors are believed to have contributed to the low vaccine uptake, including high population mobility and family size, while anecdotal evidence suggests that some parents made an active decision not to have their children immunized.

Mumps

The resurgence of mumps in the early twenty-first century was a predictable consequence of the introduction of an MMR vaccine in 1988 and the failure of the MMR vaccination programme from the late 1990s. Gaps in eligibility for MMR vaccine had resulted in a cohort of older and unprotected children who grew up in a period of

low mumps incidence. Many of the cohort, born primarily between 1981 and 1990, had been offered combined measles–rubella vaccine as part of a remedial vaccination campaign in late 1994, but remained susceptible to mumps as they progressed through secondary school and beyond in the early 2000s (Savage et al., 2005, 2006). The resulting epidemic of 2004–05 spread nationwide and was associated with some 70,000 notified cases. The majority of cases were older teenagers and young adults in university and college settings. Frequent occurrence of severe complications was a prominent feature of the epidemic.

Anti-vaccinationists have been around for over 200 years, and this is unlikely to change. And so, in anticipation of the development of many vaccines against the agent of COVID-19, a number of anti-vaccinationist narratives have already begun to develop around issues such as vaccine safety, conspiracy theories, alternative medicines, and cures (Johnson et al., 2020). Such developments have the potential to hamper efforts to exert effective control of the SARS-CoV-2 virus as effective vaccines are rolled out.

6.4.3 Ring Vaccination Strategies

The deployment of vaccines to interrupt the geographical spread of infection can take two main forms: (i) *mass vaccination* in the manner of the EPI and related programmes where, over time, the population is saturated by a vaccine or vaccines and herd immunity is reached; or (ii) *ring vaccination* to establish a 'ring of immunity' to contain local outbreaks (offensive containment in terms of **Figure 6.2**). The latter strategy has been considered by a number of workers; see, for example, Greenhalgh (1986) and Cliff and Haggett (1989). The principles involved are readily illustrated by disease outbreaks among farm animals and we draw here on Tinline's (1972) study of foot-and-mouth disease (FMD) in cattle.

Ring vaccination: epizootics

Based on data relating to the 1967–68 epizootic of FMD in the United Kingdom, Tinline demonstrated that airborne spread of FMD virus downwind of an initially infected area was an important cause of additional disease outbreaks during the epizootic. To contain the disease, Tinline investigated the possibility of implementing vaccination in areas downwind of an initial outbreak in order to create a 'buffer zone' of immunity across which the virus could not easily pass. See **Figure 6.10**. In the upper-left map of **Figure 6.10A**, the immediate ('blanket') vaccination of all herds downwind of the initial outbreak is effected on confirmation of the outbreak. Recognizing the logistical

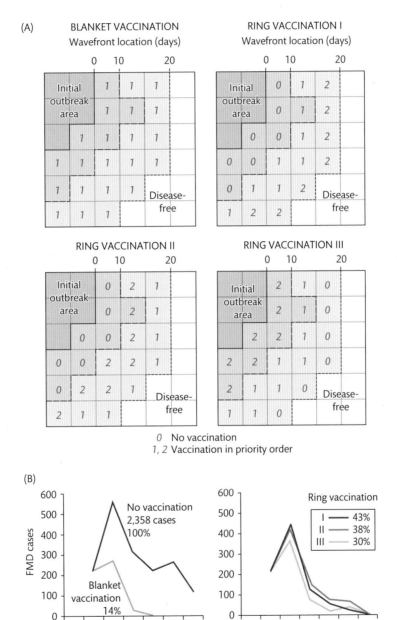

Figure 6.10 Ring vaccination schemes to control the spread of FMD virus. Tinline's simulations of alternative vaccination schemes to control the spread of the 1967–68 epizootic of FMD among cattle herds in central England. (A) Prioritization of vaccination of herds downwind of an initial outbreak area. Each cell represents a 10 km × 10 km area, with priority of vaccination indicated by codes 1 (first priority) and 2 (second priority); code 0 = no vaccination. (B) Results of simulations of the number of FMD cases with distance from the initial outbreak area for no vaccination and blanket vaccination schemes (left) and for ring vaccination schemes I–III (right). Percentage estimates of the number of FMD cases in a given vaccination scenario, relative to the no vaccination scenario (= 100 per cent), are given.

Reproduced with permission from Tinline, R.R. (1972). A Simulation Study of the 1967–68 Foot-and-Mouth Epizootic in Great Britain. Unpublished DPhil dissertation. Department of Geography, University of Bristol, UK.

difficulties involved in the implementation of such a scheme, the remaining maps provide different schemes for the priority order (cell codes 1 and 2) of vaccine delivery. The results of simulations to test the efficacy of the different schemes are summarized in **Figure 6.10B**. With the exception of blanket vaccination, which would reduce the number of FMD cases to just 14 per cent of the no vaccination scenario, Tinline identified ring vaccination scheme III as the most successful in reducing FMD transmission. The key feature of this scheme is the prioritization of vaccination from the outside, in towards the initially infected area. Practical difficulties arise, however, in the implementation of such ring vaccination strategies, including the need for accurate 20-day wind forecasts from the date of the initial onset of the FMD outbreak.

Ring vaccination in human populations

Kretzschmar et al. (2004) and Lau et al. (2005) have explored the ring vaccination approach for smallpox control in humans in the event of a bioterrorist attack. Kretzschmar and colleagues developed a stochastic model for the spread of smallpox after a small number of index cases had been introduced into a susceptible population. The model used a branching process for the spread of the infection. The different intervention measures tried included ring vaccination of direct contacts of infected persons to contain any epidemic. They concluded that ring vaccination can be successful if infectious cases are rapidly diagnosed. However, because of the inherently stochastic nature of epidemic outbreaks, both the size and duration of contained outbreaks are highly variable, so that intervention requirements would depend on the value of the basic reproduction number (R_0) which varies in different settings. The authors concluded that, considering the uncertainties connected with all parameter values of a disease diffusion process, any contingency plan for the use of ring vaccination must also identify the criteria under which switching to large-scale mass vaccination becomes justified. Lau et al. (2005) examined the impact of population density upon vaccination strategies. They concluded that mass vaccination is probably the most appropriate approach in densely populated areas and that, by implication, ring vaccination is likely to be most effective where population densities are lower.

6.5 Towards Eradication

The idea of eradicating a disease has a long history (Cliff and Smallman-Raynor, 2013, pp. 124–46). Following Edward Jenner's path-breaking work on smallpox, United States President Thomas Jefferson articulated the vision of a smallpox-free world in his well-known letter of gratitude to Jenner in 1806 (cited in Stanwell-Smith, 1996, p. 509):

> Future nations will know by history only that the loathsome smallpox has existed and by you has been extirpated.
>
> Thomas Jefferson, 'A Tribute of Gratitude' (letter)
> to Edward Jenner (14 May 1806).

Unfortunately, the world had to wait until 1979 for Jefferson's vision to be realized.

The popularity of eradication as a human disease control strategy has waxed and waned with the successes, setbacks, and failures of previous and ongoing campaigns. Many lessons have been learnt from the past (Aylward et al., 2000) and disease eradication is again at the forefront of global health policy.

6.5.1 Defining Eradication

As applied to an infectious disease agent, the term *eradication* has been defined in the literature in a variety of ways and, at times, has been confused with the related term, *elimination*. To achieve uniformity in the definition and application of terms, the Dahlem Workshop on the Eradication of Infectious Diseases, held in March 1997, defined eradication as the 'permanent reduction to zero of the worldwide incidence of infection caused by a specific disease agent as a result of deliberate efforts' (Dowdle, 1998, p. 23). The term, eradication, is reserved for the complete and permanent worldwide cessation of the natural transmission of a disease agent. Eradication thus represents a distinct stage in disease intervention. It is distinguished from the related concepts of *control* and *elimination* as defined in **Table 6.2**, where we can view control and elimination as steps on the road to eradication (cf. **Figure 6.2**). As noted previously, only one communicable disease of humans has been eradicated to date, namely smallpox in 1979.

Table 6.2 Stages in the control of infectious disease agents: definitions and their implications for control programmes

	Stages of control			
	Control	**Elimination**	**Eradication**	**Extinction**
Definition[a]	'The reduction of disease incidence, prevalence, morbidity and mortality to a locally acceptable level as a result of deliberate efforts'	*Disease*: 'Reduction to zero of the incidence of a specified disease in a defined geographical area as a result of deliberate efforts' *Infection*: 'Reduction to zero of the incidence of infection caused by a specific agent in a defined geographical area as a result of deliberate efforts'	'Permanent reduction to zero of the worldwide incidence of infection caused by a specific disease agent as a result of deliberate efforts'	'The specific infectious agent no longer exists in nature or in the laboratory'
Implication	Continued intervention measures are required to maintain reduction	Continued intervention measures are required to prevent re-establishment of infection and disease	Intervention measures no longer needed: all interventions can be halted after certification of eradication	

[a] Definitions formulated at the Dahlem Workshop on the Eradication of Infectious Diseases (March 1997), cited in Dowdle (1998, p. 23).

Indicators of eradicability

The potential of a disease agent for eradication can be assessed on the basis of three principal indicators: (i) biological and technical feasibility, (ii) costs and benefits, and (iii) societal and political considerations (Dowdle, 1998; Aylward et al., 2000):

1. *Biological and technical feasibility.* These include (i) the availability of an effective means of interrupting the transmission of the disease agent (e.g. a safe and effective vaccine); (ii) the availability of diagnostic tools of sufficient sensitivity and specificity to detect levels of infection that may result in transmission of the disease agent; and (iii) the absence of a non-human vertebrate reservoir and the inability of the disease agent to amplify in the environment.

2. *Costs and benefits.* The decision to eradicate a disease agent is contingent on the costs and benefits of the eradication programme relative to the costs and benefits arising from alternative intervention scenarios. Costs and benefits can be defined in terms of direct effects (i.e. cessation of morbidity and mortality) and consequent effects (i.e. impact on healthcare systems).

3. *Societal and political considerations.* The success or otherwise of eradication programmes is crucially dependent upon societal, political, and associated financial commitment to their success. The target disease must be recognized as being of public health importance, eradication must be recognized as a worthy goal by society, and political commitment to eradication is required at the highest level throughout the duration of the eradication programme.

6.5.2 The Road to Eradication

Once the decision to eradicate a disease has been taken, and an area is free from indigenous transmission of the associated disease agent, spatial barriers need to be established to prevent reinfection by the geographical spread of the disease agent from infected areas. Backed by vaccination, the barrier concepts of defensive isolation and offensive containment to articulate this have been illustrated in Figure 6.2. Global eradication can then be achieved by (i) progressively reducing infected areas in size using a combination of vaccination, defensive isolation, and offensive containment; and (ii) letting the disease-free areas coalesce into bigger geographical clumps. Continuous repetition of the cycle of (i) and (ii) will lead, eventually, to the worldwide eradication of the disease. For vaccine-preventable diseases, eradication ultimately rests on a globally coordinated vaccination programme to reduce the sizes of geographically distributed at-risk populations to levels at which the chains of infection cannot be maintained. In terms of the Bartlett model (see Figures 1.9 and 1.10 in Chapter 1), this means systematically reducing the epidemic waves of different communities from I to II, and from II to III, eventually bringing the type III waves into phase so that disease fade-out in all the remaining disease-active areas coincides.

6.5.3 Eradicating Poliomyelitis

The geographical road to the eradication of smallpox has been described at length in Fenner et al. (1988). After smallpox, the Forty-First World Health Assembly in May 1988 identified poliomyelitis as the vaccine-preventable disease 'most amenable' to global eradication (World Health Organization, 1988, p. 26; Hull et al., 1997; Smallman-Raynor et al., 2006, pp. 563–628). The Assembly committed the WHO to reaching this goal by 2000 through the launch of the GPEI. This initiative has four strands: (i) high routine infant immunization coverage with poliovirus-containing vaccines; (ii) supplementary immunization activities, including national immunization days, to ensure population immunity; (iii) surveillance for acute flaccid paralysis; and (iv) targeted mopping-up immunization campaigns to interrupt local chains of poliovirus transmission.

Inevitably, there has been slippage in the eradication timetable, but great progress has been made. Since 1988, five out of six WHO regions have been declared wild poliovirus free: the Americas in 1994, Western Pacific in 2000, Europe in 2002, South-East Asia in 2014, and most recently Africa in 2020. But, global eradication remains elusive with wild poliovirus type 1 remaining endemic in two countries, Afghanistan and Pakistan. Until poliovirus transmission is interrupted in these countries, all countries remain at risk of the importation of infection, especially those with weak public health and immunization services, and travel or trade links to the endemic countries.

Crucial to the eradication effort has been the use of vaccination to maintain herd immunity against the disease. The maintenance of what is effectively blanket vaccination coverage has proved extremely difficult in conflict zones where population flight to escape injury and death interrupts routine vaccination programmes and prevents strong surveillance. Indeed, wars of all types have consistently posed one of the single greatest obstacles to the effective implementation of the GPEI. In some countries, the war-related disruption of immunization services has triggered major outbreaks of poliomyelitis and other vaccine-preventable diseases. War commonly leads to the collapse of routine preventive healthcare programmes normally delivered through central governments, and the surrender of recognized government control to local interest groups and militias. In addition, the rise of Islamic fundamentalist groups in both the African and the Eastern Mediterranean Regions has added a new dimension to the problem. Such groups frequently impose their will by fear. As far as the civil population is concerned, flight to escape conflict is a common response, leading to mass refugee and internally displaced person movements. Flight may result in suboptimal immunization coverage of susceptible populations (Bush, 2000; Tangermann et al., 2000). With the general collapse of surveillance, healthcare agencies have little idea of who has been missed by vaccination programmes or where they are living.

6.6 Surveillance

6.6.1 Definition

If we are to control the spread of a communicable disease, the monitoring (surveillance) of its occurrence—where, when, and how much—is a necessary prerequisite. Although the idea of using morbidity and mortality data as a basis for public action to inhibit the spread of infection can be traced back to medieval times (section 6.3), the modern concept of disease surveillance as a basis for such action rests with the establishment of the United States Communicable Disease Center in 1946. The mandate of the Center was to initiate the investigation of health events through the systematic collection and analysis of morbidity and mortality data. In

1955, the term 'disease surveillance' was applied to these activities by Alexander D. Langmuir, chief epidemiologist, who defined disease surveillance activities as:

> the continued watchfulness over the distribution and trends of incidence through the systematic collection, consolidation and evaluation of morbidity and mortality reports and other relevant data. Intrinsic in the concept is the regular dissemination of the basic data and interpretations to all who have contributed and to all others who need to know. (Langmuir, 1963, pp. 182–3)

At the global level, Langmuir (1976) observed that the term, surveillance, was given expanded meaning in the course of the WHO's Malaria Eradication Programme and was extended to embrace active measures of control such as the administration of chemotherapy and the use of insecticides. In 1968, the Twenty-First World Health Assembly undertook an examination of surveillance as a part of public health practice and adopted the definition of surveillance as:

> the epidemiological study of a disease as a dynamic process involving the ecology of the infectious agent, the host, the reservoirs, and the vectors, as well as the complex mechanisms concerned with the spread of infection and the extent to which spread occurs. (Lucas, 1968, p. 440)

Subsequently, the United States CDC, successor to the Communicable Disease Center, defined disease surveillance as the:

> ongoing systematic collection, analysis and interpretation of health data in the process of describing and monitoring a health event. This information is used for planning, implementing, and evaluating public health interventions and programs. (Centers for Disease Control, 1988, p. 1)

Disease surveillance systems vary in method, orientation, and scope depending upon the nature of the health event being observed, and so they vary in their simplicity, acceptability, sensitivity, representativity, and timeliness (Centers for Disease Control, 1988).

In this section, which is based on Cliff and Smallman-Raynor (2013, pp. 21–62), we focus upon the role of surveillance in informing control strategies for communicable diseases. We begin by examining how morbidity and mortality are recorded and classified to form the basis of surveillance systems from the local to the global scales. Over time, collection strategies have evolved in response to changing technologies, from pen and paper, through the electric telegraph, paper tape and punch cards, to the worldwide reach and instantaneity of the Internet. The Internet age has also spawned a number of informal real-time disease surveillance mechanisms, while enhancing the opportunities for multiple-source disease tracking tools. At the same time, the global range of diseases and its population have mushroomed, so that the blanket surveillance of former times is now evolving into sampling procedures by time, disease, and geographical location. Such developments conclude this section.

6.6.2 Disease Classification

The so-called *International Classification of Diseases* (*ICD*) began formally in Chicago in 1893 with the adoption by the International Statistical Institute of Bertillon's International List of Causes of Death. In 1898, the American Public Health Association recommended the adoption of the Bertillon classification by the civil registrars of Canada, Mexico, and the United States, adding that the classification should be revised every 10 years. The first revision of the Bertillon classification appeared in 1903. Since then, the classification (now universally known as the *ICD*) has gone through 11 revisions. Currently, *ICD*-10 is in use, to be replaced by *ICD*-11 from 1 January 2022. The *ICD* is the international standard diagnostic classification for all general epidemiological and many health management purposes. It is used to classify diseases and other health problems recorded on health and vital records including death certificates and hospital records. The idea of such a classification is to ensure comparability of data recording over space and time, thus facilitating the storage and retrieval of diagnostic information for clinical and epidemiological purposes. These records also provide the basis for the compilation of national mortality and morbidity statistics by country-level surveillance organizations.

The number of epidemic-causing infectious diseases listed in the *ICD* has grown dramatically in recent decades. Thus, from a relatively stable total of around 100 diseases in the first 65 years of the *ICD*'s existence, the number included in the ninth and tenth revisions rose sharply to 350 (*ICD*-9) and over 1,000 (*ICD*-10). This growth has been driven, in part, by the discovery of many apparently new infectious diseases and their associated agents; see Chapter 3.

6.6.3 Disease Collecting Systems

In section 1.2.3 in chapter 1, we introduced the theme of disease recording in space and time. Here, we connect the theme to developments in disease surveillance and control.

Surveillance networks

A case of a particular disease may enter the statistical record at the primary (local) level by both reactive and proactive processes. In a *reactive* process, an individual may experience symptoms of a disease but may or may not be able (or inclined) to visit a medical practitioner. Such a consultation may or may not result in a correct diagnosis and the physician may or may not have to pass the record up the reporting chain. Primary data collection by general practitioners, consultants, hospital clinics, and others may or may not become part of a country's official disease records. Only diseases of major public health importance are subject to statutory notification (i.e. notifiable by law) and the quality of the data record will depend on many factors: the complexity of the disease and associated complications, the diagnostic skill of the physician, the case load of other clinical work, and so on. The routine reporting of some diseases is supplemented by a *proactive* process in which screening or surveys of 'healthy' or 'at-risk' populations may reveal evidence of infection or disease (e.g. COVID-19, HIV/AIDS, or TB) either unrecognized by the individual or for which medical advice had not been sought in the first instance. Disease-related information is channelled from the primary level, via secondary reporting routes of varying complexity, to national (e.g. CDC in the United States) and international (e.g. WHO) health agencies.

Time span of disease records

The availability of disease data varies greatly over time. A written record of the incidence of some diseases goes back to the fourteenth century in Italy, and to the eighteenth century in some European cities. Before this, historical and even prehistoric archaeological records can cast a dim and fitful light on the presence or absence of a few specific diseases (see section 3.2 in Chapter 3). With improvements in DNA testing on palaeopathological specimens, there is hope for some extension. But there is little consistent archival material until the second half of the nineteenth century. At this time, legislation was passed in the United States, Scandinavia, and the United Kingdom which ensured disease records were kept for afflictions considered to be of public health importance to national populations. As described previously, internationally endorsed classifications of causes of death (and, later, causes of morbidity) which could be used by international agencies for the compilation of disease statistics became available in the early twentieth century. From that time, agencies such as the Pan American Sanitary Bureau, the League of Nations Health Organisation, and the WHO have served as sources of international data on health and disease.

Sources of disease data

Over the centuries, many sources of disease-related data have developed at the national level—for example, in the United States, the Epidemic Intelligence Service from 1946 and *Morbidity and Mortality Weekly Report* from 1952; in the United Kingdom, the General Register Office from 1837 and the Office for National Statistics from 1996. These sources encompass mortality registration, morbidity case reporting, epidemic reporting, laboratory reporting, individual case reports, epidemic field investigations, surveys, animal reservoir and vector distribution studies, and demographic and environmental data (Declich and Carter, 1994). To these can be added hospital and medical care statistics, general practitioner records, public health laboratory reports, disease registries, drug and biologics utilization and sales data, absenteeism data, health and general population surveys, and media reports. Different data sources present their own advantages and disadvantages. Their availability varies from country to country and they differ in their level of sophistication, quality, utility, and extent.

Over and above national disease recording, international epidemiological data recording gathered pace from the middle of the nineteenth century with the first of the International Sanitary Conferences. This marked the beginning of a new phase in international health cooperation, forming a broad platform for the development of international health offices and legislative responses to infectious diseases in the next century. The primary objective of the First International Sanitary Conference, opened in Paris in 1851, was for the 12 participating states (all European) to reach agreement on the minimum quarantine requirements for cholera, plague, and yellow fever, with a view to facilitating trade and safeguarding public health. Although an international sanitary convention and associated sanitary regulations were formulated, some participants were slow to ratify the convention and it had become inoperative by 1865. Part of this failure lay in the state of medical knowledge regarding cholera and the contradictory views of the delegates regarding the role of quarantine in its control (World Health Organization, 1958).

Further International Sanitary Conferences were held in the second half of the nineteenth century, each centred on the containment of cholera, plague, and yellow fever and with their agendas dictated by epidemics of whichever disease was considered to be the most pressing at the time. The first of the effective International Sanitary Conventions, concerned with the Mecca pilgrimage, came out of the Seventh International Sanitary Conference in 1892. Subsequent conventions evolved to cover cholera (1893), plague (1897), yellow fever (1912), smallpox (1926), and louse-borne typhus fever (1926).

Of particular concern to maritime nations during the last quarter of the nineteenth century was the likelihood of the spread of communicable disease by ships trading between nations. Such concern lay, for example, behind the National Quarantine Act of 1878 in the United States. This Act legislated for the collection and publication of sanitary reports from those overseas locations with which the United States had commercial interests, mainly port cities. Its disease voice was provided by the *Weekly Abstract of Sanitary Reports* (latterly *Public Health Reports*).

The Office International D'Hygiène Publique (1907–46)

The Office International d'Hygiène Publique (OIHP) was born out of the Eleventh International Sanitary Conference, held in 1903. It was founded under the Rome Agreement on 9 December 1907 and was based in Paris. Operating on behalf of participating states, the main purpose of the OIHP was to oversee the international codification of procedures for quarantine and associated surveillance activities. Within this remit, the OIHP served three basic functions (Goodman, 1952) as:

- the body with responsibility for the revision and administration of the International Sanitary Conventions and associated Conferences
- a technical commission for the study of epidemic diseases
- an agency for the rapid exchange of epidemiological information relating to the diseases covered by the International Sanitary Conventions.

Article 9 (Annex) of the Rome Agreement of 1903 committed the OIHP to the publication, at least once a month, of the *Bulletin Mensuel de l'Office International d'Hygiène Publique*. The *Bulletin* was to include: '(1) laws and general or local regulations promulgated in the various countries respecting transmissible diseases; (2) information respecting the spread of infectious diseases; (3) information respecting the works executed or the measures taken for improving the healthiness of localities; (4) statistics dealing with public health; (5) bibliographical notes' (Goodman, 1952, p. 98). The *Bulletin* first appeared in 1909 and continued until 1946. Beginning in November 1928, information collected by the OIHP was summarized in a regular communiqué, published in the *Weekly Epidemiological Record* of the League of Nations Health Section.

Over the years, the work of the OIHP extended beyond maritime quarantine to include such issues as quarantine regulations for air traffic (an International Sanitary Convention for Aerial Navigation was drawn up in 1932 and came into force in 1935), venereal diseases in seamen, the international standardization of antidiphtheritic serum, and the control of narcotic drugs. In 1945, the United Nations Relief and Rehabilitation Administration (UNRRA) assumed responsibility for the OIHP's duties with respect to the International Sanitary Conventions; the OIHP was dissolved by protocols signed on 22 July 1946, with the epidemiological service being incorporated into the Interim Commission of the WHO on 1 January 1947 (World Health Organization, 1958).

Health Committee of the League of Nations

The period between the two world wars was also the period when the Health Committee of the League of Nations assumed a critical role in disease surveillance and morbidity and mortality recording on a systematic basis. The first meeting of the Health Committee took place in August 1921 to consider 'the question of organising means of more rapid interchange of epidemiological information' (League of Nations Health Section, 1922, p. 3). At this and subsequent meetings, it was emphasized that epidemiological intelligence work should receive immediate attention and that the most important and pressing work in this field was with regard to the submission of epidemiological information in relation to infectious diseases in Eastern Europe in general and Russia in particular. In response, the Epidemiological Intelligence Service was instituted in the Geneva Health Section and started to prepare reports on the health situation of Eastern Europe in 1921. These reports were first published in 1922 and progressively expanded to include not only Eastern Europe, but also Central Europe and all European countries. Details of the reports included in the *Epidemiological Intelligence* series and other Health Section statistical series are provided by Cliff et al. (1998, pp. 389–93). We note here that, during the inter-war period, the breadth and geographical reach of the publications evolved to include regular counts of disease-specific morbidity and mortality for a global sample of countries.

The League of Nation's concern with disease surveillance owes much to Ludwik Rajchman, the first director of the Health Organisation. Rajchman's vision was for the Health Organisation to be a global centre for epidemiological information collection and exchange (Brown, 2006). By the start of World War II, the reach of the Health Organisation's Epidemic Intelligence Service had expanded to cover some 90 per cent of the world's population. As Goodman (1952, p. 109) observes:

> By the analysis of reports coming to Geneva directly or from the Paris Office and its regional bureaux in Washington, Alexandria, Singapore and Sydney, the Health Organisation could keep a kind of sphygmographic record of the pulse of the world's epidemics and so keep governments informed of them by cable and wireless and by weekly, monthly, bi-monthly and annual publications.

When surveillance operations began in the early 1920s, the postal service represented the principal mechanism for the submission of epidemiological information from administrations to Geneva. But communications technology was developing rapidly. In October 1923, N.V. Lothian, a field epidemiologist in the Health Section of the League of Nations, could assure a meeting of the Section on Vital Statistics of the American Public Health Association that the 'question of telegraphing reports to ensure greater promptitude is under discussion' and 'that a scheme has been worked out whereby the American weekly summary can be cabled to Geneva by an ingenious code costing us only some 500 francs per year' (Lothian, 1924, p. 289). Just a few years later, the Eastern Bureau would lead the development of wireless technology as a tool in global disease surveillance.

Eastern Bureau

While the early work of the League of Nations Health Organisation was directed towards the emergency situation in Eastern Europe, the Epidemiological Intelligence Service continued to collect and publish data that provided a world view of epidemic diseases of international importance. The relative prevalence of such diseases in Asia prompted the establishment of the Health Organisation's Eastern Bureau in Singapore in March 1925. Under the initial directorship

of Gilbert E. Brooke, the Eastern Bureau provides an example of the early use of wireless communications in international health cooperation and disease surveillance (Manderson, 1995; Yach, 1998). The scope of the Bureau's operations was defined at the First Meeting of the Advisory Council of the Eastern Bureau, convened in early 1925. The 'essential task' of the Bureau was to:

> collect information on the prevalence of epidemic disease at ports in an area extending from Cape Town to Vladivostok and Alexandria, including Australia; also, to obtain intelligence on 'infected' ships to classify the information and to re-telegraph … [the] same in the form of a weekly bulletin, confirmed subsequently by mail by means of a Weekly Fasciculus, which contains also additional information on public health in various districts of the territory. (Eastern Bureau of the League of Nations Health Organisation, 1926, unpaginated)

The area under epidemiological surveillance by the Bureau, occasionally referred to in official publications as the 'Eastern Arena', covered about half the globe. For administrative purposes, the area was divided into four geographic groups: a Western group (East Coast of Africa and the Asiatic Coast from Egypt to Burma); a Central group (Malaya, Netherlands East Indies, and the administrations of Borneo and the Philippine Islands); an Eastern group (Asiatic Coast from Siam to Siberia, including Japan); and a Southern group (Australia, New Zealand, French New Caledonia, Fiji, and Honolulu). The logic behind this fourfold division was that maritime communications within each group were mainly self-contained, with connections between the groups being chiefly the concern of larger ports. Beginning with a tentative list of 35 'important ports' that were frequented by foreign trade ships, the number of ports in regular telegraphic communication with the Bureau grew rapidly to 66 (in 1926), 135 (in 1931), and, eventually, 147 (in 1938).

The information collected by the Bureau was circulated by telegram and wireless broadcasts and in the form of a *Weekly Bulletin* or resumé to countries in the Eastern Arena and the League of Nations Health Organisation in Geneva. The information was used by the administrations to inform decisions on how to prevent entry of a given disease by sea and, in later years, by air.

World Health Organization

The surveillance role of the League of Nations Health Committee was taken on *in toto* by the WHO from the latter's inception. Chapter XI of the WHO's Constitution determined that activities should be decentralized along regional lines, with the First World Health Assembly agreeing to the delineation of six world regions: Africa, Americas, Eastern Mediterranean, Europe, South-East Asia, and Western Pacific. The six Regional Offices had come into being by 1952, with the long-established Pan American Sanitary Bureau assuming the role of the Office for the Americas. This regional structure has continued through to the present day.

The inheritance of the newly created WHO included responsibility for international epidemic control in terms of (i) quarantine and the International Sanitary Conventions and (ii) epidemic intelligence and epidemiological services. One of the first major tasks of the WHO was to revise and reform the existing International Sanitary Conventions and these came into force under the new title of the International Sanitary Regulations in 1952. These Regulations represented a synthesis of existing Conventions dealing with maritime, land, and air traffic in relation to a total of six quarantine diseases (cholera, plague, smallpox, relapsing fever, typhus fever, and yellow fever). Information received under the Regulations was published in the WHO's *Weekly Epidemiological Record*. Increasingly, the WHO's work extended beyond surveillance functions for the quarantine diseases to encompass other communicable diseases including dengue haemorrhagic fever (started in 1964), salmonellosis (started in 1965), and, in cooperation with the Food and Agriculture Organization (FAO) and the World Organisation for Animal Health (OIE), rabies.

In the late 1960s, the WHO replaced 'epidemiological intelligence' with 'epidemiological surveillance' as an approach to disease control. The new approach had grown out of improved epidemiological methods (including data processing and analysis, laboratory studies, and field studies) and was defined as:

> the exercise of continuous scrutiny of and watchfulness over the distribution and spread of infections and factors related thereto, of sufficient accuracy and completeness to be pertinent to effective control. (World Health Organization, 2008, p. 175)

With this development, the Unit of Quarantine was merged with the Unit of Epidemiological Surveillance in 1968 and, by 1970, the programme was referred to as Epidemiological Surveillance. This strategy was adopted as a means of moving away from the concept that disease prevention and control could only be achieved through the application of quarantine measures. As a consequence of this development, the existing International Sanitary Regulations (1952) were revised and adopted as the International Health Regulations in 1969. Accordingly, the Committee on International Quarantine changed its name to the Committee on International Surveillance of Communicable Diseases. Information collected by the Epidemiological Surveillance programme was disseminated daily through the WHO epidemiological radiotelegraphic (later telex) bulletin and the *Weekly Epidemiological Record*. The practical reality on the ground of all this international disease surveillance activity in the six decades from the formation of the League of Nations Health Organisation was that morbidity and mortality data are available from the WHO for a wide range of communicable diseases and locations as follows:

1. *Notifiable diseases (1923–58)*. For the period 1923–58, *Annual Epidemiological Report* and its successor publication, *Annual Epidemiological and Vital Statistics*, included a chart or table which recorded in matrix format (diseases × countries) which diseases were *notifiable* in each region of the world.
2. *Reported diseases (1959–83)*. Between 1959 and 1983, the matrices of notifiable diseases were not published, but equivalent matrices of *reported* diseases by country can be constructed from the raw returns of recorded (non-zero) mortality and morbidity published in later issues of *Annual Epidemiological and Vital Statistics* and its successor publication, *World Health Statistics Annual*.

6.6.4 Developments in Programme-Oriented Surveillance

From the mid-1980s, the character of international recording of communicable disease morbidity and mortality changed fundamentally from systematic time period × disease × country surveillance of a large number of infectious conditions to a targeted surveillance

related to international health programmes. And so, in 1982, the WHO programmes on Health Statistics and Epidemiological Surveillance were merged to form the Health Situation and Trend Assessment Programme. This new programme placed emphasis on a target-oriented approach to information, with priority given to only the most essential information for the improvement of health systems (Uemura, 1988). This approach, built around vaccine-preventable and potentially globally eradicable diseases, had been presaged by the Smallpox Eradication Programme in the 1960s and 1970s and was followed by the EPI from 1974 (section 6.4.1) and the GPEI from 1988 (section 6.5.3).

6.6.5 Electronic Network Systems for Global Disease Detection

Surveillance changed radically from the mid-1980s as a result of technological developments—the rapid and widespread growth in cheap desktop computing power and software replacing a few massive mainframes, and the growth of the communications and information-rich Internet. Recent developments in this area have been shaped by the International Health Regulations which were revised in 2005 to update capacity and standards of the reporting of disease events. The 2005 Regulations expanded the traditional concerns of the International Health Regulations and provided a new framework for the management of events that may constitute a public health emergency of international concern. Under the revised Regulations, Member States are required to notify the WHO of 'all events which may constitute a public health emergency of international concern' (Article 6.1), whether naturally occurring, intentionally created, or unintentionally caused. The Regulations set minimum requirements for developing and maintaining core capacity for the detection of, and response to, public health emergencies of international concern ('core capacity requirements for surveillance response'). Internet-based systems of real-time disease surveillance lie at the heart of these developments.

The WHO Global Outbreak Alert and Response Network

The rise of newly emerging diseases, the pandemic spread of influenza, and the threat of bioterrorism have highlighted the essential function of global disease surveillance in the maintenance and promotion of international health in the early twenty-first century (Castillo-Salgado, 2010). To this end, the Global Outbreak Alert and Response Network (GOARN) for the early detection of, and rapid response to, outbreaks of diseases of international importance was formalized by the WHO in April 2000 (Heymann et al., 2001). Conceived as a 'network of networks' (Lemon et al., 2007, p. 19), and formed as an international collaboration of some 140 public, private, non-governmental, and intergovernmental institutions and organizations worldwide, GOARN is overseen by the WHO Global Alert and Response programme as the principal WHO surveillance network for international outbreak alert and response.

GOARN operates in three key areas: outbreak alert (detection, verification, and communication); outbreak response (risk assessment, technical advice and support, field investigation, research, and communication); and preparedness (assessment, planning, training, stockpiles, research, and communication). For these purposes, GOARN connects both formal and informal sources of outbreak information. Formal sources include a range of governmental agencies, universities, laboratories, and other institutions that form part of the global network of WHO collaborating centres, along with international agencies and WHO regional and country offices. Informal sources include non-governmental organizations (such as UNICEF, UNHCR, the International Committee of the Red Cross, the International Federation of Red Cross and Red Crescent Societies, and international humanitarian non-governmental organizations such as Médecins sans Frontières), along with informal Internet-based disease surveillance and scanning systems such as the Global Public Health Intelligence Network.

Real-time information gathered by GOARN is examined on a daily basis by the WHO Outbreak Verification Team. Daily reports on suspected and verified events are then distributed to specified WHO staff at Geneva and in the Regional Offices, while a weekly electronic Outbreak Verification List (including summary details of the disease, location, source of report, number of cases and deaths, and investigation status) is distributed throughout the GOARN network. Once an outbreak has been verified, situation reports are posted on the WHO website and in the *Weekly Epidemiological Record*. Outbreak responses are implemented by GOARN partners, while WHO headquarters has investigative teams for rapid dispatch to outbreak sites (Heymann et al., 2001).

6.6.6 Informal Internet-Based Global Reporting Systems

Recent years have seen the development of a spectrum of ad hoc informal Internet-based international and global disease surveillance systems and platforms. These have opened up alternative channels for the rapid detection and reporting of communicable disease outbreaks. Such Internet resources also have the potential to reduce costs and to increase the transparency of reporting. Perspectives on the broad range of operative systems and platforms are provided by Castillo-Salgado (2010) and Magid et al. (2018). For scientists whose focus is interrupting the geographical spread of communicable diseases, one of the most interesting of these informal networks is *HealthMap*. Founded in September 2006 and affiliated to the Children's Hospital Informatics Program at the Harvard-Massachusetts Institute of Technology (MIT) Division of Health Sciences and Technology, HealthMap utilizes online informal sources for disease outbreak monitoring and mapping within a geographical information system (GIS) framework. As described by Freifeld et al. (2008), HealthMap provides a global view of communicable disease outbreaks as reported by the WHO, ProMED-mail, Google News, and Eurosurveillance. The automated system operates to monitor, organize, and filter information with a view to providing real-time intelligence on emerging diseases via a website (http://www.healthmap.org) and a mobile app ('Outbreaks Near Me').

Regional disease threat tracking tools: the European Commission

An Early Warning and Response System was implemented by the European Commission in 1998 as a means of gathering and analysing data on emerging public health threats to the member states of the European Union. Since 2007, the system has been hosted in Sweden by the European Centre for Disease Prevention and Control. Notifications received from member states through the Early Warning and Response System and through other epidemic surveillance activities (including the active screening of national epidemiological bulletins and informal sources such as the media) are documented and monitored through a dedicated database (Threat Tracking Tool, or TTT) that was first activated in June 2005. Between June 2005 and December 2015, a total of 1,108 threats were monitored by the European Centre for Disease Prevention and Control, representing an average of some 100 threats per year (range 29–208) and with distinct seasonal peaks in the summer and autumn (European Centre for Disease Prevention and Control, 2010, 2017).

Sentinel practices

The legal requirements to notify critical infectious diseases are tending to be left behind by the reality of disease proliferation. As a result, blanket reporting is increasingly replaced by sampling systems in which sentinel practices are used to pick up trends in disease prevalence. Some cities have pioneered local monitoring, of which the Seattle Virus Watch programme of the 1960s is an outstanding early example (Hall et al., 1970). In the developing world, sentinel surveillance is the only cost-effective way of monitoring population health.

6.7   Conclusion

This chapter has outlined the historical development of approaches to the geographical control of infectious diseases. As we have seen, the basic tenets of approaches that have become all too familiar as the world grapples with COVID-19—lockdown, isolation, and social distancing—have their roots in medieval Italy's attempts to inhibit the spread of bubonic plague. In contrast, the practice of producing immunity by vaccination finds its early expression in the smallpox experiments of Edward Jenner in the 1790s. Ultimately, timely and accurate surveillance data that are geographically and temporally coded lie behind any control strategy which attempts to interrupt the spatial propagation of an infectious disease from one area to another. For, without such information, the development of appropriate control strategies to inhibit epidemic upturns rapidly descends into a Delphic art.

Epilogue

As we noted in the Preface, this book has been written against the background of one of the worst global pandemics of an infectious disease to have hit the human population in the last 100 years – COVID-19, caused by a new coronavirus, SARS-CoV-2, not previously identified in humans. Although details of the pandemic's first wave were discussed in Chapter 5, much has happened since the manuscript of this book went to press[1]. By the end of May 2021, confirmed cases of COVID-19 globally had reached some 175 million; the true number of cases will have been much greater because of under-reporting. By the same date, 3.5 million deaths had been recorded worldwide. **Figure E1(A)** summarises the reported pandemic history from the beginning of February 2020 to the end of May 2021. Globally, daily confirmed case numbers built steadily to late November 2020. A brief lull then followed before a resurgence from the end of March 2021. With the latter, the main geographical focus of disease activity switched from Europe and North America to Asia and South America. From June 2021, a general opening up of economic activity is anticipated, especially of hospitality and tourism which, linked to the emergence of new strains of the virus, some believe will contribute to a third global wave of disease activity in the latter part of the year. **Figure E1(B)**, which shows the instantaneous weekly reproduction rate, R_t, of

COVID-19, lends credence to this belief (Arroyo-Marioli et al., 2021). Periods when R_t exceeded 1 have been shaded red.

Vaccines to protect against severe illness and death began to come on stream from December 2020 and demonstrated that, with lockdowns, a route out of the pandemic existed. The ready transmissibility of SARS-CoV-2 from person to person and the speed with which variants of concern have emerged (13 in the United Kingdom alone) have made the rapid development of vaccines particularly difficult. Nevertheless, despite all the production and distribution problems, **Figure E1(C)** shows that some 1.5 billion doses have been administered worldwide. The geographical availability of vaccines has been predictably patchy, with the advanced economies effectively controlling supplies and poorer countries suffering.

We commented in the Preface that it remains to be seen whether the COVID-19 pandemic rolls on to become one of the truly massive pandemics to have affected the human population. But we hope that our approach in this book to the problem of understanding the underlying spatial and temporal structure of epidemics and pandemics may facilitate disease control efforts and, ultimately, enhance attempts to achieve global disease eradication. If it does, it will have achieved its purpose.

---

[1] Too late for considered inclusion even in an Epilogue, the Royal Society of London published in May 2021 an important themed issue of 21 papers on the COVID-19 pandemic entitled "Modelling that shaped the early COVID-19 pandemic response in the UK" in its journal series *Philosophical Transactions*, series B, volume 376, issue 1829; https://doi.org/10.1098/rstb.2021.0001.

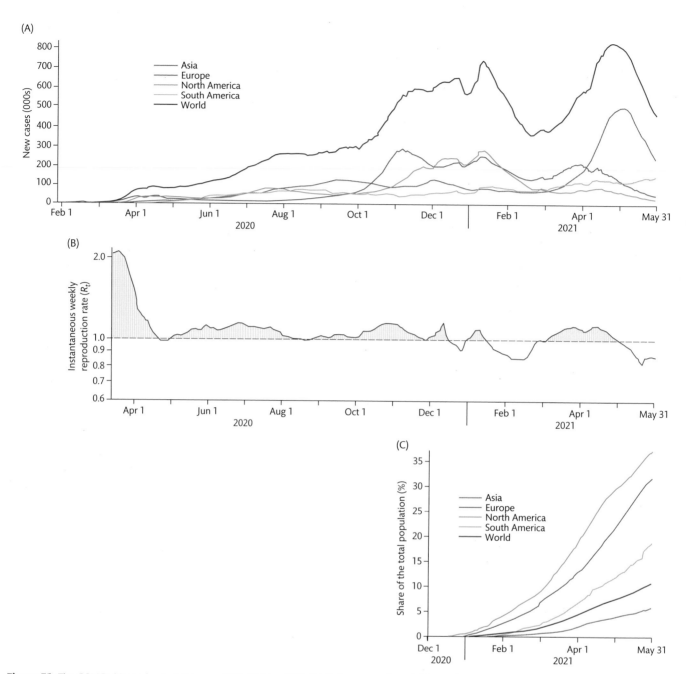

Figure E1 The COVID-19 pandemic, 1 February 2020–31 May 2021. (A) Daily new confirmed COVID-19 cases, rolling 7-day average. (B) Global estimate of the instantaneous reproduction rate, R_t, for COVID-19. The reproduction rate represents the average number of new infections caused by a single infected individual. If the rate is greater than 1, the infection is able to spread in the population. If it is below 1, the number of cases occurring in the population will gradually decrease to zero. (C) Share of people who have received at least one dose of COVID-19 vaccine, 20 December 2020–31 May 2021.

Source: Data from COVID-19 Data Repository by the Center for Systems Science and Engineering (CSSE) at Johns Hopkins University, https://github.com/CSSEGISandData/COVID-19; Our World in Data, https://ourworldindata.org/explorers/coronavirus-data-explorer, 31 May 2021.

References and Author Index

Numbers in square brackets after references indicate the section(s) in the text where the item is cited.

Ackerman, E., Elveback, L.R., Fox, J.P. (1984). *Simulation of Infectious Disease Epidemics*. Springfield, IL: C.C. Thomas. [1.6.3]

Ahmad, A., Andraghetti, R. (2007). *SARS Control: Effective and Acceptable Strategies for the Control of SARS and New Emerging Infections in China and Europe. Control Measures Implemented by the Non-European SARS Affected Countries*. Work Package 8. Hamburg: WHO EURO CSR Department. [3.4.2]

Akovali, U., Yilmaz, K. (2020). 'Polarized politics of pandemic response and the Covid-19 connectedness across the US states.' *Covid Economics*, **57**, 94–131. doi.org/10.2139/ssrn.3730712. [5.6.1]

Alvarado de la Barrera, C., Reyes-Terán, G. (2005). 'Influenza: forecast for a pandemic.' *Archives of Medical Research*, **36**, 628–36. [3.4.1]

Anderson, G.W. (1947). 'A German atlas of epidemic diseases.' *Geographical Review*, **37**, 307–22. [1.5.1]

Anderson, R.M., Fraser, C., Ghani, A.C., Donnelly, C.A., Riley, S., Ferguson, N.M., Leung, G.M., Lam, T.H., Hedley, A.J. (2004). 'Epidemiology, transmission dynamics and control of SARS: the 2002–2003 epidemic.' *Philosophical Transactions of the Royal Society London*, **B359**, 1091–105. [3.4.2]

Anderson, R.M., May, R. (1991). *Infectious Diseases of Humans: Dynamics and Control*. Oxford: Oxford University Press. [1.3.2, 1.4.3]

Angulo, J.J., Haggett, P., Megale, P., Pederneiras, A.A. (1977). 'Variola minor in Braganca Paulista county, 1956: a trend-surface analysis.' *American Journal of Epidemiology*, **105**, 272–8. [1.5.2]

Arribalzaga, R.A. (1955). 'Una nueva enfermedad a gérman desconocido: hipertermia nefrotóxica, leucopénica y enantemántica.' ['New epidemic disease due to unidentified germ: nephrotoxic, leukopenic and enanthematous hyperthermia.'] *El Día Médico*, **27**, 1204–10. [3.3.4]

Arroyo-Marioli, F., Bulano, F., Kucinskas, S., Rondon-Moreno, C. (2021). 'Tracking R of COVID-19: a new real-time estimation using the Kalman Filter.' *PLoS One*, **16**, e0244474. doi: 10.1371/journal.pone.0244474. [Epilogue]

Asaria, P., MacMahon, E. (2006). 'Measles in the United Kingdom: can we eradicate it by 2010?' *British Medical Journal*, **333**, 890–5. [6.4.1]

Aufderheide, A.C., Salo, W., Madden, M., Steitz, J., Buikstra, J., Guhl, F., Arriaza, B., Renier, C., Wittmers, L.E., Fornaciari, G., Allison, M. (2004). 'A 9,000-year record of Chagas' disease.' *Proceedings of the National Academy of Sciences USA*, **101**, 2034–9. [3.2.1]

Aylward, B., Hennessey, K.A., Zagaria, N., Olivé, J.-M., Cochi, S. (2000). 'When is a disease eradicable? 100 years of lessons learned.' *American Journal of Public Health*, **90**, 1515–20. [6.5, 6.5.1]

Bailey, N.T.J. (1957). *The Mathematical Theory of Epidemics*. London: Charles Griffin & Co., Ltd. [1.3.2, 1.3.5]

Bailey, N.T.J. (1975). *The Mathematical Theory of Infectious Diseases and Its Applications*. London: Charles Griffin & Co., Ltd. [1.3.2, 1.4.3, 1.4.4]

Barbour, A.G., Fish, D. (1993). 'The biological and social phenomenon of Lyme disease.' *Science*, **260**, 1610–16. [3.3.4]

Baroyan, O.V., Genchikov, L.A., Rvachev, L.A., Shashkov, V.A. (1969). 'An attempt at large-scale influenza epidemic modelling by means of a computer.' *Bulletin of the International Epidemiology Association*, **18**, 22–31. [1.6.4]

Bartlett, M.S. (1957). 'Measles periodicity and community size.' *Journal of the Royal Statistical Society, Series A*, **120**, 48–70. [1.4.3, 3.3.2]

Bartlett, M.S. (1960). 'The critical community size of measles in the United States.' *Journal of the Royal Statistical Society, Series A*, **123**, 37–44. [3.3.2]

Barua, D. (1992). 'History of cholera.' In: D. Barua and W.B. Greenough (eds.), *Cholera*. New York: Plenum, 1–36. [4.3.1]

Barua, D., Greenhough, W.B. (1992). *Cholera*. New York: Plenum. [4.3.3]

Bedford, J., Enria, D., Giesecke, J., Heymann, D.L., Ihekweazu, C., Kobinger, G., Lane, H.C., Memish, Z., Oh, M.D., Sall, A.A., Schuchat, A., Ungchusak, K., Wieler, L.H., WHO Strategic and Technical Advisory Group for Infectious Hazards (2020). 'COVID-19: towards controlling of a pandemic.' *Lancet*, **395**, 1015–18. [5.1]

Benach, J.L., Bosler, E.M., Hanrahan, J.P., Coleman, J.L., Habicht, G.S., Bast, T.F., Cameron, D.J., Ziegler, J.L., Barbour, A.G., Burgdorfer, W., Edelman, R., Kaslow, R.A. (1983). 'Spirochetes isolated from the blood of two patients with Lyme disease.' *New England Journal of Medicine*, **308**, 740–2. [3.3.4]

Bennett, J.V., Holmberg, J.D., Rogers, M.K., Solomon, S.L. (1987). 'Infectious and parasitic diseases.' In: R.W. Amler and H.B. Dull (eds.), *Closing the Gap: The Burden of Unnecessary Diseases*. Oxford: Oxford University Press, 100–20. [1.2.3]

Béraud, G., Abrams, S., Beutels, P., Dervaux, B., Hens, N. (2018). 'Resurgence risk for measles, mumps and rubella in France in 2018 and 2020.' *Eurosurveillance*, **23**, 1700796. doi: 10.2807/1560-7917. ES.2018.23.25.1700796. [5.2.4]

Bernard-Stoecklin, S., Rolland, P., Silue, Y., Mailles, A., Campese, C., Simondon, A., Mechain, M., Meurice, L., Nguyen, M., Bassi, C., Yamani, E., Behillil, S., Ismael, S., Nguyen, D., Malvy, D., Lescure, F.X., Georges, S., Lazarus, C., Tabaï, A., Stempfelet, M., Enouf, V., Coignard, B., Levy-Bruhl, D., Investigation Team (2020). 'First cases of coronavirus disease 2019 (COVID-19) in France: surveillance, investigations and control measures, January 2020.' *Eurosurveillance*, **25**, 2000094. doi: 10.2807/1560-7917.ES.2020.25.6.2000094. [5.3.2]

Bernoulli, D. (1760). 'Essai d'une nouvelle analyse de la mortalité causée par la vérole et des avantages de l'inoculation pour la prévenir.' *Mémoires Mathématique et Physique, Académie Royale des Sciences (Paris)*, **1**, 1–10. [1.4.3]

Berry, B.J.L. (2006). *Nihil Sine Labore: An Autobiography*. Baltimore, MD: Gateway Press. [Preface]

Birrell, P., Blake, J., van Leeuwen, E., Gent, N., de Angelis, D. (2020). 'Real-time nowcasting and forecasting of COVID-19 dynamics in

England: the first wave?' medRxiv preprint doi: https://doi.org/10.1101/2020.08.24.20180737. [5.4.2]

Böhmer, M.M., Buchholz, U., Corman, V.M., Hoch, M., Katz, K., Marosevic, D.V., Böhm, S., Woudenberg, T., Ackermann, N., Konrad, R., Eberle, U., Treis, B., Dangel, A., Bengs, K., Fingerle, V., Berger, A., Hörmansdorfer, S., Ippisch, S., Wicklein, B., Grahl, A., Pörtner, K., Muller, N., Zeitlmann, N., Boender, T.S., Cai, W., Reich, A., An der Heiden, M., Rexroth, U., Hamouda, O., Schneider, J., Veith, T., Mühlemann, B., Wölfel, R., Antwerpen, M., Walter, M., Protzer, U., Liebl, B., Haas, W., Sing, A., Drosten, C., Zapf, A. (2020). 'Investigation of a COVID-19 outbreak in Germany resulting from a single travel-associated primary case: a case series.' *Lancet Infectious Diseases*, **20**, 920–8. [5.3.2]

Bradley, D.J. (1989). 'The scope of travel medicine.' In: R. Steffen, H.O. Lobel, J. Haworth, and D.J. Bradley (eds.), *Travel Medicine: Proceedings of the First Conference on International Travel Medicine, Zürich, Switzerland, 5–8 April 1988*. Berlin: Springer Verlag, 1–9. [3.3.3]

Briand, S., Bertherat, E., Cox, P., Formenty, P., Kieny, M.-P., Myhre, J.K., Roth, C., Shindo, N., Dye, C. (2014). 'The international Ebola emergency.' *New England Journal of Medicine*, **371**, 1181–3. [3.4.3]

Briesemeister, W. (1953). 'A new oblique equal area projection.' *Geographical Review*, **43**, 260–1. [1.5.1]

Brillouin, L.N. (1964). *Scientific Uncertainty and Information*. London: Academic Press. [1.7]

Brown, T.M. (2006). 'International public health before the World Health Organization.' In: Global Forum for Health Research, *Forum 10, Cairo, Egypt, 29 October–2 November 2006*. Geneva: Global Forum for Health Research. [6.6.3]

Brownlee, J. (1907). 'Statistical studies in immunity: the theory of an epidemic.' *Proceedings of the Royal Society of Edinburgh*, **26**, 484–521. [1.4.2]

Brownstein, J.S., Wolfe, C.J., Mandl, K.D. (2006). 'Empirical evidence for the effect of airline travel on inter-regional influenza spread in the United States.' *PLoS Medicine*, **3**, e401. doi:10.1371/journal.pmed.0030401. [3.3.3]

Budd, W. (1873). *Typhoid Fever: Its Nature, Mode of Spreading, and Prevention*. London: Longmans, Green. [2.1]

Burnet, F.M., White, D.O. (1972). *Natural History of Infectious Disease* (fourth edition). Cambridge: Cambridge University Press. [1.2.1]

Bush, K. (2000). 'Polio, war and peace.' *Bulletin of the World Health Organization*, **78**, 281–2. [6.5.3]

Butler, D. (2006). 'Family tragedy spotlights flu mutations.' *Nature*, **442**, 114–15. [3.4.1]

Carrat, F., Valleron, A.J. (1992). 'Epidemiologic mapping using the "kriging" method: application to an influenza-like illness epidemic in France.' *American Journal of Epidemiology*, **135**, 1293–300. [1.5.2]

Cassel, J., Haggett, P., Lancaster, H.O., Pfanz, C., Vukanovic, C., Watson, G.S. (1969). *Advisers' Report on WHO Research in Epidemiology and Communications Science*. Geneva: United Nations (WHO, Paper RECS/69.). [1.1]

Castillo-Salgado, C. (2010). 'Trends and directions of global public health surveillance.' *Epidemiologic Reviews*, **32**, 93–109. [6.6.5, 6.6.6]

Centers for Disease Control (1988). 'Guidelines for evaluating surveillance systems.' *Morbidity and Mortality Weekly Report*, **37** (suppl. S5), 1S–10S. [6.6.1]

Centers for Disease Control and Prevention (1993). 'Update: hantavirus pulmonary syndrome – United States, 1993.' *Morbidity and Mortality Weekly Report*, **42**, 816–20. [3.3.5]

Centers for Disease Control and Prevention (1997). 'Isolation of avian influenza A (H5N1) viruses from humans – Hong Kong,

May–December 1997.' *Morbidity and Mortality Weekly Report*, **46**, 1204–7. [3.4.1]

Centers for Disease Control and Prevention (1998). 'Update: isolation of avian influenza A (H5N1) viruses from humans – Hong Kong, 1997–1998.' *Morbidity and Mortality Weekly Report*, **46**, 1245–7. [3.4.1]

Centers for Disease Control and Prevention (2007). 'Summary of notifiable diseases – United States, 2005.' *Morbidity and Mortality Weekly Report*, **56**, 1–92. [3.3.4]

Centers for Disease Control and Prevention (2008). *Hantavirus*. Atlanta, GA: CDC. http://www.cdc.gov/ncidod/diseases/hanta/hps, accessed 27 March 2021. [3.3.5]

Centers for Disease Control and Prevention (2021). *U.S. Quarantine Stations*. Atlanta, GA: CDC. https://www.cdc.gov/quarantine/quarantine-stations-us.html, accessed 27 March 2021. [6.3.3]

Chen, H., Li, Y., Li, Z., Shi, J., Shinya, K., Deng, G., Qi, Q., Tian, G., Fan, S., Zhao, H., Sun, Y., Kawaoka, Y. (2006). 'Properties and dissemination of H5N1 viruses isolated during an influenza outbreak in migratory waterfowl in western China.' *Journal of Virology*, **80**, 5976–83. [3.4.1]

Chen, Q., Yan, J., Huang, H., Zhang, X. (2021). 'Correlation of the epidemic spread of COVID-19 and urban population migration in the major cities of Hubei Province, China.' *Transportation Safety and Environment*, volume 3, pages 21–35, https://doi.org/10.1093/tse/tdaa033. [1.6.4]

Chorley, R.J., Schumm, S.A., Sugden, D.E. (1984). *Geomorphology*. London: Methuen. [1.6.2]

Chowell, G., Castillo-Chavez, C., Fenimore, P.W., Kribs-Zaleta, C.M., Arriola, L., Hyman, J.M. (2004). 'Model parameters and outbreak control for SARS.' *Emerging Infectious Diseases*, **10**, 1258–63. [5.2.4]

Christakis, N.A., Fowler, J.H. (2013). 'Social contagion theory: examining dynamic social networks and human behavior.' *Statistics in Medicine*, **32**, 556–77. [1.2.2]

Cipolla, C.M. (1976). *Public Health and the Medical Profession in the Renaissance*. Cambridge: Cambridge University Press. [6.3.3]

Cipolla, C.M. (1981). *Fighting the Plague in Seventeenth-Century Italy*. Madison, WI: University of Wisconsin Press. [6.3.2]

Claas, E.C., de Jong, J.C., van Beek, R., Rimmelzwaan, G.F., Osterhaus, A.D.M.E. (1998). 'Human influenza virus A/Hong Kong/156/97 (H5N1) infection.' *Vaccine*, **16**, 977–8. [3.4.1]

Clemow, F.G. (1889–90). 'Epidemic influenza.' *Public Health (London)*, **2**, 358–67. [4.4.2]

Clemow, F.G. (1903). *The Geography of Disease*. Cambridge: Cambridge University Press. [1.5.1]

Cliff, A.D., Haggett, P. (1981). 'Graph theory.' In: N. Wrigley and R.J. Bennett (eds.), *Quantitative Geography: A British View*. London: Routledge and Kegan Paul, 225–34. [1.4.4]

Cliff, A.D., Haggett, P. (1983). 'Changing urban-rural contrasts in the velocity of measles epidemics in an island community.' In: N.D. McGlashan and J.R. Blunden (eds.), *Geographic Aspects of Health: Essays in Honour of Andrew Learmonth*. London: Academic Press, 336–48. [1.4.2]

Cliff, A.D., Haggett, P. (1985). *The Spread of Measles in Fiji and the Pacific: Spatial Components in the Transmission of Epidemic Waves through Island Communities*. Department of Human Geography publication number HG/18. Canberra: Research School of Pacific Studies, Australian National University. [1.2.2, 1.3.5, 3.3.3]

Cliff, A.D., Haggett, P. (1988). *Atlas of Disease Distributions: Analytical Approaches to Epidemiological Data*. Oxford: Blackwell Reference. [1.4.2, 1.4.3, 1.6.4, 2.5.4]

Cliff, A.D., Haggett, P. (1989). 'Spatial aspects of epidemic control.' *Progress in Human Geography*, **13**, 315–47. [6.2, 6.3, 6.4.2]

Cliff, A.D., Haggett, P. (1990). 'Epidemic control and critical community size.' In: R.W. Thomas (ed.), *Spatial Epidemiology*. London: Pion, 93–110. [3.2.2]

Cliff, A.D., Haggett, P. (2004). 'Time, travel and infection.' *British Medical Bulletin*, **69**, 87–99. [3.3.3]

Cliff, A.D., Haggett, P. (2006). 'A swash-backwash model of the single epidemic wave.' *Journal of Geographical Systems*, **8**, 227–52. [1.5.2, 1.6.1, 1.6.2, 2.5.4]

Cliff, A.D., Haggett, P., Ord, J.K. (1979). 'Graph theory and geography.' In: R.J. Wilson and L.W. Beineke (eds.), *Applications of Graph Theory*. London: Academic Press, 293–326. [1.4.4]

Cliff, A.D., Haggett, P., Ord, J.K. (1986). *Spatial Aspects of Influenza Epidemics*. London: Pion. [2.2.3, 2.3, 2.3.2]

Cliff, A.D., Haggett, P., Ord, J.K., Bassett, K., Davies, R.B. (1975). *Elements of Spatial Structure: A Quantitative Approach*. Cambridge: Cambridge University Press. [1.1, 1.4.1, 1.6.2, 1.6.4, 2.5.2]

Cliff, A.D., Haggett, P., Ord, J.K., Versey, G.R. (1981). *Spatial Diffusion: An Historical Geography of Epidemics in an Island Community*. Cambridge: Cambridge University Press. [1.1, 1.3.4, 1.4.3, 1.4.4, 1.5.2, 1.6, 1.6.2, 2.5.2, 2.5.3, 2.5.5]

Cliff, A.D., Haggett, P., Smallman-Raynor, M.R. (1993). *Measles: An Historical Geography of a Major Human Viral Disease from Global Expansion to Local Retreat, 1840–1990*. Oxford: Blackwell Reference. [1.4.2, 2.5.1, 3.2.2]

Cliff, A.D., Haggett, P., Smallman-Raynor, M.R. (1998). *Deciphering Global Epidemics: Analytical Approaches to the Disease Records of World Cities, 1888–1912*. Cambridge: Cambridge University Press. [1.3.5, 6.6.3]

Cliff, A.D., Haggett, P., Smallman-Raynor, M.R. (2000). *Island Epidemics*. Oxford: Oxford University Press. [1.4.2, 2.1, 3.3.2]

Cliff, A.D., Haggett, P., Smallman-Raynor, M.R. (2004). *World Atlas of Epidemic Diseases*. London: Arnold. [Preface, 1.1, 1.2.1, 1.5.1, 1.6.1, 1.7, 2.5.4, 3.2.2, 4.2.3, 4.3.2]

Cliff, A.D., Haggett, P., Smallman-Raynor, M.R. (2009). 'The changing shape of island epidemics: historical trends in Icelandic infectious disease waves, 1902–1988.' *Journal of Historical Geography*, **35**, 545–67. [2.5.2, 2.5.5, 2.5.6]

Cliff, A.D., Haggett, P., Smallman-Raynor, M.R., Stroup, D.F., Williamson, G.D. (1995). 'The application of multidimensional scaling methods to epidemiological data.' *Statistical Methods in Medical Research*, **4**, 102–23. [1.5.2, 2.2.2]

Cliff, A.D., Ord, J.K. (1973). *Spatial Autocorrelation*. London: Pion. [1.6.4]

Cliff, A.D., Ord, J.K. (1975). 'Space-time modelling with an application to regional forecasting.' *Transactions of the Institute of British Geographers*, **64**, 119–28. [1.4.2]

Cliff, A.D., Smallman-Raynor, M.R. (2013). *Infectious Disease Control: A Geographical Analysis from Medieval Quarantine to Global Eradication*. Oxford: Oxford University Press. [3.4.2, 6.3.1, 6.4, 6.5, 6.6.1]

Cliff, A.D., Smallman-Raynor, M.R., Haggett, P., Stroup, D.F., Thacker, S.B. (2009). *Infectious Diseases. Emergence and Re-emergence: A Geographical Analysis*. Oxford: Oxford University Press. [1.2.2, 2.3.3, 3.1.1, 3.2, 3.2.1, 3.3.2, 3.3.3, 3.3.4, 3.3.5, 4.1.1, 4.2.4, 4.4, 4.4.2, 4.4.4, 4.5.2]

Coburn, B.J., Wagner, B.G., Blower, S. (2009). 'Modeling influenza epidemics and pandemics: insights into the future of swine flu (H1N1).' *BMC Medicine*. **7**. Article 30. doi:10.1186/1741-7015-7-30. [5.2.4]

Cockburn, W.C., Delon, P.J., Ferreira, W. (1969). 'Origin and progress of the 1968–69 Hong Kong influenza epidemic.' *Bulletin of the World Health Organization*, **41**, 345–8. [4.4.4]

Colizza, V., Barrat, A., Barthélemy, M., Valleron, A.J., Vespignani, A. (2007). 'Modeling the worldwide spread of pandemic influenza: baseline case and containment interventions.' *PLoS Medicine*, **4**, e13. doi:10.1371/journal.pmed.0040013. [3.3.3]

Colizza, V., Barrat, A., Barthélemy, M., Vespignani, A. (2006a). 'The role of the airline transportation network in the prediction and predictability of global epidemics.' *Proceedings of the National Academy of Sciences USA*, **103**, 2015–20. [3.3.3]

Colizza, V., Barrat, A., Barthélemy, M., Vespignani, A. (2006b). 'The modeling of global epidemics: stochastic dynamics and predictability.' *Bulletin of Mathematical Biology*, **68**, 1893–921. [3.3.3]

Comas-Herrera, A., Zalakaín, J., Litwin, C., Hsu, A.T., Lemmon, E., Henderson, D., Fernández, J.-L. (2020). *Mortality Associated with COVID-19 Outbreaks in Care Homes: Early International Evidence*. London: International Long Term Care Policy Network. https://ltccovid.org/international-reports-on-covid-19-and-long-term-care/, accessed 27 March 2021. [5.4.1]

Cooper, B.S., Pitman, R.J., Edmunds, W.J., Gay, N.J. (2006). 'Delaying the international spread of pandemic influenza.' *PLoS Medicine*, **3**, e212. doi:10.1371/journal.pmed.0030212. [3.3.3]

Creighton, C. (1891–94). *A History of Epidemics in Britain. From A.D. 664 to the Great Plague (Vol. I). From the Extinction of the Plague to the Present Time (Vol. II)*. Cambridge: Cambridge University Press. [3.2.1, 4.1, 4.1.1]

Crosby, A.W. (1993). 'Influenza.' In: K.F. Kiple (ed.), *The Cambridge World History of Human Disease*. Cambridge: Cambridge University Press, 807–11. [4.4.2]

Davies, R.E.G. (1964). *A History of the World's Airlines*. London: Oxford University Press. [3.3.3]

de Jong, M.D., Hien, T.T. (2006). 'Avian influenza A (H5N1).' *Journal of Clinical Virology*, **35**, 2–13. [3.3.3, 4.4.1]

de Jong, M.D., Simmons, C.P., Thanh, T.T., Hien, V.M., Smith, G.J.D., Chau, T.N.B., Hoang, D.M., Chau, N.V.V., Khanh, T.H., Dong, V.C., Qui, P.T., Cam, B.V., Ha, D.Q., Guan, Y., Peiris, J.S.M., Chinh, N.T., Hien, T.T., Farrar, J. (2006). 'Fatal outcome of human influenza A (H5N1) is associated with high viral load and hypercytokinemia.' *Nature Medicine*, **12**, 1203–7. [3.4.1]

Dean, K.R., Krauer, F., Walløe, L., Lingjærde, O.C., Bramanti, B., Stenseth, N.C., Schmid, B.V. (2018). 'Human ectoparasites and the spread of plague in Europe during the Second Pandemic.' *Proceedings of the National Academy of Sciences USA*, **115**, 1304–9. doi: 10.1073/pnas.1715640115. [4.2]

Dee, K., Goldfarb, D.M., Haney, J., Amat, J.A.R., Herder, V., Stewart, M., Szemiel, A.M., Baguelin, M., Murcia, P.R. (2021). 'Human rhinovirus infection blocks SARS-CoV-2 replication within the respiratory epithelium: implications for COVID-19 epidemiology.' *Journal of Infectious Diseases*, **224**, 31–8. [2.5.5]

Declich, S., Carter, A.O. (1994). 'Public health surveillance: historical origins, methods and evaluation.' *Bulletin of the World Health Organization*, **72**, 285–304. [6.6.3]

Dewing, H.B. (1914). *Procopius: History of the Wars, Books I and II*. London: William Heinemann. [4.2.2]

Dietz, K. (1988). 'The first epidemic model: a historical note on P.D. En'ko.' *Australian Journal of Statistics*, **30A**, 56–65. [1.1, 1.3.2]

Dietz, K. (1993). 'The estimation of the basic reproduction number for infectious diseases.' *Statistical Methods in Medical Research*, **2**, 23–41. [5.2.4]

Doherty, M., Buchy, P., Standaert, B., Giaquinto, C., Prado-Cohrs, D. (2016). 'Vaccine impact: benefits for human health.' *Vaccine*, **34**, 6707–14. [6.4.1]

Donaldson, L.J., Rutter, P.D., Ellis, B.M., Greaves, F.E., Mytton, O.T., Pebody, R.G., Yardley, I.E. (2009). 'Mortality from pandemic A/H1N1 2009 influenza in England: public health surveillance study.' *British Medical Journal*, **339**, b5213. doi: 10.1136/bmj.b5213. [4.1.1]

Dong, E., Du, H., Gardner, L. (2020). 'An interactive web-based dashboard to track COVID-19 in real time.' *Lancet Infectious Diseases*, **20**, 533–4. doi: 10.1016/S1473-3099(20)30120-1. [5.3.2]

Dorling, D. (1995). *A New Social Atlas of Britain*. Chichester: Wiley. [1.5.2]

Doshi, P. (2011). 'The elusive definition of pandemic influenza.' *Bulletin of the World Health Organization*, **89**, 532–8. [4.4.4, 4.4.5]

Dowdle, W.R. (1998). 'The principles of disease elimination and eradication.' *Bulletin of the World Health Organization*, **76** (suppl. 2), 22–5. [6.5.1]

Downs, W.G. (1993). 'Arenaviruses.' In: K.F. Kiple (ed.), *The Cambridge World History of Human Disease*. Cambridge: Cambridge University Press, 595–9. [3.3.4]

Drancourt, M., Aboudharam, G., Signoli, M., Dutour, O., Raoult, D. (1998). 'Detection of 400-year old *Yersinia pestis* DNA in human dental pulp. An approach to the diagnosis of ancient septicaemia.' *Proceedings of the National Academy of Sciences USA*, **95**, 12637–40. [3.2.1]

Du, Z., Xu, X., Wu, Y., Wang, L., Cowling, B.J., Meyers, L.A. (2020). 'Serial interval of COVID-19 among publicly reported confirmed cases.' *Emerging Infectious Diseases*, **26**, 1341–3. [5.2.2]

Du Plessis, L., McCrone, J.T., Zarebski, A.E., Zarebski, A.E., Hill, V., Ruis, C., Gutierrez, B., Raghwani, J., Ashworth, J., Colquhoun, R., Connor, T.R., Faria, N.R., Jackson, B., Loman, N.J., O'Toole, Á., Nicholls, S.M., Parag, K.V., Scher, E., Vasylyeva, T.I., Volz, E.M., Watts, A., Bogoch, I.I., Khan, K., COVID-19 Genomics UK (COG-UK) Consortium, Aanensen, D.M., Kraemer, M.U.G., Rambaut, A. (2021). 'Establishment and lineage dynamics of the SARS-CoV-2 epidemic in the UK.' *Science*, **371**, 708–12. [5.4]

Eastern Bureau of the League of Nations Health Organisation (1926). *Half-Yearly Bulletin of the Eastern Bureau, January–June 1926*. Singapore: League of Nations Health Organisation Eastern Bureau. [6.6.3]

Eichel, O.R. (1922). 'The long-term cycles of pandemic influenza.' *Journal of the American Statistical Association*, **18**, 446–54. [4.1.1, 4.4]

Eichner, M., Hadeler, K., Dietz, K. (1994). 'Stochastic models for the eradication of poliomyelitis: minimum population size for polio virus persistence.' In: V. Isham and G. Medley (eds.), *Models for Infectious Human Diseases: Their Structure and Relation to Data*. Cambridge: Cambridge University Press, 315–27. [3.2.2]

Emmerson, C., Adamson, J.P., Turner, D., Gravenor, M.B., Salmon, J., Cottrell, S., Middleton, V., Thomas, B., Mason, B.W., Williams, C.J. (2021). 'Risk factors for outbreaks of COVID-19 in care homes following hospital discharge: a national cohort analysis.' *Influenza and Other Respiratory Viruses*, **15**, 371–80. [6.3.3]

Engelthaler, D.M., Mosley, D.G., Cheek, J.E., Levy, C.E., Komatsu, K.K., Ettestad, P., Davis, T., Tanda, D.T., Miller, L., Frampton, J.W., Porter, R., Bryan, R.T. (1999). 'Climatic and environmental patterns associated with hantavirus pulmonary syndrome, Four Corners region, United States.' *Emerging Infectious Diseases*, **5**, 87–94. [3.3.5]

Enria, D.A., Briggiler, A.M., Sánchez, Z. (2008). 'Treatment of Argentine hemorrhagic fever.' *Antiviral Research*, **78**, 132–9. [3.3.4]

Epstein, J.M., Goedecke, D.M., Yu, F., Morris, R.J., Wagener, D.K., Bobashev, G.V. (2007). 'Controlling pandemic flu: the value of international travel restrictions.' *PLoS One*, **2**, e401. doi:10.1371/journal.pone.0000401. [3.3.3]

Epstein, P.R. (1995). 'Emerging diseases and ecosystem instability: new threats to public health.' *American Journal of Public Health*, **85**, 168–72. [3.3.5]

European Centre for Disease Prevention and Control (2010). *Annual Threat Report 2009*. Stockholm: ECDC. [6.6.6]

European Centre for Disease Prevention and Control (2017). *Annual Threat Report 2016*. Stockholm: ECDC. [6.6.6]

European Centre for Disease Prevention and Control (2020). *Coronavirus Disease 2019 (COVID-19) in the EU/EEA and the UK – Eleventh Update, 10 August 2020*. Stockholm: ECDC. https://www.ecdc.europa.eu/en/publications-data/rapid-risk-assessment-coronavirus-disease-2019-covid-19-eueea-and-uk-eleventh, accessed 27 March 2021. [5.2.6]

Evans, A.S. (ed.) (1984). *Viral Infections of Humans: Epidemiology and Control* (second edition). New York: Plenum. [1.2.3]

Eyler, J.M. (1987). 'Scarlet fever and confinement: the Edwardian debate over isolation hospitals.' *Bulletin of the History of Medicine*, **61**, 1–24. [6.3.3]

Farr, W. (1840). 'Causes of death in England and Wales.' In: *Second Annual Report of the Registrar General of Births, Deaths and Marriages in England*. London: HMSO, 69–98. [1.4.2]

Feldmann, H. (2014). 'Ebola – a growing threat?' *New England Journal of Medicine*, **371**, 1375–8. [3.4.3]

Fenner, F., Henderson, D.A., Arita, I., Ježek, Z., Ladnyi, I.D. (1988). *Smallpox and Its Eradication*. Geneva: WHO. [6.5.3]

Ferguson, N.M., Cummings, D.A., Fraser, C., Cajka, J.C., Cooley, P.C., Burke, D.S. (2006). 'Strategies for mitigating an influenza pandemic.' *Nature*, **442**, 448–52. [5.2.4]

Finke, L.L. (1792–95). *Versuch einer allgemeinen medicinisch-praktischen Geographie, worin der historische Theil der einheimischen Völker- und Staaten-Arzeneykunde vorgetragen wird* (three volumes). Leipzig: Weidmann. [1.5.1]

Fletcher, R.A. (1910). *Steamships: The Story of Their Development to the Present Day*. London: Sidwick and Jackson. [3.3.3]

Floret, D. (1997). 'Co-infections virus-bactéries.' *Archives de Pédiatrie*, **4**, 1119–24. [2.5.5]

Fornaciari, G., Zavaglia, K., Giusti, L., Vultaggio, C., Ciranni, R. (2003). 'Human papillomavirus in a 16th century mummy.' *Lancet*, **362**, 1160. [3.2.1]

Fraser, C., Donnelly, C.A., Cauchemez, S., Hanage, W.P., Van Kerkhove, M.D., Hollingsworth, T.D., Griffin, J., Baggaley, R.F., Jenkins, H.E., Lyons, E.J., Jombart, T., Hinsley, W.R., Grassly, N.C., Balloux, F., Ghani, A.C., Ferguson, N.M., Rambaut, A., Pybus, O.G., Lopez-Gatell, H., Alpuche-Aranda, C.M., Chapela, I.B., Zavala, E.P., Guevara, D.M., Checchi, F., Garcia, E., Hugonnet, S., Roth, C. (2009). 'WHO Rapid Pandemic Assessment Collaboration. Pandemic potential of a strain of influenza A (H1N1): early findings.' *Science*, **324**, 1557–61. [5.2.4]

Freifeld, C.C., Mandl, K.D., Reis, B.Y., Brownstein, J.S. (2008). 'HealthMap: global infectious disease monitoring through automated classification and visualization of Internet media reports.' *Journal of the American Medical Association*, **15**, 150–7. [6.6.6]

Fricker, E.J., Spigelman, M., Fricker, C.R. (1997). 'The detection of *Escherichia coli* DNA in the ancient remains of Lindow Man using polymerase chain reaction.' *Letters in Applied Microbiology*, **24**, 351–4. [3.2.1]

Gallo, R.C. (1987). 'The AIDS virus.' *Scientific American*, **256**, 39–48. [4.5.2]

Gani, R., Leach, S. (2001). 'Transmission potential of smallpox in contemporary populations.' *Nature*, **414**, 748–51. [5.2.4]

Garg, S., Kim, L., Whitaker, M., O'Halloran, A., Cummings, C., Holstein, R., Prill, M., Chai, S.J., Kirley, P.D., Alden, N.B., Kawasaki, B., Yousey-Hindes, K., Niccolai, L., Anderson, E.J., Openo, K.P., Weigel, A., Monroe, M.L., Ryan, P., Henderson, J., Kim, S., Como-Sabetti, K., Lynfield, R., Sosin, D., Torres, S., Muse, A., Bennett, N.M., Billing, L., Sutton, M., West, N., Schaffner, W., Talbot, H.K., Aquino, C., George, A., Budd, A., Brammer, L., Langley, G., Hall,

A.J., Fry, A. (2020). 'Hospitalization rates and characteristics of patients hospitalized with laboratory-confirmed coronavirus disease 2019 – COVID-NET, 14 states, March 1–30, 2020.' *Morbidity and Mortality Weekly Report*, **69**, 458–64. [5.2.5]

Giesen, C., Roche, J., Redondo-Bravo, L., Ruiz-Huerta, C., Gomez-Barroso, D., Benito, A., Herrador, Z. (2020). 'The impact of climate change on mosquito-borne diseases in Africa.' *Pathogens and Global Health*, **114**, 287–301. [3.3.5]

Gilbert, M.T., Rambaut, A., Wlasiuk, G., Spira, T.J., Pitchenik, A.E., Worobey, M. (2007). 'The emergence of HIV/AIDS in the Americas and beyond.' *Proceedings of the National Academy of Sciences USA*, **104**, 18566–70. [4.5.2]

Gilg, A.W. (1973). 'A study in agricultural disease diffusion: the case of the 1970–71 fowl-pest epidemic.' *Transactions of the Institute of British Geographers*, **59**, 77–97. [1.4.2]

Gilsdorf, A., Boxall, N., Gasimov, V., Agayev, I., Mammadzade, F., Ursu, P., Gasimov, E., Brown, C., Mardel, S., Jankovic, D., Pimentel, G., Ayoub, I.A., Elassal, E.M., Salvi, C., Legros, D., Pessoa da Silva, C., Hay, A., Andraghetti, R., Rodier, G., Ganter, B. (2006). 'Two clusters of human infection with influenza A/H5N1 virus in the Republic of Azerbaijan, February–March 2006.' *Eurosurveillance*, **11**, 122–6. [3.4.1]

Githeko, A.K., Woodward, A. (2003). 'International consensus on the science of climate and health: the IPCC Third Assessment Report.' In: A.J. McMichael, D.H. Campbell-Lendrum, C.F. Corvalan, K.L. Ebi, A. Githeko, J.D. Scheraga, and A. Woodward (eds.), *Climate Change and Human Health: Risks and Responses*. Geneva: WHO, 43–60. [3.3.5]

Glezen W.P., Couch, R.B. (1997). 'Influenza viruses.' In: A.S. Evans and R.A. Kaslow (eds.), *Viral Infections of Humans: Epidemiology and Control* (fourth edition). New York: Plenum Medical Book Company, 473–505. [4.4.1]

Goodman, N.M. (1952). *International Health Organizations and Their Work*. London: J. & A. Churchill, Ltd. [6.6.3]

Graham, R.L., Hell, P. (1985). 'On the history of the minimum spanning tree problem.' *IEEE Annals of the History of Computing*, **7**, 43–57. [2.2.2]

Grais, R.F., Ellis, J.H., Glass, G.E. (2003). 'Assessing the impact of airline travel on the geographic spread of pandemic influenza.' *European Journal of Epidemiology*, **18**, 1065–72. [3.3.3]

Greenhalgh, D. (1986). 'Optimal control of an epidemic by ring vaccination.' *Stochastic Models*, **2**, 339–63. [6.4.2]

Greenwood, M. (1935). *Epidemics and Crowd Diseases*. London: Norgate & Williams. [1.1]

Guerra, F.M., Bolotin, S., Lim, G., Heffernan, J., Deeks, S.L., Li, Y., Crowcroft, N.S. (2017). 'The basic reproduction number (R_0) of measles: a systematic review.' *Lancet Infectious Diseases*, **17**, e420–e428. [5.2.4]

Guhl, F., Jaramillo, C., Vallejo, G.A., Yockteng, R., Cardenas-Arroyo, F., Fornaciari, G., Arriaza, B., Aufderheide, A.R. (1999). 'Isolation of *Trypanosoma cruzi* DNA in 4,000-year-old mummified human tissue from Northern Chile.' *American Journal of Physical Anthropology*, **108**, 401–7. [3.2.1]

Gust, I.D., Hampson, A.W., Lavanchy, D. (2001). 'Planning for the next pandemic of influenza.' *Reviews in Medical Virology*, **11**, 59–70. [4.4]

Haas, C.J., Zink, A., Pálfi, G.Y., Szeimies, U., Nerlich, A.G. (2000). 'Detection of leprosy in ancient human skeletal remains by molecular identification of *Mycobacterium leprae*.' *American Journal of Clinical Pathology*, **114**, 428–36. [3.2.1]

Hägerstrand, T. (1953). *Innovationsförloppet ur Korologisk Synpunkt*. Lund: Gleerup. [1.4.2, 1.6.3]

Hägerstrand, T. (1967a). *Innovation Diffusion as a Spatial Process*. Chicago, IL: University of Chicago Press. [1.4.2]

Hägerstrand, T. (1967b). 'On Monte Carlo simulation of diffusion.' In: W.L. Garrison and D.F. Marble (eds.), *Quantitative Geography (Volume 1)*. Evanston, IL: Northwestern University Studies in Geography, **13**, 1–33. [1.6.3]

Haggett, P. (1976). 'Hybridizing alternative models of an epidemic diffusion process.' *Economic Geography*, **52**, 136–46. [1.6.4]

Haggett, P. (1979). *Geography: A Modern Synthesis* (third edition). New York: Harper and Row. [3.2.2]

Haggett, P. (1990). *The Geographer's Art*. Oxford: Blackwell. [1.6.3]

Haggett, P. (2000). *The Geographical Structure of Epidemics*. Oxford: Clarendon Press [Preface, 1.2.1, 1.4.2, 1.4.3, 3.3.3, 6.4.2]

Haggett, P. (2012). *The Quantocks*. Chew Magna, Somerset: The Point Walter Press. [1.3.5]

Haggett, P., Chorley, R.J. (1969). *Network Analysis in Geography*. London: Edward Arnold. [1.4.4, 1.5.2]

Haggett, P., Cliff, A.D., Frey, A. (1977). *Locational Analysis in Human Geography* (second edition). London: Edward Arnold. [1.2.2]

Hall, A.J. (1918). 'Note on an epidemic of toxic ophthalmoplegia associated with acute asthenia and other nervous manifestations.' *Lancet*, **1**, 568–9. [4.4.3]

Hall, C.E., Cooney, M.K., Fox, J.P. (1970). 'The Seattle virus watch program. I. Infection and illness experience of virus watch families during a community wide epidemic of echovirus type 30 aseptic meningitis.' *American Journal of Public Health and the Nation's Health*, **60**, 1456–65. [6.6.6]

Halloran, M.E. (1998). 'Concepts of infectious disease epidemiology.' In: K.J. Rothman and S. Greenland (eds.), *Modern Epidemiology*. Philadelphia, PA: Lippincott-Raven, 529–54. [1.3.1]

Hannesson, G. (1922). *Heilbrigðisskýrslur, 1911–1920*. Reykjavík: Fjelagsprentsmiðjan. [2.5.3]

Harb, M., Faris, R., Gad, A.M., Hafez, O.N., Ramzy, R., Buck, A.A. (1993). 'The resurgence of lymphatic filariasis in the Nile delta.' *Bulletin of the World Health Organization*, **71**, 49–54. [3.3.4]

Harris, W. (1918). 'Acute infective ophthalmoplegia or botulism.' *Lancet*, **1**, 568. [4.4.3]

Harvey, A., Kattuman, P. (2020). 'Time series models based on growth curves with applications to forecasting coronavirus.' *Harvard Data Science Review*, **Special Issue 1**. https://hdsr.mitpress.mit.edu/pub/ozgjx0yn, accessed 27 March 2021. [5.6]

Harvey, G. (1666). *Morbus Anglicus: Or, The Anatomy of Consumptions*. London: Nathaniel Brook. [4.1]

Hatcher, J. (1994). 'England in the aftermath of the Black Death.' *Past and Present*, **144**, 3–35. [4.1.1]

Hatcher, J. (2008). *The Black Death: An Intimate History*. London: Weidenfeld and Nicholson. [6.3.3]

Health Protection Agency (2006). *Communicable Disease in London 2002–05. A Review by the Health Protection Agency in London*. London: Health Protection Agency. [6.4.1]

Health Protection Agency (2008). 'Confirmed measles cases in England and Wales: an update to end-May 2008.' *Health Protection Report*, **2**, 2–3. [6.4.1]

Health Protection Agency (2009). *Pandemic Influenza Contingency Plan*. London: Health Protection Agency. [4.4.4]

Hermann, W. (1973). *Die El-Tor-Cholera-Pandemie 1961 bis 1968*. Leipzig: Johann Ambrosius Barth. [4.3.3]

Herring, D.A., Sattenspiel, L. (2007). 'Social contexts, syndemics and infectious disease in northern aboriginal populations.' *American Journal of Human Biology*, **19**, 190–202. [2.5.5]

Heymann, D.L. (ed.) (2015). *Control of Communicable Diseases Manual* (twentieth edition). Washington, DC: American Public

Health Association. [1.2.2, 1.3.1, 3.3.4, 3.3.5, 3.4.1, 3.4.3, 4.2, 4.3, 4.5.1, 5.2.3]

Heymann, D.L., Rodier, G.R., WHO Operational Support Team of the Global Outbreak Alert and Response Network (2001). 'Hot spots in a wired world: WHO surveillance of emerging and re-emerging infectious diseases.' *Lancet Infectious Diseases*, **1**, 345–53. [6.6.5]

Hirsch, A. (1883–86). *Handbook of Geographical and Historical Pathology. Vol. I. – Acute Infective Diseases. Vol. II. – Chronic Infective, Toxic, Parasitic, Septic and Constitutional Diseases. Vol. III. – Diseases of Organs and Parts*. Translated from the second German edition by C. Creighton. London: The New Sydenham Society. [1.5.1, 4.1, 4.1.1, 4.2.1, 4.3.1, 4.4, 4.4.2]

History.com (2021). *Pandemics That Changed History*. New York City: History. https://www.history.com/topics/middle-ages/pandemics-timeline, accessed 27 March 2021. [4.1.1]

Hollingsworth, T.D., Ferguson, N.M., Anderson, R.M. (2006). 'Will travel restrictions control the international spread of pandemic influenza?' *Nature Medicine*, **12**, 497–9. [3.3.3]

Hong Choi, Y., Gay, N., Fraser, G., Ramsay, M. (2008). 'The potential for measles transmission in England.' *BMC Public Health*, **8**, 338. doi: 10.1186/1471-2458-8-338. [6.4.1]

Honigsbaum, M. (2020). 'The art of medicine: revisiting the 1957 and 1968 influenza pandemics.' *Lancet*, **395**, 1824–6. [4.1.1]

Hope-Simpson, R.E. (1948). 'The period of transmission in certain epidemic diseases.' *Lancet*, **2**, 755–60. [2.3]

Hope-Simpson, R.E. (1952). 'Infectiousness of communicable diseases in the household.' *Lancet*, **2**, 549–54. [2.3]

Hope-Simpson, R.E. (1958). 'Discussion on the common cold.' *Proceedings of the Royal Society of Medicine*, **51**, 267–71. [2.3]

Hope-Simpson, R.E. (1970). 'First outbreak of Hong Kong influenza in a general practice population in Great Britain. A field and laboratory study.' *British Medical Journal*, **3**, 74–7. [2.3]

Hope-Simpson, R.E. (1978). 'Sunspots and flu: a correlation.' *Nature*, **275**, 86. [2.3]

Hope-Simpson, R.E. (1979). 'Epidemic mechanisms of type A influenza.' *Journal of Hygiene (London)*, **83**, 11–26. [2.3, 2.3.4]

Hope-Simpson, R.E., Sutherland, I. (1954). 'Does influenza spread within the household?' *Lancet*, **1**, 721–6. [2.3]

Howard, J. (1791). *An Account of the Principal Lazarettos in Europe; with Various Papers Relative to the Plague: Together with Further Observations on some Foreign Prisons and Hospitals; and Additional Remarks on the Present State of Those in Great Britain and Ireland*. London: J. Johnson. [6.3.2]

Hsu, D.C., O'Connell, R.J. (2017). 'Progress in HIV vaccine development.' *Human Vaccines and Immunotherapeutics*, **13**, 1018–30. [4.5.3]

Hufnagel, L., Brockmann, D., Geisel, T. (2004). 'Forecast and control of epidemics in a globalized world.' *Proceedings of the National Academy of Sciences USA*, **101**, 15124–9. [3.3.3]

Hughes, J.M., Peters, C.J., Cohen, M.L., Mahy, B.W. (1993). 'Hantavirus pulmonary syndrome: an emerging infectious disease.' *Science*, **262**, 850–1. [3.3.5]

Hui, E.K.-W. (2006). 'Reasons for the increase in emerging and re-emerging viral infectious diseases.' *Microbes and Infection*, **8**, 905–16. [3.3.4]

Hull, H.F., Birmingham, M.E., Melgaard, B., Lee, J.W. (1997). 'Progress toward global polio eradication.' *Journal of Infectious Diseases*, **175** (suppl. 1), S4–9. [6.5.3]

Hunter, J.M., Young, J.C. (1971). 'Diffusion of influenza in England and Wales.' *Annals of the Association of American Geographers*, **61**, 637–53. [4.4.4]

Intergovernmental Panel on Climate Change (2007). *Climate Change 2007: Fourth Assessment Report. Working Group I Report, The Physical Science Basis*. Cambridge: Cambridge University Press. [3.3.5]

Intergovernmental Panel on Climate Change (2014). *Climate Change 2014: Synthesis Report. Contribution of Working Groups I, II and III to the Fifth Assessment Report of the Intergovernmental Panel on Climate Change*. Geneva: Intergovernmental Panel on Climate Change. [3.3.5]

International Commission (1978). 'Ebola haemorrhagic fever in Zaire, 1976.' *Bulletin of the World Health Organization*, **56**, 271–93. [3.4.3]

Isard, W. (1960). *Methods of Regional Analysis: An Introduction to Regional Science*. Cambridge, MA: The MIT Press. [1.2.2]

Jahrling, P.B. (1997). 'Arenaviruses.' In: A.S. Evans and R.A. Kaslow (eds.), *Viral Infections of Humans: Epidemiology and Control* (fourth edition). London: Plenum Medical Book Company, 185–209. [3.3.4]

Jannetta, A.B. (1987). *Epidemics and Mortality in Early Modern Japan*. Princeton, NJ: Princeton University Press. [3.2.1]

Jenner, E. (1798). *An Inquiry into the Causes and Effects of the Variolæ Vaccinæ, a Disease Discovered in some of the Western Counties of England, particularly Gloucestershire, and known by the Name of the Cow Pox*. London: Sampson Low. [2.1]

Johnson, N.F., Velásquez, N., Restrepo, N.J., Leahy, R., Gabriel, N., El Oud, S., Zheng, M., Manrique, P., Wuchty, S., Lapu, Y. (2020). 'The online competition between pro- and anti-vaccination views.' *Nature*, **582**, 230–3. [6.4.1]

Johnson, N.P.A.S., Mueller, J. (2002). 'Updating the accounts: global mortality of the 1918–1920 'Spanish' influenza pandemic.' *Bulletin of the History of Medicine*, **76**, 105–15. [4.1.1, 4.4]

Jónsson, V. (1940). 'Health in Iceland. A survey of public health organization and health conditions in Iceland.' *Heilbrigðisskýrslur*, **1938**, 161–87. [2.5.2]

Jordan, E.O. (1927). *Epidemic Influenza: A Survey*. Chicago, IL: American Medical Association. [4.4]

Jung, S.M., Akhmetzhanov, A.R., Hayashi, K., Linton, N.M., Yang, Y., Yuan, B., Kobayashi, T., Kinoshita, R., Nishiura, H. (2020). 'Real-time estimation of the risk of death from novel coronavirus (COVID-19) infection: inference using exported cases.' *Journal of Clinical Medicine*, **9**, 523. doi: 10.3390/jcm9020523. [5.2.3]

Kaper, J.B., Morris, J.G. Jr., Levine, M.M. (1995). 'Cholera.' *Clinical Microbiology Reviews*, **8**, 48–86. [4.3.3]

Kelly, H. (2011). 'The classical definition of a pandemic is not elusive.' *Bulletin of the World Health Organization*, **89**, 540–1. [4.1]

Kendall, D.G. (1957). 'La propagation d'une épidémie au d'un bruit dans une population limité.' *Publications de l'Institut de Statistique de l'Université de Paris*, **6**, 307–11. [1.4.2]

Khan, A., Naveed, M., Dur-E-Ahmad, M., Imran, M. (2015). 'Estimating the basic reproductive ratio for the Ebola outbreak in Liberia and Sierra Leone.' *Infectious Diseases of Poverty*, **4**, 13. doi: 10.1186/s40249-015-0043-3. [5.2.4]

Khan, I.A. (2004). 'Plague: the dreadful visitation occupying the human mind for centuries.' *Transactions of the Royal Society of Tropical Medicine and Hygiene*, **98**, 270–7. [4.2.4]

Khunti, K., Singh, A.K., Pareek, M., Hanif, W. (2020). 'Is ethnicity linked to incidence or outcomes of covid-19?' *British Medical Journal*, **369**, m1548. doi: 10.1136/bmj.m1548. [5.2.5]

Kilbourne, E.D. (1973). 'The molecular epidemiology of influenza.' *Journal of Infectious Diseases*, **127**, 478–87. [2.2.3]

Killerby, M.E., Link-Gelles, R., Haight, S.C., Schrodt, C.A., England, L., Gomes, D.J., Shamout, M., Pettrone, K., O'Laughlin, K., Kimball, A., Blau, E.F., Burnett, E., Ladva, C.N., Szablewski, C.M., Tobin-D'Angelo, M., Oosmanally, N., Drenzek, C., Murphy, D.J., Blum, J.M., Hollberg, J., Lefkove, B., Brown, F.W., Shimabukuro, T., Midgley, C.M., Tate, J.E., CDC COVID-19 Response Clinical Team (2020).

'Characteristics associated with hospitalization among patients with COVID-19 – Metropolitan Atlanta, Georgia, March-April 2020.' *Morbidity and Mortality Weekly Report*, **69**, 790–4. [5.2.5]

Kiple, K.F. (ed.) (1993). *The Cambridge World History of Human Disease*. Cambridge: Cambridge University Press. [Preface]

Koch, T. (2005). *Cartographies of Disease: Maps, Mapping, and Medicine*. Redlands, CA: ESRI Press. [1.5.1]

Kohn, G.C. (1998). *Encyclopedia of Plague and Pestilence*. Ware, Hertfordshire: Wordsworth. [3.2.1, 4.1.1, 4.2.2]

Kolman, C.J., Centurion-Lara, A., Lukehart, S.A., Owsley, D.W., Tuross, N. (1999). 'Identification of *Treponema pallidum* subspecies *pallidum* in a 200-year-old skeletal specimen.' *Journal of Infectious Diseases*, **180**, 2060–3. [3.2.1]

Kovats, R.S. (2000). 'El Niño and human health.' *Bulletin of the World Health Organization*, **78**, 1127–35. [3.3.5]

Kovats, R.S., Bouma, M.J., Hajat, S., Worrall, E., Haines, A. (2003). 'El Niño and health.' *Lancet*, **362**, 1481–9. [3.3.5]

Kretzschmar, M., Teunis, P.F., Pebody, R.G. (2010). 'Incidence and re-production numbers of pertussis: estimates from serological and social contact data in five European countries.' *PLOS Medicine*, **7**, e1000291. doi:10.1371/journal.pmed.1000291. [5.2.4]

Kretzschmar, M., van den Hof, S., Wallinga, J., van Wijngaarden, J. (2004). 'Ring vaccination and smallpox control.' *Emerging Infectious Diseases*, **10**, 832–41. [6.4.2]

Kucharski, A. (2020). *The Rules of Contagion: Why Things Spread – And Why They Stop*. London: Profile Books. [1.2.2]

Kucharski, A., Althaus, C.L. (2015). 'The role of superspreading in Middle East respiratory syndrome coronavirus (MERS-CoV) transmission.' *Eurosurveillance*, **20**, 14–18. doi:10.2807/1560-7917.ES2015.20.25.21167. [5.2.4]

Landers, J. (1993). *Death and the Metropolis: Studies in the Demographic History of London 1670–1830*. Cambridge: Cambridge University Press. [3.2.1]

Langmuir, A.D. (1963). 'The surveillance of communicable diseases of national importance.' *New England Journal of Medicine*, **268**, 183–92. [6.6.1]

Langmuir, A.D. (1976). 'William Farr: founder of modern concepts of surveillance.' *International Journal of Epidemiology*, **5**, 13–18. [6.6.1]

Lau, C.Y., Wahl, B., Foo, W.K. (2005). 'Ring vaccination versus mass vaccination in event of a smallpox attack.' *Hawaii Medical Journal*, **64**, 34–6, 53. [6.4.2]

Lauer, S.A., Grantz, K.H., Bi, Q., Jones, F.K., Zheng, Q., Meredith, H.R., Azman, A.S., Reich, N.G., Lessler, J. (2020). 'The incubation period of coronavirus disease 2019 (COVID-19) from publicly reported confirmed cases: estimation and application.' *Annals of Internal Medicine*, **172**, 577–82. [5.2.1]

League of Nations Health Section (1922). 'Introductory note.' *Epidemiological Intelligence: Eastern Europe in 1921*, **E.I.1**, 3. [6.6.3]

Learmonth, A.T.A. (1954). 'A method of plotting on the same map health data on both intensity and variability of incidence, illustrated by three maps of cholera in Indo-Pakistan.' *Annals of Tropical Medicine and Parasitology*, **48**, 345–7. [1.5.2]

Lemon, S.M., Hamburg, M.A., Sparling, P.F., Choffnes, E.R., Mack, A. (2007). *Global Infectious Disease Surveillance and Detection: Assessing the Challenges – Finding Solutions, Workshop Summary*. Washington, DC: The National Academies Press. [6.6.5]

Levison, M., Ward, R.F., Webb, J.W. (1973). *The Settlement of Polynesia: A Computer Simulation*. Minneapolis, MN: University of Minnesota Press. [1.6.3]

Li, H.-C., Fujiyoshi, T., Lou, H., Yashiki, S., Sonoda, S., Cartier, L., Nunez, I., Munoz, I., Horai, S., Tajima, K. (1999). 'The presence of ancient human T-cell lymphotropic virus type I provirus DNA in an Andean mummy.' *Nature Medicine*, **5**, 1428–32. [3.2.1]

Li, W.H., Tanimura, M., Sharp, P.M. (1988). 'Rates and dates of divergence between AIDS virus nucleotide sequences.' *Molecular Biology and Evolution*, **5**, 313–30. [4.5.2]

Lipsitch, M., Cohen, T., Cooper, B., Robins, J.M., Ma, S., James, L., Gopalakrishna, G., Chew, S.K., Tan, C.C., Samore, M.H., Fisman, D., Murray, M. (2003). 'Transmission dynamics and control of severe acute respiratory syndrome.' *Science*, **300**, 1966–70. [5.2.4]

Liu, J., Xiao, H., Lei, F., Zhu, Q., Qin, K., Zhang, X.-W., Zhang, X.-L., Zhao, D., Wang, G., Feng, Y., Ma, J., Liu, W., Wang, J., Gao, G.F. (2005). 'Highly pathogenic H5N1 influenza virus in migratory birds.' *Science*, **309**, 1206. [3.4.1]

Liu, Y., Gayle, A.A., Wilder-Smith, A., Rocklöv, J. (2020). 'The reproductive number of COVID-19 is higher compared to SARS coronavirus.' *Journal of Travel Medicine*, **27**, taaa021. doi: 10.1093/jtm/taaa021. [5.2.4]

Liu, Y.-C., Kuo, R.-L., Shih, S.-R. (2020). 'COVID-19: the first documented coronavirus pandemic in history.' *Biomedical Journal*, **43**, 328–33. [4.1.1]

Lösch, A. (1954). *The Economics of Location*. Yale, CT: Yale University Press. [1.1]

Lothian, N.V. (1924). 'The Service of Epidemiological Intelligence and Public Health Statistics.' *American Journal of Public Health*, **14**, 287–90. [6.6.3]

Lucas, A.O. (1968). 'The surveillance of communicable diseases.' *WHO Chronicle*, **22**, 439–44. [6.6.1]

MacNamara, C. (1876). *A History of Asiatic Cholera*. London: MacMillan and Co. [4.3.2]

Macpherson, W.G., Herringham, W.P., Elliott, T.R., Balfour, A. (eds.) (1922–23). *History of the Great War Based on Official Documents: Medical Services, Diseases of the War* (two volumes). London: HMSO. [4.4.3]

Maganga, G.D., Kapetshi, J., Berthet, N., Ilunga, B.K., Kabange, F., Kingebeni, P.M., Mondonge, V., Muyembe, J.-J.T., Bertherat, E., Briand, S., Cabore, J., Epelboin, A., Formenty, P., Kobinger, G., González-Angulo, L., Labouba, I., Manuguerra, J.-C., Okwo-Bele, J.-M., Dye, C., Leroy, E.M. (2014). 'Ebola virus disease in the Democratic Republic of Congo.' *New England Journal of Medicine*, **371**, 2083–91. [3.4.3]

Magid, A., Gesser-Edelsburg, A., Green, M.S. (2018). 'The role of informal digital surveillance systems before, during and after infectious disease outbreaks: a critical analysis.' *Defence Against Bioterrorism*, 189–201. doi:10.1007/978-94-024-1263-5_14. [6.6.6]

Magistrato della sanità, Venice (1752). *An Authentick Account of the Measures and Precautions used at Venice by the Magistrate of the Office of Health for the Preservation of the Publick Health*. London: Edward Owen. [6.3.2]

Maiztegui, J., Feuillade, M., Briggiler, A. (1986). 'Progressive extension of the endemic area and changing incidence of Argentine hemorrhagic fever.' *Medical Microbiology and Immunology*, **175**, 149–52. [3.3.4]

Malek, E.A. (1975). 'Effect of the Aswan High Dam on prevalence of schistosomiasis in Egypt.' *Tropical and Geographical Medicine*, **27**, 359–64. [3.3.4]

Manderson, L. (1995). 'Wireless wars in the Eastern Arena: epidemiological surveillance, disease prevention and the work of the Eastern Bureau of the League of Nations Health Organisation, 1925-1942.' In: P. Weindling (ed.), *International Health Organisations and Movements, 1918-1939*. Cambridge: Cambridge University Press, 109–33. [6.6.3]

Marr, J.S., Malloy, C.D. (1996). 'An epidemiologic analysis of the Ten Plagues of Egypt.' *Caduceus*, **12**, 7–24. [3.2.1]

Martcheva, M. (2016). *An Introduction to Mathematical Epidemiology*. Cham: Springer. [1.3.2]

May, J. (1950–54). 'Atlas of diseases.' *Geographical Review*, **40**, 646–8; **41**, 272–3; **42**, 98–101, 283–6; **43**, 89–90, 408–10; **44**, 133–6, 408–10, 583–4. [1.5.1]

May, J. (1954). 'Map of the world distribution of leishmaniasis.' *Geographical Review*, **44**, 583–4. [1.5.1]

McEvedy, C. (1988). 'The bubonic plague.' *Scientific American*, **254**, 3–12. [4.2.3]

McKeown, T. (1988). *The Origins of Human Disease*. Oxford: Basil Blackwell. [3.2.2]

McMichael, A.J. (2001). 'Human culture, ecological change, and infectious disease: are we experiencing history's fourth great transition?' *Ecosystem Health*, **7**, 107–15. [3.3.4]

McMichael, A.J. (2004). 'Environmental and social influences on emerging infectious diseases: past, present and future.' *Philosophical Transactions of the Royal Society B*, **359**, 1049–58. [3.1.1, 3.3.4]

McMichael, A.J., Campbell-Lendrum, D.H., Corvalan, C.F., Ebi, K.L., Githeko, A., Scheraga, J.D., Woodward, A. (eds.) (2003). *Climate Change and Human Health: Risks and Responses*. Geneva: WHO. [3.3.5]

Medić, S., Katsilieris, M., Lozanov-Crvenković, Z., Siettos, C.I., Petrović, V., Milošević, V., Brkić, S., Andrews, N., Ubavić, M., Anastassopoulou, C. (2018). 'Varicella zoster virus transmission dynamics in Vojvodina, Serbia.' *PLoS One*, **13**, e0193838. doi: 10.1371/journal.pone.0193838. [5.2.4]

Mettler, N.E. (1969). *Argentine Hemorrhagic Fever: Current Knowledge*. Pan American Health Organization Scientific Publication No. 183. Washington, DC: Pan American Health Organization. [3.3.4]

Michael, E., Bundy, D.A. (1997). 'Global mapping of lymphatic filariasis.' *Parasitology Today*, **13**, 472–6. [1.5.2]

Ministry of Health (1920). *Report on the Pandemic of Influenza, 1918–19*. Reports on Public Health and Medical Subjects, No. 4. London: HMSO. [4.4.3]

Mollison, D. (1995). *Epidemic Models: Their Structure and Relationship to Data*. Cambridge: Cambridge University Press. [1.1]

Montiel, R., García, C., Cañadas, M.P., Isidro, A., Guijo, J.M., Malgosa, A. (2003). 'DNA sequences of *Mycobacterium leprae* recovered from ancient bones.' *FEMS Microbiology Letters*, **226**, 413–14. [3.2.1]

Mooney, G. (2009). 'Infection and citizenship: (not) visiting isolation hospitals in mid-Victorian Britain.' In: G. Mooney and J. Reinarz (eds.), *Permeable Walls: Historical Perspectives on Hospital and Asylum Visiting*. Amsterdam: Brill, 147–73. [6.3.3]

Morens, D.M., Folkers, G.K., Fauci, A.S. (2009). 'What is a pandemic?' *Journal of Infectious Diseases*, **200**, 1018–21. [4.1]

Morens, D.M., North, M., Taubenberger, J.K. (2010). 'Eyewitness accounts of the 1510 influenza pandemic in Europe.' *Lancet*, **376**, 1894–5. [4.4.2]

Morens, D.M., Taubenberger, J.K., Folkers, G.K., Fauci, A.S. (2010). 'Pandemic influenza's 500th anniversary.' *Clinical Infectious Diseases*, **51**, 1442–4. [4.1.1, 4.4.2]

Morse, S.S. (1995). 'Factors in the emergence of infectious diseases.' *Emerging Infectious Diseases*, **1**, 7–15. [3.3.1, 3.3.4]

Mosley, M. (2018). *The Clever Gut Diet: How to Revolutionize Your Body from the Inside Out*. New York: Atria Books. [1.2.1]

Mukerjee, S. (1963). 'Problems of cholera (El Tor).' *American Journal of Tropical Medicine and Hygiene*, **12**, 388–92. [4.3.3]

Murray, C.J.L., Lopez, A.D. (eds.) (1996) . *The Global Burden of Disease: A Comprehensive Assessment of Mortality and Disability from Diseases, Injuries, and Risk Factors in 1990 and Projected to 2020. Summary*. Cambridge, MA: Harvard School of Public Health. [1.2.3]

Nerlich, A.G., Haas, C.J., Zink, A., Szeimies, U., Hagedorn, H.G. (1997). 'Molecular evidence for tuberculosis in an ancient Egyptian mummy.' *Lancet*, **350**, 1404. [3.2.1]

Nishiura, H., Linton, N.M., Akhmetzhanov, A.R. (2020). 'Serial interval of novel coronavirus (COVID-19) infections.' *International Journal of Infectious Diseases*, **93**, 284–6. doi: 10.1016/j.ijid.2020.02.060. [5.2.2]

Olsen, S.J., Chang, H.-L., Cheung, T.Y.-Y., Tang, A.F.-Y., Fisk, T.L., Ooi, S.P.-L., Kuo, H.-W., Jiang, D.D.-S., Chen, K.-T., Lando, J., Hsu, K.-H., Chen, T.-J., Dowell, S.F. (2003). 'Transmission of the severe acute respiratory syndrome on aircraft.' *New England Journal of Medicine*, **349**, 2416–22. [3.4.2]

Ord, J.K., Getis, A. (1995). 'Local spatial autocorrelation statistics: distributional issues and an application.' *Geographical Analysis*, **27**, 286–306. [1.5.2]

Ord, K., Getis, A. (2018). 'A retrospective analysis of the spatial and temporal patterns of the West African Ebola epidemic, 2014–2015.' *Geographical Analysis*, **50**, 337–57. [5.6]

Oster, A.M., Kang, G.J., Cha, A.E., Beresovsky, V., Rose, C.E., Rainisch, G., Porter, L., Valverde, E.E., Peterson, E.B., Driscoll, A.K., Norris, T., Wilson, N., Ritchey, M., Walke, H.T., Rose, D.A., Oussayef, N.L., Parise, M.E., Moore, Z.S., Fleischauer, A.T., Honein, M.A., Dirlikov, E., Villanueva, J. (2020). 'Trends in number and distribution of COVID-19 hotspot counties – United States, March 8–July 15, 2020.' *Morbidity and Mortality Weekly Report*, **69**, 1127–32. [5.5.1]

Otterstrom, S.M., Hochberg, L. (2021). 'Relative concentrations and diffusion of COVID-19 across the United States in 2020.' *Cartographica*, **56**, 27–43. [5.5.1]

Oxenham, M.F., Kim Thuy, N., Lan Cuong, N. (2004). 'Skeletal evidence for the emergence of infectious disease in Bronze and Iron Age Northern Vietnam.' *American Journal of Physical Anthropology*, **126**, 359–76. [3.2.1]

Oxford, J.S. (2000). 'Influenza A pandemics of the 20th century with special reference to 1918: virology, pathology and epidemiology.' *Reviews in Medical Virology*, **10**, 119–33. [4.4.1, 4.4.3]

Palmer, R.J. (1978). *The Control of Plague in Venice and Northern Italy, 1348–1600*. Doctoral dissertation, University of Kent at Canterbury, UK. [6.3.2]

Panagiotakopulu, E. (2004). 'Pharaonic Egypt and the origins of plague.' *Journal of Biogeography*, **31**, 269–75. [4.2.1]

Panum, P.L. (1847). 'Iagttagelser anstillede under maeslinge-epidemien paa Faeroerne i Aaret 1846.' ['Observations made during the epidemic of measles on the Faroe Islands in the year 1846.'] *Bibliothek for Laeger*, **1**, 270–344. [2.2.2]

Parish, H.J. (1968). *Victory with Vaccines: The Story of Immunization*. Edinburgh: E. &. S. Livingstone. [6.4]

Parsons, A.C., MacNalty, A.S., Perdrau, J.R. (1922). *Report on Encephalitis Lethargica*. Reports on Public Health and Medical Subjects, No. 11. London: HMSO. [4.4.3]

Parsons, H.F. (1891). *Report on the Influenza Epidemic of 1889–90. With an Introduction by the Medical Officer of the Local Government Board*. London: HMSO. [4.1.1]

Patterson, K.D. (1986). *Pandemic Influenza, 1700–1900. A Study in Historical Epidemiology*. Totowa: Rowman and Littlefield. [4.1.1, 4.4, 4.4.2]

Patterson, K.D., Pyle, G.F. (1991). 'The geography and mortality of the 1918 influenza pandemic.' *Bulletin of the History of Medicine*, **65**, 4–21. [4.4.3]

Patz, J.A., Daszak, P., Tabor, G.M., Aguirre, A.A., Pearl, M., Epstein, J., Wolfe, N.D., Kilpatrick, A.M., Foufopoulos, J., Molyneux, D.,

Bradley, D.J., Members of the Working Group on Land Use Change and Disease Emergence (2004). 'Unhealthy landscapes: policy recommendations on land use change and infectious disease emergence.' *Environmental Health Perspectives*, **112**, 1092–8. [3.3.4]

Patz, J.A., Graczyk, T.K., Geller, N., Vittor, A.Y. (2000). 'Effects of environmental change on emerging parasitic diseases.' *International Journal for Parasitology*, **30**, 1395–405. [3.3.4]

Patz, J.A., Martens, W.J.M., Focks, D.A., Jetten, T.H. (1998). 'Dengue fever epidemic potential as projected by general circulation models of global climate change.' *Environmental Health Perspectives*, **106**, 147–53. [3.3.5]

Peiris, J.S.M., Yu, W.C., Leung, C.W., Cheung, C.Y., Ng, W.F., Nicholls, J.M., Ng, T.K., Chan, K.H., Lai, S.T., Lim, W.L., Yuen, K.Y., Guan, Y. (2004). 'Re-emergence of fatal human influenza A subtype H5N1 disease.' *Lancet*, **363**, 617–19. [3.4.1]

Pérez-López, F.R., Tajada, M., Savirón-Cornudella, R., Sánchez-Prieto, M., Chedraui, P., Terán, E. (2020). 'Coronavirus disease 2019 and gender-related mortality in European countries: a meta-analysis.' *Maturitas*, **141**, 59–62. [5.2.5]

Petitti, P. (1852). *Repertorio Administrativo ossia collezione di leggi, decreti, reali rescritti, ministeriali di massima regolamenti, ed istruzioni sull'amministrazione civile de Regno delle Due Sicilie.* Volume 3 (fifth edition). Naples: Tipografia di Gaetano Sautto. [6.3.1]

Pickles, W.N. (1939). *Epidemiology in Country Practice.* Bristol: John Wright. [1.4.1, 2.1, 2.2, 2.2.2, 2.2.3, 2.2.4]

Pickles, W.N., Burnet, F.M., McArthur, N. (1947). 'Epidemic respiratory infection in a rural population with special reference to the influenza A epidemics of 1933, 1936–7 and 1943–4.' *Journal of Hygiene (London)*, **45**, 469–73. [2.2.3]

Pollán, M., Pérez-Gómez, B., Pastor-Barriuso, R., Oteo, J., Hernán, M.A., Pérez-Olmeda, M., Sanmartín, J.L., Fernández-García, A., Cruz, I., Fernández de Larrea, N., Molina, M., Rodríguez-Cabrera, F., Martín, M., Merino-Amador, P., León Paniagua, J., Muñoz-Montalvo, J.F., Blanco, F., Yotti, R., ENE-COVID Study Group (2020). 'Prevalence of SARS-CoV-2 in Spain (ENE-COVID): a nationwide, population-based seroepidemiological study.' *Lancet*, **396**, 535–44. [5.2.6]

Pollitzer, R. (1954). *Plague.* Geneva: WHO. [4.1.1, 4.2.4]

Pollitzer, R. (1959). *Cholera.* Geneva: WHO. [4.3.1, 4.3.2]

Porta, M. (ed.) (2008). *A Dictionary of Epidemiology* (fifth edition). Oxford: Oxford University Press. [4.1]

Public Health England (2020a). *Country and PHE Region HIV Data Tables to End December 2018. Tables No. 2. 2019.* London: Public Health England. https://www.gov.uk/government/statistics/hiv-annual-data-tables, accessed 27 March 2021. [4.1.1]

Public Health England (2020b). *Weekly Coronavirus Disease 2019 (COVID-19) Surveillance Report. Summary of COVID-19 Surveillance Systems. Week 33.* London: Public Health England. https://www.gov.uk/government/publications/national-covid-19-surveillance-reports, accessed 27 March 2021. [5.4.2]

Pybus, O., Rambaut, A., du Plessis, L., Zarebski, A.E., Kraemer, M.U.G., Raghwani, J., Gutiérrez, B., Hill, V., McCrone, J., Colquhoun, R., Jackson, B., O'Toole, A., Ashworth, J., COG-UK Consortium (2020). 'Preliminary analysis of SARS-CoV-2 importation and establishment of UK transmission lineages.' https://virological.org/t/preliminary-analysis-of-sars-cov-2-importation-establishment-of-uk-transmission-lineages/507, accessed 27 March 2021. [5.4]

Raettig, H. (1954–61). 'The plague pandemic of the 20th century.' In: E. Rodenwaldt and H.J. Jusatz (eds.), *Welt-Seuchen-Atlas: World-Atlas of Epidemic Diseases. Parts II and III.* Hamburg: Falk-Verlag, III/33. [4.2.4]

Rafferty, S., Smallman-Raynor, M.R., Cliff, A.D. (2018). 'Variola minor in England and Wales: the geographical course of a smallpox epidemic and the impediments to effective disease control, 1920–1935.' *Journal of Historical Geography*, **59**, 2–14. [6.4.1]

Rafi, A., Spigelman, M., Stanford, J., Lemma, E., Donoghue, H., Zias, J. (1994). '*Mycobacterium leprae* DNA from ancient bone detected by PCR.' *Lancet*, **343**, 1360–1. [3.2.1]

Raoult, D., Aboudharam, G., Crubézy, E., Larrouy, G., Ludes, B., Drancourt, M. (2000). 'Molecular identification by "suicide PCR" of *Yersinia pestis* as the agent of Medieval Black Death.' *Proceedings of the National Academy of Sciences USA*, **97**, 12800–3. [4.2.3]

Ravenholt, R.T. (1993). 'Encephalitis lethargica.' In: K.F. Kiple (ed.), *The Cambridge World History of Human Disease.* Cambridge: Cambridge University Press, 708–12. [4.4.3]

Ravenholt, R.T., Foege, W.H. (1982). '1918 influenza, encephalitis lethargica, parkinsonism.' *Lancet*, **2**, 860–4. [4.4.3]

Ravenstein, E.G. (1885). 'The laws of migration.' *Journal of the Royal Statistical Society*, **48**, 167–235. [1.6.4]

Ravenstein, E.G. (1889). 'The laws of migration. Second paper.' *Journal of the Royal Statistical Society*, **52**, 241–305. [1.6.4]

Registrar-General for England and Wales (1920). *Report on the Mortality from Influenza in England and Wales During the Epidemic of 1918–19: Supplement to the Eighty-first Annual Report of the Registrar-General of Births, Deaths, and Marriages in England and Wales.* London: HMSO. [4.1.1]

Reid, A.H., Fanning, T.G., Hultin, J.V., Taubenberger, J.K. (1999). 'Origin and evolution of the 1918 'Spanish' influenza hemagluttinin gene.' *Proceedings of the National Academy of Sciences USA*, **96**, 1651–5. [3.2.1, 4.4.3]

Rivers, C.M., Lofgren, E.T., Marathe, M., Eubank, S., Lewis, B.L. (2014). 'Modeling the impact of interventions on an epidemic of Ebola in Sierra Leone and Liberia.' *PLoS Currents*, **6**, Outbreaks. Edition 2. doi: 10.1371/currents.outbreaks.4d41fe5d6c05e9df30dd ce33c66d084c. [5.6]

Rocklöv, J., Dubrow, R. (2020). 'Climate change: an enduring challenge for vector-borne disease prevention and control.' *Nature Immunology*, **21**, 479–83.

Rodenwaldt, E. (ed.) (1952–61). *Welt-Seuchen-Atlas: World-Atlas of Epidemic Diseases. Parts I–III.* Hamburg: Falk-Verlag. [1.5.1, 4.2.4]

Rogers, E.M. (1995). *Diffusion of Innovations* (fourth edition). New York: The Free Press. [1.1]

Roller, D.W. (2010). *Eratosthenes' Geography.* Princeton, NJ: Princeton University Press. [1.1]

Rothstein, M.A., Alcalde, M.G., Majumder, M.A., Palmer, L.I., Stone, T.H., Hoffman, R.E. (2003). *Quarantine and Isolation: Lessons Learned from SARS.* Louisville, KY: University of Louisville School of Medicine, Institute for Bioethics, Health Policy and Law. Report to the Centers for Disease Control and Prevention, Atlanta. [3.4.2]

Rowland, K.T. (1970). *Steam at Sea: A History of Steam Navigation.* Newton Abbot: David and Charles. [3.3.3]

Russell, J.C. (1972). 'Population in Europe 500–1500.' In: C.M. Cipolla, (ed.), *The Fontana Economic History of Europe: The Middle Ages.* London: Fontana, 25–70. [4.2.2]

Salo, W.L., Aufderheide, A.C., Buikstra, J., Holcomb, T.A. (1994). 'Identification of *Mycobacterium tuberculosis* DNA in a pre-Columbian Peruvian mummy.' *Proceedings of the National Academy of Sciences USA*, **91**, 2091–4. [3.2.1]

Sattenspiel, L. (2009). *The Geographic Spread of Infectious Diseases: Models and Applications.* Princeton, NJ: Princeton University Press. [1.2.2, 1.3.2, 1.4.4]

Sattenspiel, L., Herring, D.A. (1998). 'Structured epidemic models and the spread of influenza in the central Canadian subarctic.' *Human Biology*, **70**, 91–115. [1.2.2]

Savage, E., Ramsay, M., White, J., Beard, S., Lawson, H., Hunjan, R., Brown, D. (2005). 'Mumps outbreaks across England and Wales in 2004: observational study.' *British Medical Journal*, **330**, 1119–20. [6.4.1]

Savage, E., White, J.M., Brown, D.E.W., Ramsay, M.E. (2006). 'Mumps epidemic – United Kingdom, 2004–2005.' *Morbidity and Mortality Weekly Report*, **55**, 173–5. [6.4.1]

Shally-Jensen, M. (ed.) (2010). *Encyclopedia of Contemporary American Social Issues. 2.* Santa Barbara, CA: ABC-CLIO. [4.1.1]

Shannon, G.W., Pyle, G.F., Bashshur, R.L. (1991). *The Geography of AIDS.* New York: The Guilford Press. [4.5.2]

Sharp, P.M., Bailes, E., Chaudhuri, R.R., Rodenburg, C.M., Santiago, M.O., Hahn, B.H. (2001). 'The origins of acquired immune deficiency syndrome viruses: where and when?' *Philosophical Transactions of the Royal Society of London. Series B, Biological Sciences*, **356**, 867–76. [4.5.2]

Sharp, P.M., Hahn, B.H. (2011). 'Origins of HIV and the AIDS pandemic.' *Cold Spring Harbor Perspectives in Medicine*, **1**, a006841. doi: 10.1101/cshperspect.a006841. [4.5.2]

Shereen, M.A., Khan, S., Kazmi, A., Bashir, N., Siddique, R. (2020). 'COVID-19 infection: origin, transmission, and characteristics of human coronaviruses.' *Journal of Advanced Research*, **24**, 91–8. doi: 10.1016/j.jare.2020.03.005. [5.2]

Shortridge, K.F. (1992). 'Pandemic influenza: a zoonosis?' *Seminars in Respiratory Infections*, **7**, 11–25. [4.4.1]

Shortridge, K.F., Stuart-Harris, C.H. (1982). 'An influenza epicentre?' *Lancet*, **2**, 812–13. [4.4.1]

Shousha, A.T. (1948). 'Cholera epidemic in Egypt: a preliminary report.' *Bulletin of the World Health Organization*, **1**, 353–81. [4.1.1]

Simpson, W.J. (1905). *A Treatise on Plague, Dealing with the Historical, Epidemiological, Clinical, Therapeutic and Preventive Aspects of the Disease.* Cambridge: Cambridge University Press. [4.2.1]

Singer, M. (2020). 'Deadly companions: COVID-19 and diabetes in Mexico.' *Medical Anthropology*, **39**, 660–5. [2.5.5]

Smallman-Raynor, M.R., Cliff, A.D. (2004). *War Epidemics: An Historical Geography of Infectious Diseases in Military Conflict and Civil Strife, 1850–2000.* Oxford: Oxford University Press. [3.2.1, 4.1.1]

Smallman-Raynor, M.R., Cliff, A.D. (2007). 'Avian influenza A (H5N1) age distribution in humans.' *Emerging Infectious Diseases*, **13**, 510–12. [3.4.1]

Smallman-Raynor, M.R., Cliff, A.D. (2008). 'The geographical spread of avian influenza A (H5N1): panzootic transmission (December 2003–May 2006), pandemic potential and implications.' *Annals of the Association of American Geographers*, **98**, 553–82. [3.4.1]

Smallman-Raynor, M.R., Cliff, A.D. (2012). *Atlas of Epidemic Britain: A Twentieth Century Picture.* Oxford: Oxford University Press. [4.2.4, 4.4.4, 6.4]

Smallman-Raynor, M.R., Cliff, A.D. (2013). 'The geographical spread of the 1947 poliomyelitis epidemic in England and Wales: spatial wave propagation of an enigmatic epidemiological event.' *Journal of Historical Geography*, **40**, 36–51. [1.5.2]

Smallman-Raynor, M.R., Cliff, A.D. (2018). *Atlas of Refugees, Displaced Populations, and Epidemic Diseases. Decoding Global Geographical Patterns and Processes since 1901.* Oxford: Oxford University Press. [3.4.3]

Smallman-Raynor, M.R., Cliff, A.D., Barford, A. (2015). 'Geographical perspectives on epidemic transmission of cholera in Haiti, October

2010 through March 2013.' *Annals of the Association of American Geographers*, **105**, 665–83. [5.6]

Smallman-Raynor, M.R., Cliff, A.D., Haggett, P. (1992). *London International Atlas of AIDS.* Oxford: Blackwell Reference. [3.3.3, 4.5.2]

Smallman-Raynor, M.R., Cliff, A.D., Trevelyan, B., Nettleton, C., Sneddon, S. (2006). *Poliomyelitis. A World Geography: Emergence to Eradication.* Oxford: Oxford University Press. [3.2.2, 6.5.3]

Sogoba, N., Doumbia, S., Vounatsou, P., Bagayoko, M.M., Dolo, G., Traoré, S.F., Maïga, H.M., Touré, Y.T., Smith, T. (2007). 'Malaria transmission dynamics in Niono, Mali: the effect of the irrigation systems.' *Acta Tropica*, **101**, 232–40. [3.3.4]

Song, Z., Xu, Y., Bao, L., Zhang, L., Yu, P., Qu, Y., Zhu, H., Zhao, W., Han, Y., Qin, C. (2019). 'From SARS to MERS, thrusting coronaviruses into the spotlight.' *Viruses*, **11**, 59. doi:10.3390/v11010059. [3.4.2]

Soper, G.A. (1918). 'The pandemic in the army camps.' *Journal of the American Medical Association*, **71**, 1899–909. [4.4.3]

Spielman, A. (1994). 'The emergence of Lyme disease and human babesiosis in a changing environment.' *Annals of the New York Academy of Sciences*, **740**, 146–56. [3.3.4]

Spiteri, G., Fielding, J., Diercke, M., Campese, C., Enouf, V., Gaymard, A., Bella, A., Sognamiglio, P., Sierra Moros, M.J., Riutort, A.N., Demina, Y.V., Mahieu, R., Broas, M., Bengnér, M., Buda, S., Schilling, J., Filleul, L., Lepoutre, A., Saura, C., Mailles, A., Levy-Bruhl, D., Coignard, B., Bernard-Stoecklin, S., Behillil, S., van der Werf, S., Valette, M., Lina, B., Riccardo, F., Nicastri, E., Casas, I., Larrauri, A., Salom Castell, M., Pozo, F., Maksyutov, R.A., Martin, C., Van Ranst, M., Bossuyt, N., Siira, L., Sane, J., Tegmark-Wisell, K., Palmérus, M., Broberg, E.K., Beauté, J., Jorgensen, P., Bundle, N., Pereyaslov, D., Adlhoch, C., Pukkila, J., Pebody, R., Olsen, S., Ciancio, B.C. (2020). 'First cases of coronavirus disease 2019 (COVID-19) in the WHO European Region, 24 January to 21 February 2020.' *Eurosurveillance*, **25**, 2000178. doi: 10.2807/1560-7917.ES.2020.25.9.2000178. [5.3.2]

Stanwell-Smith, R. (1996). 'Immunization: celebrating the past and injecting the future.' *Journal of the Royal Society of Medicine*, **80**, 509–13. [6.5]

Steere, A.C. (1998). 'Lyme disease.' In: R.M. Krause (ed.), *Emerging Infections: Biomedical Research Reports.* San Diego, CA: Academic Press, 219–37. [3.3.4]

Steere, A.C., Grodzicki, R.L., Kornblatt, A.N., Craft, J.E., Barbour, A.G., Burgdorfer, W., Schmid, G.P., Johnson, E., Malawista, S.E. (1983). 'The spirochetal etiology of Lyme disease.' *New England Journal of Medicine*, **308**, 733–40. [3.3.4]

Steere, A.C., Malawista, S.E., Snydman, D.R., Shope, R.E., Andiman, W.A., Ross, M.R., Steele, F.M. (1977). 'Lyme arthritis: an epidemic of oligoarticular arthritis in children and adults in three Connecticut communities.' *Arthritis and Rheumatism*, **20**, 7–17. [3.3.4]

Strahler, A.N. (1952). 'Hypsometric (area-altitude) of erosional topography.' *Geological Society of America Bulletin*, **63**, 1117–42. [1.6.2]

Streeck, H., Schulte, B., Kümmerer, B.M., Richter, E., Höller, T., Fuhrmann, C., Bartok, E., Dolscheid-Pommerich, R., Berger, M., Wessendorf, L., Eschbach-Bludau, M., Kellings, A., Schwaiger, A., Coenen, M., Hoffmann, P., Stoffel-Wagner, B., Nöthen, M.M., Eis-Hübinger, A.M., Exner, M., Schmithausen, R.M., Schmid, M., Hartmann, G. (2020). 'Infection fatality rate of SARS-CoV2 in a super-spreading event in Germany.' *Nature Communications*, **11**, 5829. doi: 10.1038/s41467-020-19509-y. [5.3.2]

Stuart-Harris, C.H., Schild, G.C., Oxford, J.S. (1985). *Influenza: The Viruses and the Disease* (second edition). Baltimore, MD: Edward Arnold. [4.4.3]

Sun, J., He, W.T., Wang, L., Lai, A., Ji, X., Zhai, X., Li, G., Suchard, M.A., Tian, J., Zhou, J., Veit, M., Su, S. (2020). 'COVID-19: epidemiology, evolution, and cross-disciplinary perspectives.' *Trends in Molecular Medicine*, **26**, 483–95. [5.3.1]

Süss, J., Klaus, C., Gerstengarbe, F.-W., Werner, P.C. (2008). 'What makes ticks tick? Climate change, ticks, and tick-borne diseases.' *Journal of Travel Medicine*, **15**, 39–45. [3.3.4]

Tangermann, R.H., Hull, H.F., Jafari, H., Nkowane, B., Everts, H., Aylward, R.B. (2000). 'Eradication of poliomyelitis in countries affected by conflict.' *Bulletin of the World Health Organization*, **78**, 330–8. [6.5.3]

Tansley, E.M., Christie, D.A., Reynolds, L.A. (1998). *Wellcome Witnesses to Twentieth Century Medicine. Volume II, Research in General Practice.* London: Wellcome Institute for the History of Medicine/Wellcome Trust. [2.3, 2.6]

Taubenberger, J.K., Morens, D.M. (2009). 'Pandemic influenza – including a risk assessment of H5N1.' *Revue Scientifique et Technique (International Office of Epizootics)*, **28**, 187–202. [4.1.1]

Tauxe, R.V. (1998). 'Cholera.' In: A.S. Evans and P.S. Brachman (eds.), *Bacterial Infections of Humans: Epidemiology and Control* (third edition). New York: Plenum Medical Book Company, 223–42. [4.3]

Taylor S.J., Eckles, D. (2018). 'Randomized experiments to detect and estimate social influence in networks.' In: S. Lehmann and Y.Y. Ahn (eds.), *Complex Spreading Phenomena in Social Systems: Influence and Contagion in Real-World Social Networks.* Cham: Springer, 289–22. [1.2.2]

Than, K. (2014). 'Two of history's deadliest plagues were linked, with implications for another outbreak.' *National Geographic.* https://www.nationalgeographic.com/news/2014/1/140129-justinian-plague-black-death-bacteria-bubonic-pandemic/#:~:text=The%20Justinian%20plague%20struck%20in,Africa%2C%20Arabia%2C%20and%20Europe, accessed 27 March 2021. [4.1.1]

The Health Foundation (2021). *NHS Test and Trace Performance Tracker.* London: The Health Foundation. https://www.health.org.uk/news-and-comment/charts-and-infographics/nhs-test-and-trace-performance-tracker, accessed 27 March 2021. [6.3.3]

Thompson, T. (1852). *Annals of Influenza or Epidemic Catarrhal Fever in Great Britain from 1510 to 1837.* London: Sydenham Society. [4.1.1, 4.4.2]

Tinline, R.R. (1972). *A Simulation Study of the 1967–68 Foot-and-Mouth Epizootic in Great Britain.* Unpublished DPhil dissertation. Department of Geography, University of Bristol, UK. [1.6.3, 1.6.4, 6.4.2]

Tomić, Z.B., Blažina, V. (2015). *Expelling the Plague: The Health Office and the Implementation of Quarantine in Dubrovnik, 1377–1533.* Montreal: McGill-Queen's University Press. [6.3.2]

Tornqvist, G. (1967). *Growth of TV Ownership in Sweden, 1956–65.* Uppsala: Uppsala University Press. [1.4.2]

Trevisanato, S.I. (2004). 'Did an epidemic of tularemia in Ancient Egypt affect the course of world history?' *Medical Hypotheses*, **63**, 905–10. [3.2.1]

Trevisanato, S.I. (2007a). 'The biblical plague of the Philistines now has a name, tularemia.' *Medical Hypotheses*, **69**, 1144–6. [3.2.1]

Trevisanato, S.I. (2007b). 'The 'Hittite plague', an epidemic of tularemia and the first record of biological warfare.' *Medical Hypotheses*, **69**, 1371–4. [3.2.1]

Truelove, S.A., Keegan, L.T., Moss, W.J., Chaisson, L.H., Macher, E., Azman, A.S., Lessler, J. (2020). 'Clinical and epidemiological aspects of diphtheria: a systematic review and pooled analysis.' *Clinical Infectious Diseases*, **71**, 89–97. [5.2.4]

Tumpey, T.M., Basler, C.F., Aguilar, P.V., Zeng, H., Solórzano, A., Swayne, D.E., Cox, N.J., Katz, J.M., Taubenberger, J.K., Palese, P., Garcia-Sastre, A. (2005). 'Characterization of the reconstructed 1918 Spanish influenza pandemic virus.' *Science*, **310**, 77–80. [3.2.1]

Twain, M. (1884). *The Adventures of Huckleberry Finn.* London: Chatto & Windus. [1.1]

Uemura, K. (1988). 'World health situation and trend assessment from 1948 to 1988.' *Bulletin of the World Health Organization*, **66**, 679–87. [6.6.4]

UNAIDS (2020). *UNAIDS Data 2020.* Geneva: UNAIDS. [4.5.3]

United Kingdom Government (2020). *Coronavirus (COVID-19) in the UK.* London: UK Government. https://coronavirus.data.gov.uk/, accessed 27 March 2021. [4.1.1]

Van Heuverswyn, F., Peeters, M. (2007). 'The origins of HIV and implications for the global epidemic.' *Current Infectious Disease Reports*, **9**, 338–46. [4.5.2]

Viboud, C., Grais, R.F., Lafont, B.A., Miller, M.A., Simonsen, L. (2005). 'Multinational impact of the 1968 Hong Kong influenza pandemic: evidence for a smoldering pandemic.' *Journal of Infectious Diseases*, **192**, 233–48. [2.3.2, 2.3.3, 4.4.4]

Viboud, C., Miller, M.M., Grenfell, B.T., Bjørnstad, O.N., Simonsen, L. (2006). 'Air travel and the spread of influenza: important caveats.' *PLoS Medicine*, **3**, e41. doi: 10.1371/journal.pmed.0030503. [3.3.3]

Viglizzo E.F., Pordomingo, A.J., Castro, M.G., Lértora, F.A., Bernardos, J.N. (2004). 'Scale-dependent controls on ecological fluctuations in agroecosystems of Argentina.' *Agriculture, Ecosystems and Environment*, **101**, 39–51. [3.3.4]

Vynnycky, E., White, R. (2010). *An Introduction to Infectious Disease Modelling.* Oxford: Oxford University Press. [1.2.1, 1.3.1, 1.3.2, 1.4.4, 1.6.3]

Walker, A., Houwaart, T., Wienemann, T., Vasconcelos, M.K., Strelow, D., Senff, T., Hülse, L., Adams, O., Andree, M., Hauka, S., Feldt, T., Jensen, B.E., Keitel, V., Kindgen-Milles, D., Timm, J., Pfeffer, K., Dilthey, A.T. (2020). 'Genetic structure of SARS-CoV-2 reflects clonal superspreading and multiple independent introduction events, North-Rhine Westphalia, Germany, February and March 2020.' *Eurosurveillance*, **25**, 2000746. doi: 10.2807/1560-7917.ES.2020.25.22.2000746. [5.3.2]

Watts, D.J., Muhamad, R., Medina, D.C., Dodds, P.S. (2005). 'Multiscale, resurgent epidemics in a hierarchical metapopulation model.' *Proceedings of the National Academy of Sciences USA*, **102**, 11157–62. [1.2.2]

Webster, R.G. (1999). '1918 Spanish influenza: the secrets remain elusive.' *Proceedings of the National Academy of Sciences USA*, **96**, 1164–6. [4.4.3]

Weiss, R.A. (2001). 'The Leeuwenhoek Lecture 2001. Animal origins of human infectious disease.' *Philosophical Transactions of the Royal Society B*, **356**, 957–77. [3.2]

Whaley, F. (2006). 'Flight CA112: facing the spectre of in-flight transmission.' In: WHO (ed.), *SARS: How a Global Epidemic was Stopped.* Manila: WHO (Western Pacific Region), 149–54. [3.4.2]

Wheatley, P. (1971). *The Pivot of the Four Quarters: A Preliminary Enquiry into the Origins and Character of the Ancient Chinese City.* Edinburgh: University of Edinburgh Press. [3.2.2]

WHO/International Study Team (1978). 'Ebola haemorrhagic fever in Sudan, 1976.' *Bulletin of the World Health Organization*, **56**, 247–70. [3.4.3]

Wilson, A.G. (2000). *Complex Spatial Systems.* Harlow: Prentice Hall. [1.6.4]

Wilson, G.S., Miles, A.A. (1975). *Topley and Wilson's Principles of Bacteriology, Virology and Immunity* (sixth edition). London: Edward Arnold. [4.1.1]

Wilson, M.L. (1994). 'Rift Valley fever ecology and the epidemiology of disease emergence.' *Annals of the New York Academy of Sciences*, **740**, 169–80. [3.3.4]

World Health Organization (1958). *The First Ten Years of the World Health Organization*. Geneva: WHO. [6.6.3]

World Health Organization (1988). *41st World Health Assembly. WA41/1988/REC/1: Resolutions and Decisions. Annexes*. Geneva: WHO. [6.5.3]

World Health Organization (1995). *International Travel and Health: Vaccination Requirements and Health Advice*. Geneva: Epidemiological Surveillance and Statistical Services. [3.3.3]

World Health Organization (2000). *WHO Report on Global Surveillance of Epidemic-prone Infectious Diseases*. Geneva: WHO (WHO/CDS/CSR/ISR/2000.1). [4.1.1]

World Health Organization (2004). *Avian Influenza A(H5N1) in Humans and Poultry in Viet Nam*. Geneva: WHO. https://www.who.int/csr/don/2004_01_13/en/, accessed 27 March 2021. [3.4.1]

World Health Organization (2005a). 'Avian influenza: frequently asked questions (updated on 19 October 2005).' *Weekly Epidemiological Record*, **80**, 377–84. [3.4.1]

World Health Organization (2005b). *Avian Influenza: Assessing the Pandemic Threat*. Geneva: WHO (WHO/CDS/2005:29). [3.4.1, 4.4]

World Health Organization (2005c). *Summary of Probable SARS Cases with Onset of Illness from 1 November 2002 to 31 July 2003*. Geneva: WHO. [3.4.2]

World Health Organization (2005d). *WHO Global Influenza Preparedness Plan: The Role of WHO and Recommendations for National Measures Before and During Pandemics*. Geneva: WHO (WHO/CDS/CSR/GIP/2005.5). [4.4.4]

World Health Organization (2006a). *SARS: How a Global Epidemic was Stopped*. Manila: WHO Regional Office for the Western Pacific. [3.4.2]

World Health Organization (2006b). 'Epidemiology of WHO-confirmed human cases of avian influenza A(H5N1) infection.' *Weekly Epidemiological Record*, **81**, 249–57. [3.4.1]

World Health Organization (2008). *The Third Ten Years of the World Health Organization, 1968–1977*. Geneva: WHO. [6.6.3]

World Health Organization (2009). *World Now at the Start of 2009 Influenza Pandemic*. Geneva: WHO. https://www.who.int/mediacentre/news/statements/2009/h1n1_pandemic_phase6_20090611/en/, accessed 27 March 2021. [4.1]

World Health Organization (2015a). *Ebola Situation Report, 6 May 2015*. Geneva: WHO. http://apps.who.int/ebola/en/current-situation/ebola-situation-report-6-may-2015, accessed 27 March 2021. [3.4.3]

World Health Organization (2015b). *Ebola Situation Report, 27 May 2015*. Geneva: WHO. http://apps.who.int/ebola/current-situation/ebola-situation-report-27-may-2015, accessed 27 March 2021. [3.4.3]

World Health Organization (2017). *Pandemic Influenza Risk Management: A WHO Guide to Inform & Harmonize National & International Pandemic Preparedness and Response*. Geneva: WHO (WHO/WHE/IHM/GIP/2017.1). [4.4.5]

World Health Organization (2020a). *Avian Influenza Weekly Update Number 763. 16 October 2020*. Geneva: WHO. https://www.who. int/docs/default-source/wpro---documents/emergency/surveillance/avian-influenza/ai-20201015.pdf?sfvrsn=30d65594_78#:~:text=Globally%2C%20from%20January%202003%20to,30%20April%202019%20(source), accessed 27 March 2021. [3.4.1]

World Health Organization (2020b). *Current WHO Phase of Pandemic Alert (Avian Influenza H5N1)*. Geneva: WHO. https://www.who.int/influenza/human_animal_interface/h5n1phase/en/, accessed 27 March 2021. [3.4.1]

World Health Organization (2020c). *MERS Situation Update January 2020*. Cairo: WHO Regional Office for the Eastern Mediterranean. [3.4.2]

World Health Organization (2020d). 'Ebola virus disease – Democratic Republic of the Congo. Update, 26 June 2020.' *Weekly Epidemiological Record*, **95**, 301–6. [3.4.3]

World Health Organization (2020e). *Prioritizing Diseases for Research and Development in Emergency Contexts*. Geneva: WHO. https://www.who.int/activities/prioritizing-diseases-for-research-and-development-in-emergency-contexts, accessed 27 March 2021. [3.5]

World Health Organization (2020f). *WHO Director-General's Opening Remarks at the Media Briefing on COVID-19 – 11 March 2020*. Geneva: WHO. https://www.who.int/director-general/speeches/detail/who-director-general-s-opening-remarks-at-the-media-briefing-on-covid-19---11-march-2020, accessed 27 March 2021. [4.1]

World Health Organization (2020g). *Global Health Observatory Data: HIV/AIDS*. Geneva: WHO. https://www.who.int/gho/hiv/en/, accessed 27 March 2021. [4.1.1]

World Health Organization (2020h). *WHO Coronavirus Disease (COVID-19) Dashboard*. Geneva: WHO. https://covid19.who.int/, accessed 27 March 2021. [4.1.1]

World Health Organization (2020i). *Novel Coronavirus (2019-nCoV) Situation Report – 22*. Geneva: WHO. https://www.who.int/emergencies/diseases/novel-coronavirus-2019/situation-reports, accessed 27 March 2021. [5.1]

World Health Organization (2020j). *Statement on the Second Meeting of the International Health Regulations (2005) Emergency Committee Regarding the Outbreak of Novel Coronavirus (2019-nCoV)*. Geneva: WHO. https://www.who.int/news/item/30-01-2020-statement-on-the-second-meeting-of-the-international-health-regulations-(2005)-emergency-committee-regarding-the-outbreak-of-novel-coronavirus-(2019-ncov), accessed 27 March 2021. [5.1]

Yach, D. (1998). 'Telecommunications for health – new opportunities for action.' *Health Promotion International*, **13**, 339–47. [6.6.3]

Zeiss, H. (ed.) (1942–45). *Seuchen Atlas. Herausgabe im Auftrag des Chefs des Wehrmacht Sanitätswesen*. Gotha: Perthes. [1.5.1]

Zhu, Q.Y., Qin, E.D., Wang, W., Yu, J., Liu, B.H., Hu, Y., Hu, J.F., Cao, W.C. (2006). 'Fatal infection with influenza A (H5N1) virus in China.' *New England Journal of Medicine*, **354**, 2731–2. [3.4.1]

Zink, A.R., Reischl, U., Wolf, H., Nerlich, A.G. (2002). 'Molecular analysis of ancient microbial infections.' *FEMS Microbiology Letters*, **213**, 141–7. [3.2.1]

Zink, A.R., Reischl, U., Wolf, H., Nerlich, A.G., Miller, R.L. (2001). 'Corynebacterium in ancient Egypt.' *Medical History*, **45**, 267–72. [3.2.1]

Živanović, S. (1982). *Ancient Diseases: The Elements of Palaeopathology*. New York: Pica Press. [3.2.1]

Index